Essential Skills for Dentis

Essential Skills for Dentists

Edited by

Peter A. Mossey

Gareth J. Holsgrove

David R. Stirrups

and

Elizabeth S. Davenport

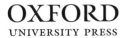

OXFORD
UNIVERSITY PRESS

Great Clarendon Street, Oxford OX2 6DP

Oxford University Press is a department of the University of Oxford.
It furthers the University's objective of excellence in research, scholarship,
and education by publishing worldwide in

Oxford New York

Auckland Cape Town Dar es Salaam Hong Kong Karachi
Kuala Lumpur Madrid Melbourne Mexico City Nairobi
New Delhi Shanghai Taipei Toronto
With offices in
Argentina Austria Brazil Chile Czech Republic France Greece
Guatemala Hungary Italy Japan South Korea Poland Portugal
Singapore Switzerland Thailand Turkey Ukraine Vietnam

Oxford is a registered trade mark of Oxford University Press
in the UK and in certain other countries

Published in the United States
by Oxford University Press Inc., New York

ISBN 978-0-19-852619-3

Printed and bound by CPI Group (UK) Ltd,
Croydon, CR0 4YY

Contents

Introduction ix

List of abbreviations xv

List of editors and contributors xvii

Part 1: Generic skills

1.1   History taking and examination 1
       Bernard McCartan and Christine McCreary

1.2   Ethics and law, consent and professionalism 19
       Jennifer King

1.3   Communication skills 37
       Jennifer King

1.4   Health and safety 49
       David Stirrups

1.5   Infection control in dentistry 59
       Mike Martin

1.6   Dental public health 71
       Cynthia Pine and Rebecca Harris

1.7   Medical emergencies including therapeutics 85
       Farida Fortune

1.8   Human disease 95
       Farida Fortune

1.9   Pharmacological management of pain and anxiety 111
       Andrew Mason

1.10   The identification and behavioural management of the dentally anxious adult
       and child patient 131
       Ruth Freeman

1.11   Dental radiology 151
       Laetitia Brocklebank

1.12 Prevention and interception 173
Anne Maguire

1.13 Patient referral 189
Peter Mossey

1.14 Isolation and moisture control 195
Francis Burke

1.15 Impression-making: general and special circumstances 207
Francis Burke

Part 2: Discipline specific skills

1.16 Dental materials science 219
Garry Fleming

2.1a Paediatric dentistry: treatment of primary and mixed dentition 233
Elizabeth Davenport and Patricia Baxter

2.1b Pulp therapy in the primary dentition 251
Paula Jane Waterhouse

2.1c Paediatric dentistry: dental trauma 273
Dafydd Evans

2.2 Special care dentistry 283
June Nunn

2.3 Orthodontics 297
Peter Mossey and David Stirrups

2.4 Periodontology 313
Mike Milward and Iain Chapple

2.5 Restorative dentistry 333
Francis Burke and Finbarr Allen

2.6 Endodontics 371
Bill Saunders

2.7 Prosthodontics 385
Damien Walmsley and John Drummond

2.8 Surgical dentistry 421
Jonathan Pedlar

2.9 Oral medicine 441
Mike Lewis

2.10 Oral pathology 459
Edward Odell

Part 3: Integrated skills

3.1   Key skills in integrated dental care 469
       Gareth Holsgrove, David Stirrups, Peter Mossey and Elizabeth Davenport

3.2   Assessment 481
       Gareth Holsgrove, Peter Mossey, Elizabeth Davenport and David Stirrups

3.3   Teamwork 497
       Elizabeth Davenport, Gareth Holsgrove, Peter Mossey and David Stirrups

       Index 509

Introduction

The concept and context of essential skills for the new dentist

Key points

- This is a book directed primarily at undergraduate dental students and the newly qualified dentist, but may also be used by educationalists.

- It is a comprehensive text achieved through consultation with leading academics in a range of dental specialties and covers all disciplines and facets in the practice of clinical dentistry.

- Facilitating learning is the core function of the book, and by clearly defining the learning outcomes, using check lists for in course formative assessment, and facilitating revision through the use of the mind maps, this can be achieved.

- It highlights key competencies in the clinical context with a view to delivering a curriculum aimed to produce a self-reflective and competent professional who can respond to the challenge in an evolving, team-orientated profession.

- The topic-orientated layout of the book allows the graduate or trainee to dip into specific topics on a stand-alone basis.

- Systematic assessment of competencies in dental education is a desirable objective and this publication is designed to assist with its achievement.

Introduction

The term 'competent' may be defined as 'capable of successful completion of a task' and in the context of the professions refers to the acquisition of special skills, combined with appropriate knowledge and attitude derived from training and experience. The level of competence is an outcome measure of the quality of the educational process and this can be applied at all levels in the profession, from pre-graduation, continuing professional development and including specialization. Competencies are reflective of professional development in its entirety, and the competent dentist will possess academic and clinical skills in all relevant scientific, biological, behavioural and clinical science aspects of the practice of dentistry. Furthermore, competence implies the capability of a professional to integrate knowledge, skills and attitudes in an appropriate context in a new scenario.

This text is aimed primarily at undergraduate dental education, bearing in mind that this is the beginning of a continuum of education preparing the graduate for postgraduate and a life-long career in the profession. On graduation it is expected that the knowledge, attitude and skills conferred through undergraduate dental education will underpin the training and the skills required in postgraduate general professional (GPT) or senior house officer (SHO) grades and facilitate success in a career in any aspect of general or specialist practice.

While the inspiration for the book has been the recommendations of the UK's General Dental Council on the undergraduate dental curriculum, and much of the text takes note of these learning outcomes, it refers also to similar and parallel developments in the US and European contexts.

The Dearing Report

In the UK, in May 1997 the first major review of higher education since the Robins Report in 1963 was published. This report is entitled 'Higher Education in the Learning Society'. Sir Ron Dearing, Chairman of the Committee, stated that the purpose of education is to contribute to the quality of life and that in the next century the economically successful nations will be those where all are committed through effective education and training to life-long learning. Appropriately defined competencies might be one way of measuring the effective outcomes of education and training in the dental profession.

Undergraduate dental training

In 1997 the GDC issued a document entitled *The First Five Years* containing recommendations on which skills should be included in the core undergraduate dental curriculum. In 2001/2002, this has undergone extensive revision, with the explicit introduction of 'learning outcomes' for undergraduate dental training in the revised version (www.gdc-uk.org/ffy.html). For Dental Schools to proceed with the implementation of the GDC recommendations, the learning outcomes for the undergraduate curriculum can be converted to competency described 'aims and objectives' statements. Assessment of competencies might be looked upon as a redefinition and standardization of what we have been doing for years.

The concept of levels of competency is important when devising courses for the development of both core and specialist clinical skills. Core clinical skills would be those essential to the practice of dentistry and can be taught and acquired in a general, nonspecialist forum, and for the dental graduate, it will be necessary to ensure competence in these. Competence in other skills will be outside the scope of the undergraduate curriculum, but it will be necessary for graduates to 'have knowledge of' or to be *au fait* with them so that they can be managed appropriately, and for more specialist skills, to have observed them, and to 'be familiar with' them so that they have an awareness of their place in the context of overall dental care. Essential skills for the graduate in this respect will be an awareness of the scope of evidence-based dental care, an awareness of their own limitations, and the ability to ensure optimal care for every patient by appropriate referral.

The next two years

The dental profession introduced a one-year period of mandatory Vocational Training (VT) in 1993. This is seen as a supplementary year post-graduation in general dental practice to reinforce existing competencies and learn new competencies (e.g. practice management skills).

In 1996 the General Professional Training Committee of the GDC considered the concept of a two-year post-qualification training scheme entitled General Professional Training (GPT). GPT is defined as the structured further development of knowledge skills and attitudes common to all branches of the dental profession, which will provide a basis for informed career choice and improved patient care. The concept of general professional training within dentistry as a voluntary, flexible and broadly based system is now well established, and the SHO grade is a component part. More recently the Standing Dental Advisory Committee (SDAC) at the Department of Health has indicated that the educational and clinical curricula in both SHO and GPT programmes require refinement and standardization. Part of this review will be to affirm the requirement that progress through these programmes be determined by assessment, and there is an interest in the concept of clinical competence-based methods for this.

Re-certification

The GDC established the Re-certification Review Group in 1996 with the remit 'to consider appraisal and re-accreditation and other matters relevant to any future re-certification system for registered dentists'. The Faculty of General Dental Practitioners has already developed proposals for a career pathway in general dental practice which includes, as one of its features, a five-year re-accreditation process. The dental faculties of the surgical Royal Colleges, in co-operation with specialist societies, have developed a continuing professional education scheme for the dental specialities.

The use of agreed competencies in qualitative analysis of process and outcome might provide a more versatile and acceptable tool in performance review. A competency-based system in undergraduate and postgraduate training would not only enable progression to be monitored, but revisiting of key competencies would also make it possible to assess and define an appropriate development programme on an individual basis.

Specialization

The Specialist Training Advisory Committee (STAC) of the GDC has established specialist lists for thirteen distinctive branches of dentistry, enabling patients to identify registered dentists who have met certain requirements. These are defined on the EDC website www.gdc-uk.org and the list is a follows:

Oral Surgery, Surgical Dentistry, Orthodontics, Paediatric Dentistry, Endodontics, Periodontics, Prosthodontics, Restorative Dentistry, Dental Public Health, Oral Medicine, Oral Microbiology, Oral Pathology and Dental and Maxillofacial Radiology.

The prescribed training programmes in each specialty will lead to the award of a Certificate of Competence in Speciality Training (CCST). The STAC is charged with development of the detailed procedures that support the introduction and maintenance of these specialist lists, and the Specialist Advisory Committees that oversee such specialty training are developing competency described outcomes for approved programmes.

The European and American dimension

The methods and standards of undergraduate dental education in Europe have been under scrutiny by virtue of a thematic network project (TNP) funded by the EU's Directorate on Education and Culture. This project, called 'DentEd' (www.dented.org), was designed to promote higher standards of dental education and training throughout Europe by promoting better communication and sharing best practices. The structures being developed in the UK will conform to the regulations produced by the member states of the European economic area, the European Dental Directives.

Undergraduate dental education in the UK is governed by a dental directive, and two specialties, orthodontics and oral surgery, are recognized under the European Dental Directive. The implications of establishing specialist registrar grades and the award of Certificates of Completion of Specialty Training (CCST), followed by the introduction of specialist, lists will be topics for debate within the specialty in the immediate future. There is a level of skill beyond competency known as 'proficiency' which is acquired through increased experience or advanced training leading to specialization.

Competency-defined curricula have been the norm in the USA and Canada for over a decade, the increasing emphasis on competencies in dentistry being based on a recognition of the need for a hands-on approach to dental education. Chambers (1994) defines professional competence in the context of observed behaviour. This behaviour incorporates understanding, skill and value in an integrated response to the full range of requirements presented in clinical practice. It is also emphasized that competence should be viewed as dynamic and responsive to any clear need for change. An individual competency is the demonstrated ability to perform a clinical task or to explain and discuss a clinical concept, and Chambers states that competencies must be acquired in a clinical setting or in the context of patient care.

Professional attitude – competence and conduct

The GDC, as the statutory body for upholding professional standards, is increasing its remit in this role. This is being seen as necessary in the fast-changing world of modern dentistry. It is regarded as unacceptable that a dentist on qualifying can practise for the rest of his or her career without a requirement to keep his or her skills and knowledge updated and to be accountable for the upholding of professional standards. This applies not only to the provision of clinical services but also to financial and lifestyle matters as far as these affect patient care. Abuse of alcohol or drugs and unprofessional attitudes affect the delivery of care and there will be increasing emphasis on the importance of identifying poorly performing practitioners. Litigation goes hand in hand with the delivery of professional services and a competency-based system would not only be a means of ensuring delivery of a high quality of dental care, but also of protecting the practitioner and the profession.

Summary

Competencies are the descriptors around which dental learning and practice are based. They are the means by which dental education outcomes can be assessed and thus high-quality dental care can be achieved. They may be seen as the common thread. This book aims to provide explicit details of what have been identified as key competencies in the practice of dentistry and thereby provide guidance to those who are engaged in the delivery of the undergraduate dental curriculum and beyond. The discussions on whether and how key competencies evolve at all levels in dental education must take place in the context of the ongoing developments alluded to above.

References

Chambers D.W. (1994) Competencies: a new view of becoming a dentist. *J Dent Educ* 58(5), 342–5.
General Dental Council (2002) *The First Five Years: a framework for undergraduate dental education*, 2nd edn. London, General Dental Council.
Shanley D. B. (ed.) (2001) *Dental Education in Europe – Towards Convergence*. DentEd: A Thematic Network project funded by the EU Directorate for Education and Culture, Dental Press Kft.
Unfinished business. Proposal for reform of the Senior House Officer grade (2002). Available at: http://www.rcgp.org.uk/information/publications/summaries/SUMMPDF02/0213.pdf

Acknowledgements

The editors and publishers gratefully acknowledge those who have granted permission to include copyrighted material in this book. Particular reference is made to the General Dental Council's *The First Five Years: a framework for undergraduate dental education*, 2nd edn. and the Quality Assurance Agency for Higher Education's Subject Benchmarking Statements for Dentistry 2002 (1–85824–656–3).

List of abbreviations

ART	atraumatic restorative treatment
AVPU	alert, verbal response, pain response, or unresponsive
BASCD	British Association for the Study of Community Dentistry
BDA	British Dental Association
BNF	*British National Formulary*
BPE	basic periodontal examination
BSP	British Society of Periodontology
BSPD	British Society for Paediatric Dentistry
C/O	complaining of
CCD	charge-coupled device
CJD	Creutzfeldt-Jakob disease
CME	continuing medical education
CMOS	complementary metal-oxide semiconductor
COSHH	Control of Substances Hazardoous to Health
CPITN	Community Periodontal Index of Treatment Need
CPR	cardiopulmonary resuscitation
DAS	Dental Anxiety Scale
DCP	Dental Care Professionals
DMFT	decayed, missing, filled teeth
DNF	*Dental National Formulary*
DOB	date of birth
DPT	dental panoramic tomogram
EMQs	extended matching questions
EO	extra-oral
FBC	full blood count
FOTI	fibre-optic transillumination
FWS	free way space
GA	general anaesthetic
GCF	gingival crevicular fluid
GDC	General Dental Council
GIC	glass ionomer cement
HIV	human immunodeficiency virus
HPC	history of presenting complaint
IARC	International Agency for Cancer Research
IO	intra-oral

IOTN	index of orthodontic treatment needed
LA	local anaesthetic
MCQs	multiple choice questions
MDAS	Modified Dental Anxiety Scale
MELS	maximum exposure limits
MMPA	maxillary-mandibular planes angle
MOCDO	missing, overjet, cross-bite, displacement, overbite
MRSA	methicillin-resistant *Staphlycoccus aureus*
N/A	not applicable
NUG	necrotizing ulcerative gingivitis
NUP	necrotizing ulcerative periodontitis
OCSE	objective structured clinical examination
ODP	operating department practitioner
OES	occupational exposure standards
OVD	Occluso-Vertical Dimension
PC	presenting complaint
PDH	past dental history
PMPs	patient management plans
PSP	photo-stimulable phosphor
RAST	radio-allergen sorbert test
RBCs	resin-based composites
RFA	reason for attendance
RFH	relevant family history
RIDDOR	Reporting of Injuries, Diseases and Dangerous Occurences
RMH	relevant medical history
RVD	Resting Vertical Dimension
SCOT	Structured Clinical Operative Test
SH	social history
SLS	sodium lauryl sulphate
SNA	Sella-Nasion A-point
SNB	Sella-Nasion B-point
SPP	storage phosphor plate
SSCS	stainless steel crowns
TMJ	temporomandibular joint
TTP	tender to percussion
TTV	Transfusion Transmission Virus
vCJD	variant Creutzfeldt-Jakob disease

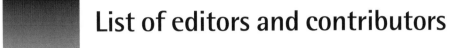

List of editors and contributors

Editors

Professor Peter A. Mossey is Professor of Craniofacial Development and Honorary Consultant in Orthodontics, Orthodontic Section at the Dundee Dental Hospital and School.

Dr Gareth J. Holsgrove is Medical Education Adviser to the Royal College of Psychiatrists.

Professor David R. Stirrups is Head of Orthodontics at the Dundee Dental Hospital and School.

Professor Elizabeth S. Davenport is Professor of Dental Education at Barts and the London Queen Mary's School of Medicine and Dentistry, Queen Mary, University of London.

Contributors

Dr Finbarr Allen is Senior Lecturer/Consultant in Restorative Dentistry at the University Dental School and Hospital, National University of Ireland, Cork.

Dr Patricia Baxter is Specialist in Paediatric Dentistry and Orthodontics at the Victoria Hospital, Kirkcaldy.

Dr Laetitia Brocklebank is Senior Lecturer in Oral Radiology at the Glasgow Dental Hospital and School.

Dr Francis Burke is Senior Lecturer/Consultant in Restorative Dentistry at the University Dental School and Hospital National University of Ireland, Cork.

Professor Iain Chapple is Professor of Periodontology and Consultant in Restorative Dentistry at the Birmingham School of Dentistry, University of Birmingham.

Dr John Drummond is Senior Lecturer/Consultant in Restorative Dentistry at the Dundee Dental Hospital and School.

Dr Dafydd Evans is Senior Lecturer in Paediatric Dentistry at the Dundee Dental Hospital and School.

Dr Garry Fleming is Senior Lecturer in Dental Materials Science in the Division of Oral Biosciences, Dublin Dental School and Hospital.

Professor Farida Fortune is Professor of Medicine in relation to Oral Health at Barts and the London School of Medicine and Dentistry, Queen Mary College, University of London.

Professor Ruth Freeman is Professor of Dental Public Health and Behavioural Sciences at the Queen's University Belfast.

Dr Rebecca Harris is Senior Lecturer in Dental Public Health at the Liverpool University Dental Hospital and School of Dental Studies.

Dr Jennifer King is Lecturer in Ethics and Law Applied to Dentistry at Barts and the London School of Medicine and Dentistry, Queen Mary College, University of London.

Professor Mike Lewis is Professor of Oral Medicine and Head of Oral Surgery, Medicine, and Pathology at the School of Dentistry, Wales College of Medicine, Cardiff University.

Professor Bernard McCartan is Professor and Director of Specialist Training in Dentistry, Royal College of Surgeons in Ireland, and Visiting Professor in Oral Medicine, Trinity College, Dublin.

Dr Christine McCreary is Consultant in Oral Medicine at the University Dental School and Hospital, National University of Ireland, Cork.

Dr Anne Maguire is Senior Lecturer in Child Dental Health at the School of Dental Sciences, University of Newcastle.

Dr Mike Martin is Professor and Honorary Consultant in Oral Microbiology at the Liverpool University Dental Hospital and School of Dental Studies.

Dr Andrew Mason is Lecturer in Oral Biology at the Dundee Dental Hospital and School.

Dr Mike Milward is Clinical Lecturer in Periodontology at the Birmingham School of Dentistry, University of Birmingham.

Professor June Nunn is Professor of Special Care Dentistry at the School of Dental Sciences, Trinity College, Dublin.

Professor Edward Odell is Professor of Oral Pathology and Medicine at King's College London Dental Institute at Guy's, King's, and St Thomas' Hospital.

Dr Jonathan Pedlar is Senior Lecturer in Oral Surgery at the University of Leeds.

Professor Cynthia Pine is Dean of Dental Studies and Professor of Dental Public Health and Primary Dental Care at the Liverpool University Dental Hospital and School of Dental Studies.

Professor Bill Saunders is Professor of Endodontology and Dean of Dentistry at the Dundee Dental Hospital and School.

Professor Damien Walmsley is Professor of Restorative Dentistry at the University of Birmingham.

Dr Paula Jane Waterhouse is Clinical Lecturer in Child Dental Health at the University of Newcastle.

1.1 History taking and examination
Bernard McCartan and Christine McCreary

Key points

Case notes and record keeping:

- Sign and date every entry.
- Write legibly and use sketches or diagrams where appropriate.
- Keep it brief.
- Write contemporaneously – don't trust your memory.
- Be discreet.

Taking a history

- The process should be methodical and systematic.
- The patient should be put at ease.
- The clinician should be friendly but not familiar.
- Avoidance of jargon, leading questions and judgemental remarks is important.
- The clinician must **LISTEN**.

Format of examination

- The process should be methodical and systematic.
- The patient must have consented to the examination and must be put at ease.
- The clinician should be careful to avoid anything that the patient might interpret as impropriety.
- The examination must be systematic and comprehensive.
- Special tests must be selected using your judgement; over-testing is to be avoided.
- The information obtained by examination should be consistent with the history; inconsistencies must be explored.

Introduction

The revised edition of *The First Five Years – A Framework for Undergraduate Dental Education* sets out in detail the aim of undergraduate dental education (GDC 2002). In paragraph 19, under the heading of Generic Learning Outcomes, the first skill specifically alluded to is the ability: 'to obtain and record a comprehensive history, perform an appropriate physical examination, interpret the findings and organize appropriate further investigations'.

Documents from the Quality Assurance Agency (QAA 2002) and from the European Commission Advisory Committee on the Training of Dental Practitioners (EC 2000) mention similar skills. The QAA makes the following specific points in relation to the graduating dentist's abilities under the heading of history, examination, and diagnosis:

- obtain and record a relevant medical history which identifies both the possible effects of oral disease on medical well-being and the medical conditions that affect oral health and dental treatment;

- assess and appraise contemporary information on the significance and effect of drugs and other medicaments, taken by the patient, on dental management;

- obtain a detailed dental history to include chief complaint and history of present illness;

- make a general evaluation of a patient's appearance, including the identification of abnormalities in their physical, emotional or mental status;

- recognize signs of physical, emotional and substance abuse and seek advice from appropriate authorities;

Table 1 Intended learning outcomes for history taking and examination.

Be competent at	Have knowledge of	Be familiar with
Obtaining a detailed history of the patient's dental state	Managing patients from different social and ethnic backgrounds	
Obtaining a relevant medical history	Dental problems that may manifest themselves in older patients and of the principles involved in the management of such problems	
Using laboratory and imaging facilities appropriately and efficiently		
Clinical examination and treatment planning		

- perform a physical and oral examination to include head and neck, oral hard and soft tissues, vital signs and recognize disease states and abnormalities including detrimental oral habits;
- establish and maintain accurate patient records.

The European Commission Advisory Committee on the Training of Dental Practitioners (EC 2000) includes 'taking a proper case history, including a medical history' as the first of the procedures at which a dentist practising in the EU should be clinically competent.

From the above it is apparent that the licensing authorities and the various watchdog organizations are becoming much more aware of what is required of the graduating dentist in the twenty-first century. It is therefore incumbent on the dental undergraduate to be come familiar and proficient both with the process of history taking and in carrying out a clinical examination.

Case notes and record keeping

History and examination are valueless unless recorded. Notes must be contemporary (i.e. they must be written up at the time, not from memory) and they must be dated. Where entries carry over to further pages, each should be dated and the abbreviation 'cont.' (continued) written after the date. Illegible notes are of no use to the clinician or to those who will treat the patient in later years. Both student and supervisor must sign notes. Since students pass quickly through dental schools (and, therefore, perhaps out of memory when they have left) the student's name should be printed clearly along with the signature. A rubber stamp of the name might seem pretentious but is invaluable.

Follow the format of any clinical stationery in use locally. Otherwise lay out the notes in standard order of a history and examination (see below), giving each heading (abbreviated in standard form if you wish). Important findings should stand out clearly.

Avoid abbreviations that are not widely accepted in dentistry (note that many dental schools accept 'local' abbreviations: these are undesirable). Where an error occurs in the notes, the incorrect entry should be deleted by drawing a single line through it. The correct entry should be made and the correction initialled and dated. The error should not be obliterated by use of any opaque material (e.g. correcting fluids) or ink. It should remain readable.

Nothing should be written in the notes that the clinician does not want the patient to read (patients are entitled to see their notes) or that would be inappropriate if read out in court. The entries should be detailed without being unduly wordy.

Photographs, diagrams and sketches are very useful to illustrate the location, size, shape etc. of localized lesions such as lumps and ulcers. Make full use of any pro forma diagrams included in the clinical stationery. Remember that a picture is worth a thousand words.

At the end of this chapter there is a mind map which illustrates the key points of taking a history and examining a patient.

Taking the history

The taking of the history and the clinical examination make up the two components of the diagnostic process and are inextricably linked. Obtaining a history from the patient is essential before it is possible to consider a diagnosis, and in many situations the diagnosis may be made solely from the history. However, history taking is an art, improved and refined by experience, and is therefore a difficult task for the novice. History taking as part of the clinical assessment is an exercise in eliciting, assembling and processing all the relevant information about the patient and their complaint. This, of necessity, takes place over a limited time, therefore it must be methodical, systematic and painstaking. As it is a logical procedure it must be performed in a step-by-step manner.

At the beginning of the dental student's clinical experience there is much to learn and remember. The first meeting and interaction between the student clinician and the patient is an anxious time for the student, although often the patient remains unaware of this.

The case history should be a planned, professional, well-organized and structured conversation that enables the patient to communicate their symptoms, feelings and fears to the clinician. From this information the clinician obtains insight into the nature of the patient's condition and their attitude to it. The level of knowledge and understanding that the student has will, of course, influence the degree of insight obtained following the conversation with the patient.

It is important to position the patient correctly for history taking. The position for history taking is not the same as that for examination or for the delivery of dental treatment. The patient should be sitting comfortably at the same level as the clinician in a position where eye contact can be made, with no physical barriers (such as the bracket table) between them. Only in unusual circumstances should it be necessary to wear a mask while taking a history.

The patient should be encouraged to tell their own story in their own words and, in general, should not be interrupted while they are talking. Occasionally it may be necessary to intervene to clarify particular points or to obtain further information but if possible the patient should be allowed to complete their 'story'. Initial questions should therefore allow the patient to speak at some length and to gain confidence as they settle into the interaction. Medical jargon should be avoided as even those patients who appear to understand medical terminology may use it wrongly and cause misunderstanding. Questions should be phrased sensitively and the clinician must be careful to avoid comment that may be perceived by the patient as critical or judgemental. If possible, open questions should be used throughout the conversation, as this allows patients to use their own words and to summarize their view of the problem. It also gives them confidence, as they feel they are partly directing the interaction and this helps to generate rapport. In this situation, however, the clinician must listen attentively and avoid interruptions to extract the relevant detail.

Some closed questions may be helpful to focus the patient's thoughts, to elicit specific information quickly and to fill in gaps in the information given in response to open questions. Closed questions also prevent vague historians from rambling away too far from the complaint but they do restrict the patient's opportunities to talk. If you ask leading questions the patient may infer that you are not really interested in the problem. Avoid leading questions that suggest a particular answer because patients often feel compelled to agree with your statement.

The history should be of the patient and by the patient but the history taker must direct it. Some patients are better historians than others. The good ones require little help; the poor historians may need to be led but this should be done cautiously. Many patients are nervous, some are inarticulate and others are confused. History taking needs to be tailored to suit the individual patient. Sometimes the patient may find it difficult to speak freely or be may reluctant to divulge certain facts, particularly when it is necessary to discuss personal or psychological details or embarrassing medical conditions. This is when the questioning technique is most critical and will require encouragement and empathy from the clinician, often in the form of a visual or verbal expression of understanding.

Empathy as part of the history-taking process is an important skill to develop as it helps the clinician to establish effective communication. Empathy is a complex multidimensional concept and has moral, cognitive, emotional, and behavioural components that are difficult to define. Clinical empathy may be considered to have three stages. The first is in understanding the patient's situation, perspective and feelings (and their attached meanings). The second is in communicating that understanding back to the patient while confirming its accuracy and the last is in acting on that understanding in a way that is helpful to the patient. The experienced clinician is working on the development of clinical empathy and rapport with the patient from the very first moment of their meeting.

During history taking, the clinician must take the opportunity to assess the patient's mental and emotional state. Rarely there may be an element of psychosomatic disease but more commonly unreasonable and unrealistic expectations may be expressed by the patient, and it is important to try to modify them during the initial consultation otherwise no treatment may be satisfactory.

The student should be competent to demonstrate the ability to take a case history in a planned, professional, well-organized and structured way:

♦ introduce himself to the patient in a friendly but professional manner;

♦ position the patient and himself so that eye contact can be comfortably maintained and so that the patient is not at a disadvantage;

♦ elicit the patient's name, address and date of birth;

♦ ask the patient to describe in their own words their reason for attending;

♦ demonstrate an ability not to interrupt and to allow the patient to tell their story;

♦ avoid the use of medical jargon;

♦ be able to find out all the relevant details relating to the presenting problem by the appropriate use of open and closed questions;

- assess the patient's motivation for attending and their expectations from treatment;
- show that they have, where at all possible, tried to relate to the patient as an individual and had an empathetic encounter;
- elicit a comprehensive medical history;
- elicit a comprehensive dental history;
- elicit a relevant family history;
- elicit relevant details relating to their personal/social circumstances.

Checklist 1 illustrates the overall format of the essential elements for taking a history from a patient. However, it is important to allow the patient to describe in their own words the current problem or reason for attending taking into account the following.

History of the presenting complaint

- record the description of the complaint in *the patient's own words*;
- elicit the meaning of those words;
- record the duration and time course of any changes in symptoms;
- include any relevant facts in the patient's medical history;
- note any temporal relationship between them and the presenting complaint;
- consider any previous treatments and their effectiveness.

Relevant medical history

- attending the doctor for anything at present;
- any history of allergies to drugs such as penicillin or aspirin;
- currently taking any medicine, tablets, pills, injections including oral contraceptive and over the counter preparations or homeopathic medicines;
- had any recent illnesses;
- previous serious illnesses;
- any operations in the past;
- previous hospitalization;
- heart trouble: rheumatic fever, congenital heart lesions, heart murmurs, myocardial infarct, etc.;
- chest trouble: asthma, bronchitis, pneumonia;
- hay fever, eczema or other allergic conditions;
- any problems or family history of problems relating to general anaesthesia;
- any history of epilepsy, diabetes or jaundice.

Past dental history

- attendance: regular, symptomatic or emergency attendance only;
- previous extractions: uncomplicated, dry socket, haemorrhage;
- previous anaesthetic: local anaesthesia with or without sedation, general anaesthesia.

Social history

- occupation
- marital status: if relevant
- children: number, age, health
- smoking: how much per day, for how long
- alcohol consumption: units per week
- other habits
- living arrangements.

Family history (and inherited disease)

- father
- mother
- siblings (brothers/sisters)
- children
- other relatives.

The elements above form the basis for the written record of the clinical interview.

If the patient presents with a history of pain, then there is an additional set of questions and answers relating to the pain history that it is important to include (see **Checklist 2**).

- Type (character): verbal descriptor of pain; aching, throbbing, stabbing, shooting, dull, sharp, etc.
- Severity: mild, moderate, severe.
- Duration: time since onset; minutes, hours, days, weeks, months, years; duration of pain or attacks.
- Frequency/nature: how many attacks; continuous, paroxysmal; is pain present between attacks?
- Periodicity and pattern: night time, meal times etc.
- Exacerbating and relieving factors.
- Localization: get the patient to map out the distribution of the pain if possible; well or poorly defined?

- ◆ Referral: is the pain referred to any other area?

- ◆ Associated features and any other symptom or sign noticed by the patient or physician when they have the pain.

Examination of the patient

When we take a history, examine a patient, or request special tests, we are asking questions. Some of our questions are asked verbally, some with the eyes and hands, and some with the assistance of sophisticated equipment. The skill lies in asking the correct questions and in interpreting the responses.

In theory, as one should ask the same basic questions of all patients, it should not matter which comes first, the history or the examination. Conventionally the history is taken first. This seems an obvious way of doing things. However, there is more than simple convention involved. A patient would probably be more than a little startled to be examined without any attempt at obtaining details of the problem. More importantly, the examination may have to be conducted differently as a result of information obtained during the examination (for example, the patient's cardiac status).

As with the history, the examination must be conducted according to a routine. If this routine is followed for every patient, it should eventually become second nature and the clinician will rarely omit an important part of the examination process. On the other hand, if each examination is approached as a new experience to be carried out in whatever order seems appropriate to the particular patient, then the clinician may become caught up in the detail of examining the obvious and may omit some less obvious but significant part of the process. For this reason it is important not to begin by examining the region of the complaint but by carrying out a full examination that will include this region in its turn. Be methodical: record findings as they are made and do not rely on memory. Recording findings on diagrams may be helpful at future appointments.

Remember that the patient must be expecting to be examined and must have given consent at least by implication. Be sensitive to cultural differences; remember to explain what is about to happen and why; ensure that the patient is comfortable with this.

The routine described here may seem complicated, but with practice the soft tissue examination it is carried out in a couple of minutes on most patients.

When recording size of lesions, use actual measurements in millimetres (mm) rather than by general descriptions such as 'the size of a pea'. When recording the sites of lesions do so by reference to anatomical landmarks rather than by general descriptions such as 'on the side of the face'. Learn to elicit the anatomical planes in which lesions lie. Remember that some anatomical terms cause problems in relation to the oral cavity. For example, 'deeper' implies further from the body surface and hence, in some cases, closer to the surface of the mouth; 'distal' in relation to a tooth implies the surface furthest away from the front of the mouth while in relation to many anatomical structures such as nerves and ducts it may imply the end nearest the front of the mouth.

When recording the consistency of a swelling, use standard terms such as bony, hard (the consistency of contracted muscle), firm (relaxed muscle or fibrous tissue), soft (as in fat tissue) or crepitation. This latter sensation is an eggshell cracking that implies a very thin plate of bone over the swelling. Air trapped in the tissues may give a similar sensation. To determine if there is fluid in a swelling, try to elicit fluctuation by palpation; the index finger of one hand is placed on the swelling, but not centrally, while the index finger of the other hand is placed diametrically opposite on the swelling. Each index finger in turn is pressed lightly into the swelling and the other finger is closely observed to see if it lifts. If so, the test must immediately be repeated in a second plane at right angles to the first. The fluctuation is real only if it is felt in both planes; it is possible, for example, to elicit a pseudo-fluctuation across the body of a muscle but this cannot be done along the muscle.

If a pulse or thrill is felt in the swelling, place the fingers as when detecting fluctuation. If there is a pulse the fingers will move with the pressure wave. If they move radially outwards from the swelling, this is expansile pulsation and the swelling may have an arterial connection; if the fingers rise and fall, then the pulsation is transmitted and the lesion may lie over an artery.

With some swellings it may be useful to place one finger inside the mouth and a finger of the other hand outside; this is called bimanual palpation.

When examining an ulcer note the size (in mm) and position, using anatomical landmarks. Describe the surrounding tissues and the edge of the ulcer: is it a crater (inflammatory ulcer), or are the edges raised (typically due to malignancy), or punched out (syphilis) or undermined (tuberculosis)? Describe the base. Palpate the base. What is its colour and consistency? Is it attached to the underlying tissues?

Examination of the regional lymph nodes must be carried out properly and systematically if it is to be of any use in diagnosis. Position the patient properly. They should be seated upright: this often means seated away from the reclining back of the dental chair. The area to be examined must not be obstructed. Ask the patient to remove any headwear (check if this is acceptable to the patient). Ensure that the button of a tight collar is opened and that a necktie is loosened.

During the intra-oral examination it is useful to have two mouth mirrors. They can be used as retractors, illuminators and reflectors and allow you to make an efficient examination of the soft tissues.

When percussing teeth, remember that the tooth is likely to be tender. If a tender tooth is struck too firmly it may be severely painful. One way to avoid this is to use a pulled blow. Using a mirror as the percussive instrument, hold the mirror neck lightly between thumb and forefinger. Tap the tooth lightly with the handle and pull the handle away immediately rather than letting it fall on the tooth as a dead blow. A mirror is preferable for this purpose as it has no sharp angles at the working end and is unlikely to tear your examination glove.

Vitality testing with hot and cold is sometimes used to elicit pain rather than 'vitality'. In such a case, remember to ask the patient if the sensation that they feel is the same as the pain of which they have been complaining.

The examination routine described here may seem complicated, but with practice it is carried out in a couple of minutes on most patients (see **Checklist 3**). Remember when recording findings that others, including the patient, may read these notes later.

Format of the examination

General

◆ Observe the patient's appearance, demeanour (and gait, if patient has not been seated in the dental chair at first encounter).

Extra-oral

Position the patient correctly for extra-oral examination.

◆ Look at facial appearance, including skin colour, pigmentation, facial expression and facial asymmetry.

◆ Examine swelling: site, size, shape, anatomical planes, appearance of overlying skin, consistency, fluctuence, pulsation or thrill (differentiate between expansile and transmitted pulsation).

◆ Examine ulcers: site, size, shape, edge, floor, base, attachments to underlying tissues.

◆ Prepare and position patient for examination of the regional lymph nodes:

  ▪ Examine the regional lymph nodes: enlargement (lymphadenopathy), tenderness (lymphadentitis).

◆ Examine the parotid and submandibular salivary glands: enlargement, tenderness.

◆ Elicit normal jaw movements and note deviations from normality:

  ▪ Palpate the accessible muscles of mastication for tenderness

  ▪ Palpate the temporomandibular joints for tenderness and clicking.

◆ Examine the lips for swelling and other abnormalities.

Intra-oral examination

Position the patient correctly for intra-oral examination. Examine the soft tissues in the following order:

◆ Lips, buccal mucous membranes, oropharynx, tongue (all surfaces), floor of mouth, hard palate, soft palate, edentulous regions of alveolus, salivary orifices). This order of examination is not the only order that can be adopted but it is important to follow the same order each time to avoid missing important structures or lesions.

◆ Examine the gingivae (see Chapter 2.4 for detailed periodontal examination).

◆ Examine the periodontal tissues as follows: bleeding, pocketing, suppuration (see Chapter 2.4 for detailed periodontal examination).

Examine the teeth

◆ Teeth present, plaque scores, abnormalities of form and structure, abrasion, erosion, attrition, faceting, calculus, fracture (with fracture classification), caries, discolourations, restorations and their condition, mobility, tenderness to percussion, vitality.

◆ Look at any prostheses and note their condition.

Special tests

◆ Take (or arrange to have taken) appropriate radiographic examinations: record projections and radiation doses, process radiographic films, access digital radiographic images (if appropriate), interpret radiographic images and record significant findings.

◆ Select and institute appropriate special tests for haematology, microbiology, histopathology, immunology, take biopsies, obtain blood specimens, take swabs for special tests, label specimens appropriately, complete request forms for laboratory tests, ensure correct transportation of specimens, interpret laboratory results as appropriate.

Checklist 1 **History taking competence**

Task	Yes	No	N/A
Introduces self in professional manner			
Positions patient and self appropriately			
Elicits or checks patient's demographic details			
Starts the interview by asking the patient to describe the problem in their own words			
Allows the patient to tell their story			
Does not interrupt unnecessarily			
Avoids use of technical terms and medical jargon			
Uses open and closed questions appropriately			
Determines patient's motivation			
Determines patient's expectations			
Elicits a comprehensive medical history			
Elicits a comprehensive dental history			
Elicits a relevant family history			
Elicits relevant details relating to the patient's personal and social circumstances			

For the student to be recorded as competent not more than two N/A categories must be marked as N/A (implying unsuitability for this competence test) and all other categories must be marked as YES. Any category marked as NO fails.

Checklist 2 **Pain history competence**

Task	Yes	No	N/A
Asks regarding the character of the pain			
Asks regarding its severity			
Asks regarding the duration			
Asks regarding the frequency/nature			
Asks regarding the periodicity			
Asks regarding any exacerbating and relieving factors			
Asks regarding localization of the pain			
Asks regarding referral of the pain			
Asks regarding associated features or phenomena			

For the student to be recorded as competent not more than two N/A categories must be marked as N/A (implying unsuitability for this competence test) and all other categories must be marked as YES. Any category marked as NO fails.

Checklist 3 **For examination competence***

	Yes	No	N/A
Positions patient correctly for extra-oral examination			
Records patient's general appearance and demeanour			
Records facial appearance			
Examines and records any facial swelling and asymmetry			
Examines and records any facial ulceration			
Positions patient correctly for lymph node examination			
Examines and records the condition of the regional lymph nodes			
Examines and records the condition of the temporomandibular joint (TMJ), jaw movements and muscles of mastication as appropriate			
Examines and records the condition of the lips			
Positions patient correctly for intra-oral examination			
Examines and records condition of the soft tissues			
Examines and records condition of gingivae			
Examines and records condition of the periodontium			
Examines and records the condition of the teeth			
Examines and records the condition of any prostheses			
Selects and prescribes appropriate special tests			
Selects and prescribes appropriate diagnostic imaging			
Maintains an appropriate record of all findings			

For the student to be recorded as competent not more than two N/A categories must be marked as N/A (implying unsuitability of the case for this competence test) and all other categories must be marked as YES. Any category marked as NO fails.

* Some of these categories may be superseded or examined in more detail as competences in specific clinical subject areas. In this checklist a general level of competence is expected rather than the level of examination competence required as a prerequisite for specialist treatment.

References and further reading

EC (2000) *Advisory Committee on the Training of Dental Practitioners Report and recommendations on core knowledge and understanding – prerequisites to achieving clinical proficiencies (competencies)*. Document XV/E/8011/3/97-EN. Brussels, European Commission.

GDC (2002) *The First Five Years: a framework for undergraduate dental education*, 2nd edn. London, The General Dental Council.

QAA (2002) *Dentistry: academic standards*. Subject benchmark statements. Gloucester, Quality Assurance Agency for Higher Education.

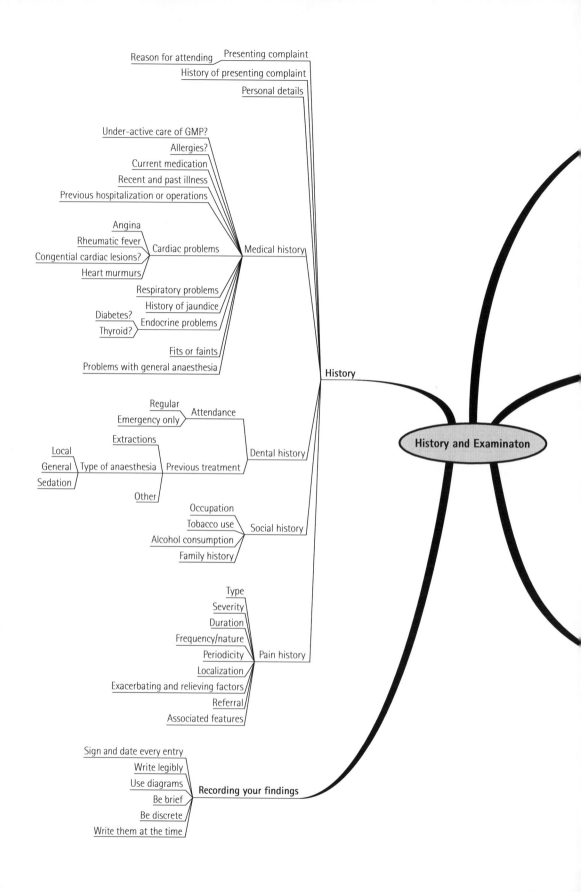

History and Examinaton

History

Presenting complaint
- Reason for attending
- History of presenting complaint
- Personal details

Medical history
- Under-active care of GMP?
- Allergies?
- Current medication
- Recent and past illness
- Previous hospitalization or operations
- Cardiac problems
  - Angina
  - Rheumatic fever
  - Congental cardiac lesions?
  - Heart murmurs
- Respiratory problems
- History of jaundice
- Endocrine problems
  - Diabetes?
  - Thyroid?
- Fits or faints
- Problems with general anaesthesia

Dental history
- Attendance
  - Regular
  - Emergency only
- Previous treatment
  - Extractions
  - Type of anaesthesia
    - Local
    - General
    - Sedation
  - Other

Social history
- Occupation
- Tobacco use
- Alcohol consumption
- Family history

Pain history
- Type
- Severity
- Duration
- Frequency/nature
- Periodicity
- Localization
- Exacerbating and relieving factors
- Referral
- Associated features

Recording your findings
- Sign and date every entry
- Write legibly
- Use diagrams
- Be brief
- Be discrete
- Write them at the time

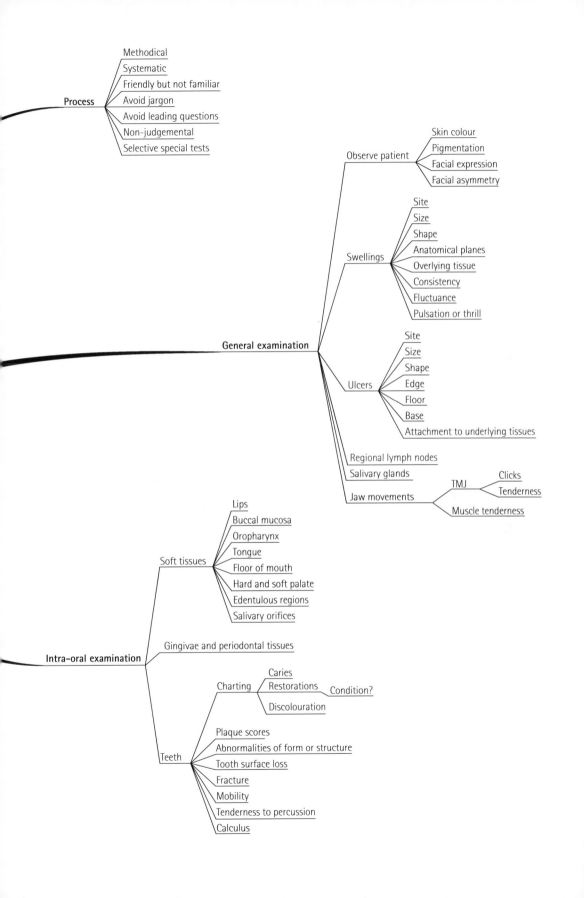

Process
- Methodical
- Systematic
- Friendly but not familiar
- Avoid jargon
- Avoid leading questions
- Non-judgemental
- Selective special tests

General examination
- Observe patient
  - Skin colour
  - Pigmentation
  - Facial expression
  - Facial asymmetry
- Swellings
  - Site
  - Size
  - Shape
  - Anatomical planes
  - Overlying tissue
  - Consistency
  - Fluctuance
  - Pulsation or thrill
- Ulcers
  - Site
  - Size
  - Shape
  - Edge
  - Floor
  - Base
  - Attachment to underlying tissues
- Regional lymph nodes
- Salivary glands
- Jaw movements
  - TMJ
    - Clicks
    - Tenderness
  - Muscle tenderness

Intra-oral examination
- Soft tissues
  - Lips
  - Buccal mucosa
  - Oropharynx
  - Tongue
  - Floor of mouth
  - Hard and soft palate
  - Edentulous regions
  - Salivary orifices
- Gingivae and periodontal tissues
- Teeth
  - Charting
    - Caries
    - Restorations
      - Condition?
    - Discolouration
  - Plaque scores
  - Abnormalities of form or structure
  - Tooth surface loss
  - Fracture
  - Mobility
  - Tenderness to percussion
  - Calculus

1.2 Ethics and law, consent and professionalism

Jennifer King

Key points

- Dentists must understand the ethical, legal and professional basis of good dental care. They must act to protect patients' life and health by always maintaining high standards of care.

- Respect for the other person's right to autonomy establishes trust: therefore obtaining consent, telling the truth and keeping confidentiality are moral imperatives in the dental consultation.

- Dental care should be provided fairly and without prejudice.

- Dentists should be aware of the moral principles that apply to treating vulnerable patients, such as the very young, and people with disabilities.

- Dentistry is regulated by the General Dental Council.

- Ethical practice increases professional satisfaction and reduces the likelihood of complaint or litigation.

- The teaching of ethics and law as applied to the practice of dentistry must be a systematic component of the curriculum and integrated throughout.

Introduction

Law and ethics, consent and professionalism are a related set of subjects that have only recently begun to be taught systematically as an essential part of the dental curriculum. Each is a subject in its own right but they are integrated in their clinical application within health care. These subjects are also closely linked with communication skills in their chair-side application. For instance, the moral principle of respect for autonomy is worked out in dental practice by giving good explanations to people before obtaining their consent to be treated. This in turn requires good communication skills on the part of the dentist. The behavioural sciences are also important here. An understanding of sociology shows, for example, how ethnicity, social class and gender influence health beliefs and behaviour; and an understanding of psychology is important in the recognition and management of pain and anxiety. An example of how these subjects are integrated for a dental patient can be found at the end of this chapter. Competency in these subjects is an essential part of every dental student's personal and professional development.

Dental students must take considerable responsibility in providing dental treatment for patients as a necessary part of their clinical training. In doing so they must form professional relationships with patients and with the dental team. Good relationships are based on trust. Students must therefore learn about the ethical and legal principles on which trust is based. They must develop the necessary communication skills to build trusting relationships with the people they treat. There is now a greater emphasis on people's rights and the importance of patient-centred care. This means sharing information and decision-making rather than the paternalism of the past where dentists took decisions based on their own specialist knowledge.

The professional conduct expected of dentists, and dental students, is outlined by the General Dental Council in *Standards for Dental Professionals* (GDC 2005). Students should maintain high moral standards because it is good practice, rather than simply to avoid complaint. Showing respect for others promotes mutual satisfaction by reducing anxiety and stress for all concerned.

Educational guidelines

Attaining appropriate knowledge, attitudes and skills in law and ethics and professionalism is a necessary part of the undergraduate dental curriculum. These key competencies are outlined in the educational guidance from the General Dental Council, *The First Five Years* (GDC 2002), which gives guidelines for the teaching of these subjects in paragraphs 63–69, and identifies specific learning outcomes:

LAW, ETHICS AND PROFESSIONALISM

Paragraph 63 Dental students should understand the legal and ethical obligations of registered dental practitioners, the permitted activities of DCPs and the regulatory functions of the GDC. Every student should be aware of the principles and practice involved in dental audit, of the ethical responsibilities of the dental profession in clinical investigation and research and in the development of new therapeutic procedures, including the concept of risk assessment and management. The ethical aspects of professional relationships should also be drawn to students' attention and their reconciliation with personal and public morality. Dental students need to have some familiarity with the specific requirement of contemporary general dental practice, including reference to relevant regulations and the valuable role played by the dental defence organisations. Students should recognise and act upon the obligations of membership of the dental profession, as outlined in the GDC's publication *Maintaining Standards*. The Disability Discrimination Act and the Human Rights Act are examples of how this area is rapidly changing and influencing many facets of professional life. Issues of professionalism such as student behaviour with respect to alcohol and the use of recreational drugs should be addressed.

Paragraph 64 The legal basis under which patients are treated should be discussed and the ethical responsibilities that the student assumes under these circumstances examined. No student should proceed to treat patients without a proper understanding of these matters, especially consent, assault, duty of care and confidentiality. The legal requirement to maintain full, accurate clinical records should also be appreciated by the student.

Paragraph 65 Students should understand the importance of communication between practitioner and patient. This helps to develop attitudes of empathy and insight in the student and provides the opportunity for discussion of contemporary ethical issues. Students should also be encouraged to understand their own responses to work pressures and their management. There may be opportunities for integrated or complementary teaching with other basic sciences on topics such as pain, stress and anxiety, and with clinical specialities on topics such as social class, poverty, and the needs of children and the elderly.

Paragraph 66 There should be guidance on the key ethical and legal dilemmas confronting the contemporary practitioner and on the basics of employment law. Students should also have opportunities to consider the ethical and legal dimensions of day to day practice. For example, students should learn how to:

- handle patient complaints;
- ensure that patients' rights are protected;
- provide appropriate care for vulnerable patients;
- confront issues concerning treatment planning and the practice of medicine and dentistry within the context of limited financial resources;
- maintain confidentiality;
- deal with gender and racial issues;
- deal with colleagues failing their professional responsibilities.

Paragraph 67 Students should also understand the practical and ethical considerations that should be taken into account when seeking patients' consent, such as:

- providing sufficient information about conditions and possible treatments;
- responding to questions;
- knowing who is the most appropriate person to give consent;
- gaining consent in emergencies;
- establishing a patient's capacity to give consent;
- statutory requirements that may need to be taken into account;
- gaining valid consent.

> **Paragraph 68** Ethical and safety issues should form an important part of the 'Introduction to Clinical Dentistry' element of the curriculum. The course material must not ignore the moral and ethical dilemmas which confront the dentist in practice.
>
> **Paragraph 69** The ethical approach to patient care will subsequently be reinforced in the clinical dental course, being broadened as time passes to encompass the legal obligations of the practitioner. In that regard, special attention must be paid to the regulatory mechanisms of dentistry, particularly as they apply to general dental practice. Stress should be placed on good record keeping.

Dental students should have opportunities to learn about these subjects throughout the dental course from the beginning to the end as they take increasing responsibility for patient care. They should be competent to apply them in the clinic as they prepare for independent practice on qualification.

It is just as important that the educational institute and its staff should have the highest ethical standards in its organization. If students are to learn professional standards of care they must do so from the examples of good practice that they encounter on the clinic as well as from the more formal curriculum.

Table 1.2.1 Specific learning outcomes for law, ethics and professionalism

Be competent at	Have knowledge of	Be familiar with
Maintaining full accurate clinical records	Responsibilities of consent, duty of care and confidentiality	The legal and ethical obligations of registered dental practitioners with the obligation to practice in the best interests of patients at all times
	Patient rights	
	The permitted activities of DCPs	The need for life-long learning and professional development
	The regulatory functions of the General Dental Council	

Law and ethics applied to dentistry

The law

Dentistry is practised within a legal framework but apart from the Dentists Act itself there in no specific dental law in the United Kingdom. Dentists are subject to the law of the land and increasingly to international law that is evolving in the European Union, for instance in human rights law. The law in Scotland and Ireland, both north and south, is slightly different from the law in England and Wales. There are professional codes of conduct agreed by the dental profession and outlined by the General Dental Council (GDC). There are sanctions if the law is breached through the courts, and disciplinary action may be taken by the GDC.

If a dentist causes harm to a patient they may be open to a civil charge of negligence or assault and damages claimed for financial compensation. This is the most usual route if legal action is taken against a dentist. However a criminal charge may also be brought, for example if a dentist makes fraudulent NHS claims. Any conviction in a court of law, other than for a very minor offence, will automatically be reported to the General Dental Council. A dentist may be charged with professional misconduct and if the charge is upheld then they risk having their name removed from the dental register and losing their license to practice.

Medico-legal decisions are based on the professional standard, sometimes called the Bolam Test, from case law, and a court ruling in the case of Bolam v. Friern Hospital Management Committee (1957). This standard states that in a medico-legal dispute a doctor or dentist will be judged on whether or not their conduct is found by the courts to conform with an accepted body of medical or dental opinion.

Dental students should not be expected to have a detailed knowledge of the law, but they must be aware of the legal framework in which they operate and be familiar in outline with relevant statute and case law and with professional codes of practice.

Dental students must be aware of the legal aspects of dental practice and they should:

◆ Understand that dentistry operates within a legal framework and be aware of the legal sanctions that operate;

◆ Understand that dentists and dental students are subject to the requirements of the General Dental Council, and government through the National Health Service and Department of Health;

◆ Know in outline how the courts function, the difference between criminal and civil actions, and appreciate the difference between case and statute law;

◆ Understand in general terms the law in relation to negligence and assault as it relates to dental practice;

◆ Know the law in relation to consent and data protection as it relates to dental practice;

◆ Be aware of key statute law and professional requirements such as, The Dentists Act (1984), Human Rights Act (1998), Mental Health Act (1983), Children Act (1989), Family Law Reform Act (1969), Data Protection Act (1998), Health and Safety Regulations, General Dental Council Requirements, NHS regulations governing dentistry, relevant Department of Health directives;

◆ Be aware of the relevance of landmark case law, such as Bolam v Friern HMC (1957) (sets the professional standard for judging medico-legal issues): Canterbury v SpenceUSA (1972) (sets a reasonable person standard for consent): Sidaway v Board of Governors Maudsley Hospital (1984) (upholds the professional standard for consent): F v West Berkshire HA (1989) (outlines how treatment is carried out for incompetent adults): Gillick *v* West Norfolk and Wisbech HA (1985) (defines conditions for treating mature children without parental consent): Re C (1994) (outlines legal conditions for judging competence).

Ethics

Ethical principles, unlike the law, do not carry sanctions. Dentists practise ethically because it is an essential part of what it means to be a good dentist. Ethical principles are more general and have wider application than the specific requirements of the law. The standards of a dentist who acts ethically are likely to be higher than those of a dentist who acts to avoid litigation; although adopting ethical standards will undoubtedly meet legal requirements too.

Dentists must always act in ways that are in the best interest of patients. Dental care should be provided on the basis of dental health needs. A dentist has professional duties of care to protect life and health to an acceptable professional standard, to respect autonomy, and to do so justly and fairly. A dentist would be in breach of these duties of care if, for example, they did not employ proper cross-infection control procedures; if they did not obtain informed consent before carrying out treatment; or if they were to discriminate in any way against patients on the grounds of race or gender or age.

Professional duties of care in dentistry

1. To protect life and health
   - Protecting the airway
   - Cross-infection control
   - Only doing necessary treatment
   - Relieving pain
   - Treating infection
   - Restoring function
   - Promoting oral health
   - Meeting health and safety requirements

2. To respect autonomy
   - Respecting patients' rights
   - Obtaining informed consent
   - Explaining options and risks
   - Checking patients have understood
   - Not coercing patients
   - Respecting confidentiality
   - Being open and truthful

3. To act justly and fairly

   ◆ Respecting people of whatever age, race, gender or status

   ◆ Not discriminating e.g. because of blood-borne infections or disability

   ◆ Having dental services accessible to all.

Vulnerability

Some of the most difficult moral dilemmas for dentists arise in the provision of treatment for those who for some reason are especially vulnerable and have limited understanding or reasoning capacity, such as young children, adults with disabilities or psychiatric illness. Understanding the particular moral and legal issues that arise in treating vulnerable patients is essential in the successful management of their dental care.

The dental profession has responsibilities towards the whole community as well as to individual patients. There are important ethical issues that concern equity in resource allocation and in the provision of services that are affordable, accessible and available for all members of the community, including children, people with disabilities and elderly people. Dental students must be aware of the moral debates about prevention versus cure and the need for oral health promotion.

Learning opportunities in ethics should equip dental students to be competent to:

◆ State a dentist's professional duties of care and how they relate to good dental practice, to protect life and health, to respect autonomy, to act justly and fairly;

◆ Be aware of the moral importance of respect for people's rights and patient-centred approaches to dental care;

◆ Understand the difference between moral and legal negligence;

◆ Understand the importance of moral reciprocity in building health-promoting relationships: the golden rule is to do as you would be done by;

◆ Be able to formulate commonly accepted moral arguments and how they may lead to different interpretations in what is acceptable dental practice;

◆ Know how to obtain informed consent from competent adult patients;

◆ Say why confidentiality is such an important principle for maintaining trust and state those circumstances where it may be broken;

◆ Understand the importance of being open and honest with patients;

◆ Know how to obtain consent from children and their proxies;

◆ Know the moral basis for treating vulnerable incompetent adults;

◆ Outline the different ways of providing dental care and the moral arguments for and against each contractual arrangement;

◆ Be aware of the debates about the equitable organization of dental services and resource allocation and the moral arguments for health promotion and prevention versus cure.

Consent

There is an increasing emphasis in all health care on the importance of obtaining consent from patients before any active treatment is started. In 2001 the UK Department of Health published detailed guidance on consent. People's right to consent to or to refuse any treatment should always be respected. Only in an emergency, such as if a person is unconscious, should treatment proceed in the patient's best interests as a matter of necessity. Although a level of consent is clearly implied when a patient makes and keeps an appointment, consent for any tests, intervention or treatment needs to be made more explicit, including information about alternative treatments and any associated risks.

> Graduating dentists must be aware of the necessity for provision of information to patients on the variety of treatment options that might be available, including the risks involved so that informed consent can be obtained.
>
> QAA (2002, paragraph 1.7)

Principles of informed consent require a competent adult patient to be informed, to understand the information and to give their consent freely. The information should include explanations of the dental condition, treatment and what it involves, alternative treatment options including no treatment, any material risks or side effects balanced against the expected benefits, and any cost and time implications.

For some forms of treatment, general anaesthesia and surgery, written consent is required. But consent in writing, especially if there is an extensive treatment plan, is becoming increasingly important for all dental treatment. Then both dentists and patients can be clear about the nature of the proposed treatment and any cost. The information and the options given, the risks explained and the agreed decision should all be documented. For some adults, although they may be legally competent to give their consent, differences in culture and language may necessitate the involvement of health advocates or interpreters.

Informed consent as outlined above applies to competent adult patients who can understand and reason about their treatment, but for vulnerable adults who do not have the necessary mental capacity to consent for themselves clinicians must act in the patient's best interest. The capacity to consent is judged by a person's ability to understand, reason about, remember and apply the information they are given to themselves. Capacity is specific to the task, for instance a person with a mild learning disability may be judged to be able to consent for a dental examination but not for a general anaesthetic.

There is no legal provision for adult proxy for consent to medical or dental treatment in England and Wales at present. Although good practice is to involve carers and the patient as far as they are able in the decision-making process, it is the clinician who ultimately makes treatment decisions for incompetent adults. In Scotland there are new forms of incapacity certification and provisions for proxy decision-making. In England similar mental health law comes into force in 2007.

Consent for children under the age of sixteen must be obtained from a parent or someone who has been granted legal parental responsibility, but a child should not be forced to co-operate against their will. Morally their evolving autonomy should be respected by involving them in explanations and choices about their dental treatment. Mature children not yet sixteen may in some circumstances be judged to be competent and treated as adults and give their own consent. This follows the judgment in the case of Gillick v West Norfolk and Wisbech HA (1985).

Consent is a process that is an essential part of clinical history taking and treatment planning. Any changes in treatment plans should be consented to. Consent should ideally be obtained by the clinician carrying out the treatment. Providing good explanations and offering choices is an important part of good patient management. It respects personal autonomy and helps to create confidence and trust and so improve co-operation.

Obtaining consent is a process that opens up a dialogue between dentists and patients. It is a necessary part of treatment planning that helps to establish a greater partnership.

The process consists of a logical sequence of stages from listening to a patient's history, giving explanations, outlining treatment options and risks, checking understanding and responding to questions to finally obtaining freely given consent.

Informed consent is of benefit to patients and to dentists. It informs the relationship between them respecting patients' rights to information and choice. Taking informed consent seriously establishes mutually beneficial and mature professional relationships that promote good health.

Checklist 4 Stages in the process of obtaining consent

Task	Yes	No
Introductions		
Finding out what the person already understands		
Explaining the nature of the person's dental condition		
Outlining treatment options and procedures		
Explaining risks and benefits, including time and cost		
Checking what has been understood		
Inviting further questions		
Confirming preferred treatment options		
Giving and gaining explicit consent		

There are particular conditions for obtaining informed consent in experimental research that involves human subjects. These have been internationally agreed in the Declaration of Helsinki. Subjects should be told about the research, what it will involve and any potential risks. Participation should be voluntary. Local ethics committees must review all research proposals.

Dental students should learn about the principles of consent and develop skills in their clinical application. They should be competent to:

Table 1.2.2 The value of informed consent

Benefits to patient	Benefits to dentist	Benefits to relationship
• Provides information	• Reduces stress	• Increases mutual understanding
• Offers choices	• Encourages realistic treatment planning	• Establishes common aims
• Reduces anxiety		
• Increases empowerment	• Increases co-operation	• Shares responsibility
• Enhances dignity	• Helps to avoid litigation	• Fosters mature relationships
• Increases motivation	• Saves time and money in the long run	
• Increases satisfaction		• Promotes confidence and trust

- ◆ Know that people have a right to consent to or refuse any dental treatment, and recognize the importance of obtaining informed consent from a legal, ethical and professional standpoint;

- ◆ Understand the doctrine of necessity for treatment in an emergency;

- ◆ Know the criteria for judging legal competence and that competence is task-specific;

- ◆ Appreciate the difference between implied and explicit consent and understand the value of written consent and the importance of documentation;

- ◆ Understand that obtaining consent is a process within the dental consultation;

- ◆ Know the conditions for obtaining informed consent;

  - ▪ Patient is competent to give their consent;

  - ▪ Relevant information is given;

  - ▪ The information is reasonably well understood;

  - ▪ That consent is not coerced or manipulated in any way;

- ◆ Know the categories of information that are required;

  - ▪ The nature of the condition

  - ▪ The reasons for treatment

  - ▪ Any alternative treatment options, including no treatment

  - ▪ Any material risks or possible side effects

  - ▪ The benefits of treatment

  - ▪ Cost and timescale

- ◆ Be aware of the issues of cross-cultural communication in obtaining consent and the need for health advocacy;

- ◆ Know the conditions for obtaining consent from adult patients who are judged to be either temporarily or permanently incompetent to give their own consent by reason

of psychiatric illness or mental disability. Be aware of changes in mental health
law;

◆ Know the particular conditions for obtaining consent for children from their
  parents, and understand the circumstances when mature children may be legally
  able to consent for themselves;

◆ Be aware of the function of ethics committees and the need to obtain informed
  consent for research involving human subjects as stated in the Helsinki Declaration;

◆ Develop clinical and communication skills in obtaining consent for all categories of
  patients.

Professionalism

Professionalism concerns the standards of conduct that all dentists are expected to
maintain. This includes the individual conduct of dentists, the dental team and also the
conduct of the dental profession as a whole. Students of dentistry must know the professional behaviour that is expected of them as they prepare to enter the dental profession.

Dentistry is a self-regulating profession and is governed by the General Dental
Council, a statutory body that has both dental and lay representation. To practise dentists
must be qualified from a recognized dental school and must be registered with the GDC.
Students must be aware that their own conduct must be acceptable if they are
to be registered when they qualify. The GDC has powerful and legally binding disciplinary functions. The Council can warn or remove a dentist's name from the register
if they break the law or if they fail to maintain accepted professional standards. All
qualified dentists are required to have professional indemnity through a protection
society.

Dental students are expected to develop a reflective approach to their work and continue in life-long education and be aware of the GDC requirements for re-certification.
Students must be aware of the principles of clinical governance and of procedures for
dealing with complaints. When qualified they must understand their own limitations
and make specialist referrals when appropriate. Students should understand the health
impact of stress and of drug and alcohol use. Dentists are expected to take appropriate
action if they find for any reason that patients' welfare is put at risk because of poor
standards of performance, of either themselves or a colleague.

Dentists must keep an accurate and confidential record of all patient treatment. All
patient information must be kept safely stored in accordance with the Data Protection
Act. Dental premises must comply with health and safety regulations, especially with
regard to cross-infection control and radiological safety.

Dentists must keep up to date with any changes in the law and any new professional
or government directives that effect dental practice. An example would be recent
changes regarding general anaesthesia in dental practice.

Dentists work as part of a team and they should be familiar with the role and functions of dental care professionals (DCPs) as members of the team.

In learning about professionalism students should:

- ✦ Understand that they are entering a profession and be aware the standards of conduct that are expected of them;

- ✦ Appreciate the role of the GDC as the governing body of dentistry;

- ✦ Know how to handle complaints and be aware of the need for professional indemnity;

- ✦ Develop a reflective approach, be aware of their limitations and continue with life-long education; be aware of the requirements of clinical governance;

- ✦ Be aware of the health implication of stress, and drug and alcohol use. Be prepared to take appropriate action if their own or colleagues standards of work are poor;

- ✦ Keep full, accurate and confidential patient records;

- ✦ Keep all health and safety requirements;

- ✦ Know the role of DCPs;

- ✦ Keep up to date with changes in legislation and health directives that are relevant to dental practice.

All that has been outlined about learning dental ethics and law and professionalism in the dental curriculum must be supported by the collective professional conduct of the educational institute in which students learn. This requires clear policies, for example about consent, confidentiality and the management of dental records. The organizational systems must be user friendly, there is a need for clear disciplinary procedures and for appropriate staff training. Students learn most of all by example and from the conduct of others, especially from their peers and their teachers. Good practice is learnt by observing good practice. Dental schools therefore have particular responsibilities for ensuring that all teaching is ethically conducted and that the organisation and management of the school, especially in its clinical teaching, conforms with acceptable professional practice.

Applying human science and dental ethics to a case

Dental students must not only understand the philosophical arguments, the legal requirements and the behavioural science theory that underpins ethical dental practice, they must be able to apply what they have learnt to specific cases. The following example case shows how these subjects are integrated in a human science and medical ethics integrated examination question for third year dental students.

Case scenario

Mrs Jackson is 75 years old. She has lived alone since her husband died six years ago. She sometimes finds hearing difficult now. She has lost all of her natural teeth and has been wearing upper and lower dentures for the past eight years. She has noticed that her dentures have become rather loose and there is some brown staining which she can't remove with a toothbrush. She has been putting off going to the dentist because she is very nervous. Her first words to you are, 'I don't really like dentists.'

Sociology

Question 1 Mrs Jackson is 75 years old. How does sociology describe different categories of elderly people? What do you understand by the word ageism? Give three examples from research studies of variations in levels of complete tooth loss in different social groups in the UK. You should include evidence from the research literature in you answer.

Answer 1 Many new elderly people are fit and well but others are the frail elderly, they may be sick or have mobility problems or be house-bound or hospitalized. Ageism means discrimination against a person on the grounds of age. Figures for edentulousness vary with social factors such as age, class, ethnicity, and geographical regions in the UK. Students should refer to the adult dental health surveys.

Psychology

Question 2 Mrs Jackson says she is very nervous. Describe two psychological factors which might influence the amount of distress that Mrs Jackson feels in the dental clinic. What are four things that you could do to minimize her anxiety? You should refer to psychological theory and research in your answer.

Answer 2 Previous experience, feeling that what is happening to her is not in her control, are factors that might influence Mrs Jackson's anxiety. Her fear may be alleviated by giving good explanations, involving her in decision-making, reassurance of professional expertise, creating a comfortable and attractive environment (pictures on the ceiling, music), not keeping her waiting, and possible pharmacological options. Psychological theory suggests that negative experiences and lack of control are important in many situations. This is backed up by evidence from research studies of dental anxiety.

Ethics and law

Question 3 What are your ethical duties of confidentiality to Mrs Jackson? Give three examples of when it would be acceptable to speak to another person about her dental condition. Describe four practical steps you would take to ensure her confidentiality. Give three reasons why keeping confidentiality is morally and legally important in dentistry.

Answer 3 Nothing learnt about Mrs Jackson in the dental surgery should be divulged. Information may only be passed to another member of the dental team treating her, if she gives her permission for you to speak to someone else, if a court of law requires information, if a person is in danger of causing serious harm. Practical steps to ensure confidentiality would include closing the door, asking others to leave the room, not speaking about a person in public areas, filing notes securely, having a practice policy on confidentiality. Confidentiality is morally and legally important because it respects a person's rights, respects their autonomy, (the second duty of care) it maintains trust in the dental profession, it increases patient satisfaction and is good business ethics, it is a GDC requirement, and it respects the Data Protection Act.

Communication skills

Question 4 What do you understand by the word empathy? Give an empathetic response to Mrs Jackson's comment that she doesn't like dentists. Mrs Jackson is rather deaf. Describe five communication skills that you could use to overcome the communication challenges raised by Mrs Jackson's deafness.

Answer 4 Empathy means putting your self in the other person's place. Empathetic responses acknowledge the person's feelings, e.g. 'yes dentists can be very frightening', or 'this must make you feel very anxious.' (A non-empathetic response would be 'don't worry'.) Communication skills which would help to overcome her deafness would be non-verbal, i.e. good eye contact, writing things down, using pictures, showing her instruments, materials etc., or verbal, i.e. speaking slowly and clearly, repeating, checking she has understood, attentive listening, using lip reading, or sign language if appropriate.

Conclusion

Dental students must develop skills to be able to relate to patients in ways that are both ethical and empathetic so that people can have confidence in the dental profession. These interpersonal skills compliment a dentist's technical competence.

In conclusion

+ Learning about ethics and law and professionalism must span the whole of the dental curriculum and be systematically taught and assessed. It applies to all clinical subjects.

+ Dental schools must recognize that students need continued support throughout their undergraduate training to establish and maintain the professional conduct that is necessary for them to treat patients and to become good dental practitioners when they qualify.

+ Students learn by example from the organization of the institute in which they study and from the attitudes and conduct of the dentists who teach them. It is therefore essential that high ethical standards inform all that makes up dental teaching and learning.

References and further reading

Beauchamp T. and Childress J. (2001) *Principles of Biomedical Ethics*, 5th edn. Oxford, Oxford University Press.

Brazier M. (2003) *Medicine Patients and the Law*. Harmondsworth, Penguin Books.

Bridgman A., Collier A., Cunningham J., Doyal L., Gibbons D. and King J. (1999) Teaching and assessing ethics and law in the dental curriculum. *Br Dent J* 187(4), 217–19.

Department of Health (2001) *Reference Guide to Consent for Examination or Treatment*. Available at: http://www.dh.gov.uk/consent. London, Department of Health.

General Dental Council (2002) *The First Five Years: a framework for undergraduate dental education*, 2nd edn. London, The General Dental Council.

General Dental Council (2005) *Standards for Dental Professionals*. Available at www.gdc-org.uk.

Humphries G. and Ling M. (2000) *Behavioural Sciences for Dentistry*. Edinburgh, Churchill Livingstone.

King J., Doyal L. and Hillier S. (2000) *Consent in Dental Care*. London, Kings Fund.

Lambden P. (ed.) (2002) *Dental Ethics and Law*. Washington, DC, Radcliffe Medical Press.

Montgomery J. (2001) *Health Care Law*, 2nd edn. Oxford, Oxford University Press.

Ozar D. and Sokol D. (2002) *Dental Ethics at Chairside: professional principles and practical applications*, 2nd edn. Washington, DC, Georgetown University Press.

QAA (2002) *Dentistry: academic standards*. Subject benchmark statements. Gloucester, Quality Assurance Agency for Higher Education.

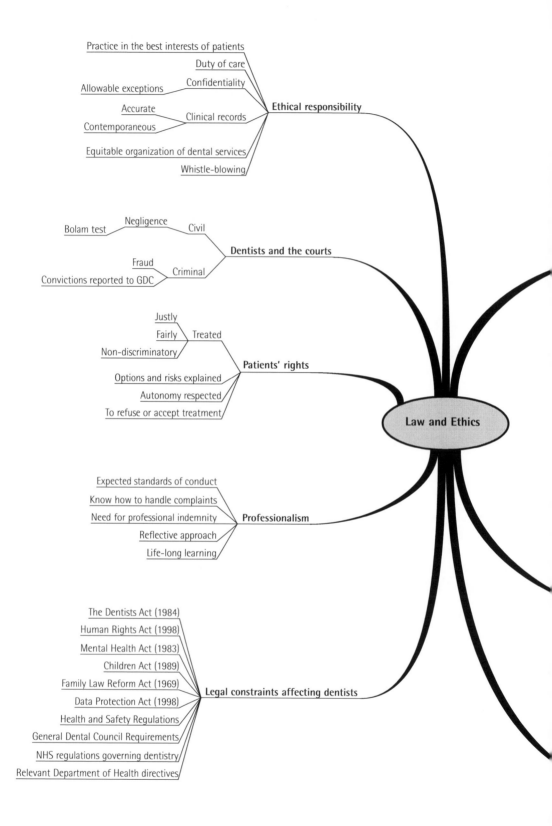

Practice in the best interests of patients
Duty of care
Allowable exceptions — Confidentiality
Accurate
Contemporaneous — Clinical records
Equitable organization of dental services
Whistle-blowing

Ethical responsibility

Negligence
Bolam test — Civil
Fraud
Convictions reported to GDC — Criminal

Dentists and the courts

Justly
Fairly — Treated
Non-discriminatory
Options and risks explained
Autonomy respected
To refuse or accept treatment

Patients' rights

Expected standards of conduct
Know how to handle complaints
Need for professional indemnity
Reflective approach
Life-long learning

Professionalism

The Dentists Act (1984)
Human Rights Act (1998)
Mental Health Act (1983)
Children Act (1989)
Family Law Reform Act (1969)
Data Protection Act (1998)
Health and Safety Regulations
General Dental Council Requirements
NHS regulations governing dentistry
Relevant Department of Health directives

Legal constraints affecting dentists

Law and Ethics

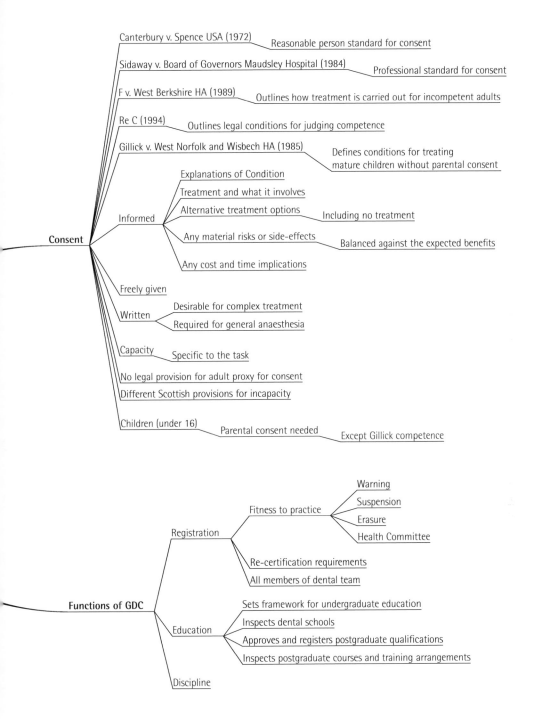

Consent
- Canterbury v. Spence USA (1972) — Reasonable person standard for consent
- Sidaway v. Board of Governors Maudsley Hospital (1984) — Professional standard for consent
- F v. West Berkshire HA (1989) — Outlines how treatment is carried out for incompetent adults
- Re C (1994) — Outlines legal conditions for judging competence
- Gillick v. West Norfolk and Wisbech HA (1985) — Defines conditions for treating mature children without parental consent
- Informed
  - Explanations of Condition
  - Treatment and what it involves
  - Alternative treatment options — Including no treatment
  - Any material risks or side-effects — Balanced against the expected benefits
  - Any cost and time implications
- Freely given
- Written
  - Desirable for complex treatment
  - Required for general anaesthesia
- Capacity — Specific to the task
- No legal provision for adult proxy for consent
- Different Scottish provisions for incapacity
- Children (under 16) — Parental consent needed — Except Gillick competence

Functions of GDC
- Registration
  - Fitness to practice
    - Warning
    - Suspension
    - Erasure
    - Health Committee
  - Re-certification requirements
  - All members of dental team
- Education
  - Sets framework for undergraduate education
  - Inspects dental schools
  - Approves and registers postgraduate qualifications
  - Inspects postgraduate courses and training arrangements
- Discipline

DCPs
- Teamworking
- Permitted activities

1.3 Communication skills
Jennifer King

Key points

- Skill in communication is essential in establishing good relationships between dentists and patients.
- When people have their dental condition explained to them they have more control, redressing some of the imbalances of power that have often characterized clinical relationships in the past.
- Patients want to be listened to; to be understood; to have more information; to have their questions addressed; and to have choices.
- By being empathetic and non-judgemental the dentist can do much to avoid future misunderstanding or complaint.
- Consultations that are patient-centred help to reduce anxiety and bring greater satisfaction to all concerned.
- Communication skills can be learnt and they should be a systematic part of all dental education.

Introduction

Respect for other people is the basis for confident professional relationships in dental practice. Much misunderstanding can be avoided if information is honestly shared and explanations given in an empathetic way so that the other person's perspective is taken properly into account. This includes relationships with people receiving dental care, with the dental team, and with the dental profession.

There are many times when good communication is needed, for instance taking a history, responding to questions, motivating people, calming an anxious child, explaining a procedure to someone who speaks another language and obtaining a person's consent to be treated.

Complaints and litigation are often the result of poor communication. Good communication, on the other hand, increases confidence and satisfaction. Dentists must develop skills in talking to the people they treat so that people feel comfortable in the dental environment.

The General Dental Council, in *The First Five Years* states that 'the key to the provision of good dental care is the ability to communicate with patients from all backgrounds. An understanding of the social issues must be an important part of the undergraduate curriculum' (GDC 2002, paragraph 52).

Learning about communication skills is grounded in a study of the behavioural sciences. Sociology for example provides important insights into health behaviour and the different social groups in the community and helps dentists to understand about how factors such as class, age, gender, ethnicity, and disability influence dental health. Psychological theory explores pain, anxiety and behaviour modification, all of which are very important in the practice of dentistry. The ethical and legal principles of honesty, consent and confidentiality are put into practice using good communication.

Students entering dental school will already have well developed social skills but they must learn to put these skills into practice in a professional setting. As part of their clinical education they will provide dental care for a wide variety of people. They must be competent to recognize communication challenges and identify helpful behaviours in overcoming these challenges. Good communication skills are therefore as important to the practice of dentistry as good technical skills. These are all skills that can be learned.

Educational guidelines

Key competencies in communication are outlined in the educational guidance from the General Dental Council, *The First Five Years,* which gives guidelines for the teaching of communication skills in paragraph 53, and identifies specific learning outcomes:

> Communication skills are an essential aspect of the education of the dental student. As with teaching in psychology and sociology, it can best be undertaken on a collaborative basis both by individuals dedicated to the subject and by clinical dental teachers. Initially, it may be taught in role-playing situations and with simulated patients. Eventually, however, it will be the basis of students' care of their own patients. This is also an appropriate stage to introduce complaints handling procedures. There should be emphasis on the need to communicate to patients the knowledge and understanding of treatment proposed or advice given. The patient's involvement in treatment planning must be stressed. Communication skills must be taught longitudinally throughout the programme so that all students achieve good communication skills before they graduate.
>
> GDC (2002, paragraph 53)

Students will inevitably learn communication skills whilst treating patients in the clinic. In the past this has been the informal way that dentists have learnt how to talk to patients. However, there is much that can be done more systematically to help students to be confident in making clinical relationships by exploring the principles of good communication and putting theoretical principles and research findings into practice. Practical methods of experiential learning, such as working in small groups and role-play with simulated patients, are powerful ways for students to discover for themselves what works well, and what does not work well, when communicating with another person.

Table 1.3.1 Specific learning outcomes for communication skills

Be competent at	Be familiar with
Communication with patients, other members of the dental team and other health professionals	The social and psychological issues relevant to the care of patients

Patient-centred communication

Patient-centred communication recognizes that dentists and patients bring different perspectives to the dental consultation. The patient is concerned about how their dental problem is impinging on their life and making them feel ill, whilst the dentist must consider the disease and its treatment. In the consultation the dentist needs good communication skills to initiate dialogue in order to reach a common understanding that takes proper account of each person's agenda and bridges the gap between the patient's and the dentist's understanding.

Figure 1.3.1 The patient-centred dental interview: schematic representation

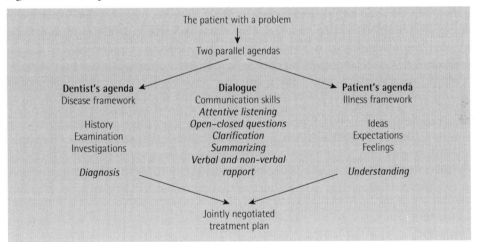

Putman and Lipkin (1995) reviewing research on the outcomes of the patient-centred interview suggest that this approach allows patients to express their concerns, seeks patients specific requests, elicits patients' own understanding of their illness, helps patients to express their feelings, and involves patients in the planning of treatment.

Bridging the communication gap

When a person enters the dental clinic all of their senses – sight, sound, touch and smell – pick up messages, whether consciously or unconsciously. Communication is both verbal and non-verbal, and dental consultations will normally include both.

Non-verbal communication

Communication starts from when a person first enters the dental clinic. Friendly attitudes and courteous staff will help to make a person feel welcome. Whether the clinic is clean and well maintained, whether it is light and well designed, will have an immediate impact. Conversely a poorly maintained clinic and inattentive staff will have a negative impact.

In the dental consultation non-threatening body language, such as sitting at a comfortable distance, at an equal level and having a face to face conversation, encourages good communication. Eye contact is important when talking to some one else and indicates that two people are paying attention to each other. It is very difficult to establish a good relationship with someone who is standing behind you or whilst you are lying flat in a dental chair.

Sensitive use of touch, showing people radiographs and models, looking in a mirror, drawing pictures, and offering literature, are all important means of non-verbal communication which complement the conversational exchange.

Factors that impede communication

People may be nervous and in pain when they visit the dentist, making them feel very vulnerable. Pain and anxiety must be acknowledged and addressed at the outset of the dental consultation because otherwise these factors impede good communication. A patient is unlikely to take in the details of a long and complex treatment plan if their most pressing need is to be relieved of their toothache.

The dentist may take a paternalistic approach and simply tell the patient what they are going to do, whilst the patient blindly accepts what the dentist says. The dentist is seen as the expert and the patient as the passive receiver of care. This is an imbalance of power that often characterizes professional relationships. As a result a person no longer feels that they are in control of their situation. Good communication skills, on the other hand, can help to establish more equal and autonomous relationships, involving people more, in what is after all happening to their mouth, by giving understandable information, offering choices and sharing decision-making.

Empathy

Empathy means putting oneself in the other person's place and acknowledging their feelings. For instance, if a person says that they feel nervous about coming to the dentist then an empathetic response would be to say, 'I can see that this worries you': a non-empathetic response would be 'don't worry about it'. Empathy helps the other person to know that the dentist recognizes their perspective.

The shape of the consultation

Every consultation has a beginning, middle, and end. The substance of the consultation is in the middle but greetings and endings are very important in good communication. A greeting by name helps to develop rapport from the start. Then it is important at the end to say goodbye and arrange further appointments if they are required so that both dentist and patient are clear about what will happen next.

Attentive listening

Listening to a person's account of their dental problem and past medical and social histories requires that dentists are attentive listeners. Being a good listener is a skill that will help dentists to appreciate the other person's point of view and enhance the relationship between them. The dentist will discover what the person already understands about their condition and the vocabulary that they are comfortable with. The dentist can then use the same words in return. It is very reassuring for the other person to know that they are being listened to attentively. Making gestures and facilitating by nodding, and making encouraging remarks such as, 'yes' or, 'please go on', shows that the dentist is listening and encourages people to continue with their account.

Asking questions

Dentists will need to ask questions in the consultation to gather information to enable them to reach a better understanding of a person's dental condition. An open question at the start of a consultation, such as 'how are you today?', helps people to express their concerns. Later in the consultation a closed question will help to focus the consultation and elicit specific information, for example 'how often do you brush your teeth?'

Inviting questions

People too will need to voice their own concerns and queries. Inviting questions and being prepared to listen to and to answer those questions is important if two people are to reach a reasonable understanding. Concerns may be very different. Whilst the dentist may be interested in technical details of dental treatment, the patient may have questions about the cost and time treatment may take and whether it will hurt.

Giving information

The dentist has specialist dental knowledge and expertise that should be shared with a patient so that they are better able to understand their dental condition. Explanations should be simple and avoid the use of technical terms. They should be repeated if necessary and backed up by visual aids and literature. People can only take in limited amounts of information: complex information should therefore be broken down and given in small amounts at a time.

Checking understanding

Assumptions cannot be made that what has been said in the consultation has been fully understood by the patient or that it will be remembered. It is helpful to clarify what the other person does understand and then to summarize what has been said. It is often possible to judge from a person's facial expression whether they do understand or whether they remain puzzled.

Behaviour modification

Dentists must be good teachers as well as good technicians. Non- judgmental explanations and reinforcement support and encourage people to take their own personal responsibility for setting goals and making positive behaviour change to improve their dental health.

Models of behaviour change, for example that proposed by Prochaska and DiClemente (1986), suggests that people must contemplate change before taking action, and then maintain the desired change. At different stages people need a different health education input. It is no good giving a person details of tooth-brushing techniques if they do not even realize that there is a problem. The first task is to help them to become aware of the problem, let them have a chance to think about it, provide information to develop their motivation to make changes, and only then give them any instructions they may need in order to take the appropriate action. This action then needs reinforcement and monitoring to maintain the behaviour change so that it becomes a regular habit.

Figure 1.3.2 Model of change

Based on a model described by Prochaska and DiClemente (1986).

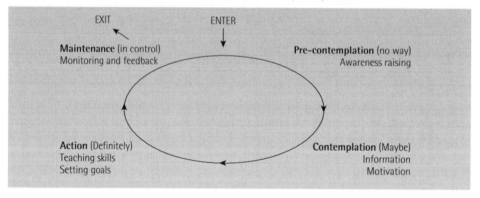

Assertive behaviour

Assertive behaviour aids communication. This is not aggressive, in an angry, arrogant or manipulative way, nor is it passive, rather an assertive person takes personal responsibility and communicates openly and directly. Assertive behaviour says to the other person, 'I'm OK and you're OK'. Accepting and not in any way judging others is the key to nurturing that critical autonomy that enables the other person to feel comfortable in the dental clinic and empowers them to make any desired behaviour changes. If a person has a good relationship with the dentist then they are more likely to be co-operative with treatment, they are more likely to keep appointments and they are more likely to be motivated to look after their own teeth

Cultural competence

Dentists must be aware of cultural diversity and the factors that help to overcome the communication challenges of cultural differences. Cultural competence starts by first recognizing the dentist's own personal background and how that may influence the relationship. Then it is important to be aware of the perspectives of others and the dental health expectations that they may have. Dentists must develop an empathy with people from different cultures. This cultural competence should then become a natural part of all communication between dentists and patients. This applies to differences in gender, education, ethnicity and so on. There may be particular communication challenges when patients and dentists do not share the same language and it may be necessary to work with a translator. Students should understand the role of health advocates and their role in cross-cultural communication.

Vulnerability

Dentists must learn to adapt to the communication needs of a wide variety of people. For instance, they must be particularly aware of the emotions of people who are vulnerable because they are very young or very old or because they have a disability. Communication with people who have a sensory impairment requires skills in communication to be adapted to their needs. A blind person may need to be guided to the dental chair. A deaf person may need to have explanations and instructions written down for them.

Complaints

Dentists may sometimes encounter difficult communication situations and complaints. These need to be handled ethically and sensitively. Should something go wrong, people want to be told the truth, to receive an apology and prevent the same mistakes happening to others. Dealing with complaints promptly and locally helps to resolve the situation quickly and to avoid any further action. It is however always better to minimize any misunderstandings by good communication in the first place.

Building a therapeutic relationship

All communication between dentists and patients aims to build respectful relationships that promote health. Listening to people, giving them appropriate information and involving them in decision-making helps them to feel in control of their situation. This reduces anxiety and gives people greater confidence. The psychologist Carl Rogers (1957) speaks of unconditional positive regard for the other as the necessary requirement for therapeutic change. A trusting, open, friendly and autonomous relationship will help to motivate people and encourage them to take good care of their own dental health.

The broad objectives of our course in communication skills are that students should be competent to:

◆ Understand the importance of good communication skills in creating trust and increasing rapport and mutual satisfaction in clinical relationships, and within the dental team.

◆ Understand how empathetic non-judgemental communication helps to build health-promoting relationships with patients, and encourages co-operation.

◆ Understand how poor communication can have a negative effect on health outcomes and lead to complaints.

◆ Appreciate the value of attentive listening in order to understand the patients perspective, their experiences and expectations.

◆ Discuss the importance of verbal and non-verbal communication and the value of written information and use appropriate non-technical language.

◆ Recognize and use appropriate assertive behaviour and encourage others to do so.

◆ Understand challenges to good communication, such as pain, anxiety cultural differences, and what helps to reduce them.

◆ Be able to describe theories of behavioural change and support patients in developing favourable dental health behaviours.

◆ Deal with complaints and difficult communication situations in a sensitive and ethical way.

◆ Identify behaviours which help communication across cultural barriers and understand the role of health advocates.

A case used in an OSCE assessment of communication skills

Behavioural sciences and ethics and law and communication skills teaching can be integrated as part of a students' personal and professional development programme.

This integration is illustrated in the following objective structured clinical examination (OSCE) station for fifth year dental students. An examiner works with a simulated patient to assess students personal and professional skills using a case scenario, in this example the case concerns obtaining consent for treatment of an impacted wisdom tooth.

Case scenario

You must speak to Jane Wright, a 21-year-old college student, who has pain associated with an impacted wisdom tooth. This is the second time this has happened. You must provide enough information to obtain written consent for treatment. You have a consent form.

Examiner please mark ONE response for each item

Checklist 5 **Obtaining consent for dental treatment for a 21-year-old student**

	Good	Adequate	Not done
Communication skills			
• Introduces self			
• Invites questions and clarification			
• Uses appropriate language			
Giving information			
• Explains the problem			
• Explains treatment options			
• Explains what would happen with no treatment			
• Explains risks associated with the extraction			
• Explains the risks associated with local and general anaesthetic			
• Outlines time it will take			
• Explains benefits			
Obtaining consent			
• Check patient has understood			
• Confirms patient choice			
• Consent form signed			

Conclusion

Building up good professional relationships takes much of the stress and anxiety out of dental care. Both dentists and patients feel more satisfied and misunderstandings and potential complaints or litigation can be avoided.

◆ Communication skills can be learned and they should be systematically taught and assessed throughout the dental curriculum as part of the personal and professional development of dental students.

◆ Communication should be patient-centred and empathetic. This requires listening as well as explaining and giving information or offering advice. Dental treatment can be very daunting, but open honest and non-judgemental approaches can help to overcome anxiety and create more equal relationships in the dental clinic.

◆ Forming good relationships builds up the trust necessary for dental care to be provided in ways that are mutually satisfying and health promoting.

References and further reading

Cole S. and Bird J. (2000) *The Medical Interview*, 2nd edn. St Louis, Mosby.

GDC (2002) *The First Five Years: a framework for undergraduate dental education*, 2nd edn. London, The General Dental Council.

Humphries G. and Ling M. (2000) *Behavioural Sciences for Dentistry*. Edinburgh, Churchill Livingstone.

Jacob J. and Plamping D. (1989) *The Practice of Primary Dental Care*. London, Wright.

Kent G. G. and Croucher R. (1998) Helping patients to achieve oral health. In G. G. Kent and R. Croucher *Achieving Oral Health*, pp. 57–81. London, Wright.

Levinson W. *et al.* (1997) The relationship with malpractice claims among primary care physicians and surgeons. *Journal American Medical Association* 277, 553–9.

Locker D. (2003) Psychosocial consequences of dental fear and anxiety. *Community Dentistry and Oral Epidemiology* 31(2), 144–51.

Maguire P. (2000) *Communication Skills for Doctors*. London, Arnold.

Novak D. (1995) Therapeutic aspects of the clinical encounter. In M. Lipkin, S. Putnam and A. Lazare (eds) *The Medical Interview*, pp. 32–49. New York, Springer.

Prochaska J. and DiClemente C.C. (1986) Towards a comprehensive model of change. In W. R. Miller and N. Heather (eds) *Treating Addictive Behaviour: processes of change*, pp. New York, Plenum Press.

Putman S. and Lipkin M. (1995) The patient-centred interview: research support. In M. Lipkin, S. Putnam and A. Lazare (eds) *The Medical Interview*, pp. 530–7. New York, Springer.

QAA (2002) *Dentistry: academic standards*. Subject benchmark statements. Gloucester, Quality Assurance Agency for Higher Education.

Rogers C. (1957) The necessary and sufficient conditions of therapeutic personality change. *Journal of Consulting and Clinical Psychology* 21, 95–103.

Simpson M. *et al.* (1991) Doctor patient communication; the Toronto consensus statement. *BMJ* 303, 1385–7.

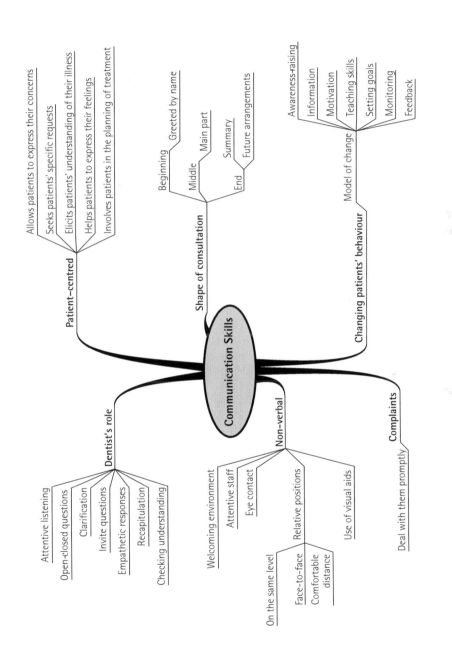

Communication Skills

Patient-centred
- Allows patients to express their concerns
- Seeks patients' specific requests
- Elicits patients' understanding of their illness
- Helps patients to express their feelings
- Involves patients in the planning of treatment

Shape of consultation
- Beginning — Greeted by name
- Middle — Main part
- End — Summary
- Future arrangements

Changing patients' behaviour
- Model of change
  - Awareness-raising
  - Information
  - Motivation
  - Teaching skills
  - Setting goals
  - Monitoring
  - Feedback

Dentist's role
- Attentive listening
- Open-closed questions
- Clarification
- Invite questions
- Empathetic responses
- Recapitulation
- Checking understanding

Non-verbal
- Welcoming environment
- Attentive staff
- Eye contact
- Relative positions
  - On the same level
  - Face-to-face
  - Comfortable distance
- Use of visual aids

Complaints
- Deal with them promptly

1.4 Health and safety

David Stirrups

Key points

It is a legal necessity to have in place systems to ensure as safe a working environment as practical to:

◆ ensure health, safety and welfare at work of all employees.

◆ provide and maintain plant and systems of work that are safe and without risk to health.

◆ make arrangements to ensure the safe use, storage, handling and transport of equipment and materials.

◆ maintain the workplace and its access in a safe condition.

These requirements also extend to others who may be affected e.g. patients.

Introduction

It is not the purpose of this chapter to cover aspects of clinical activity such as infection control and radiological matters that are covered in Chapter 1.5 and Chapter 1.11 respectively, but rather to look at those other aspects of the practice organization where it is appropriate and in some instances, a legal necessity, to have in place systems to ensure as safe a working environment as practical.

The General Dental Council (GDC 2002) expects that new graduate will be familiar with the principles that lead to safe dental practice:

Paragraph 72 With the introduction to clinical dentistry, even though working under close supervision, the student takes responsibility for the safety of patients. Wider aspects of this include the safety of staff and fellow students. Therefore topics which must be discussed at this stage include infection control, substances hazardous to health, fire regulations and safety problems associated with dental equipment, including dental radiographic equipment. A modern approach to health and safety in the workplace should be an essential component of this part of the curriculum. Students must be able to:

- adhere to health and safety legislation as it affects dental practice;

- understand the legal basis of radiographic practice;

- implement and perform satisfactory infection control and prevent physical, chemical or microbiological contamination in the practice of dentistry;

- arrange and use the working practice environment in the most safe and efficient manner for all patients and staff.

GDC (2002, paragraph 72)

In addition the QAA Benchmarking Statement for Dentistry (QAA 2002) stated, in relation to the working environment:

Paragraph 3.23 Graduating dentists should:

- Adhere to health and safety legislation as it affects dental practice;

- Arrange and use the working practice environment in the most safe and efficient manner for all staff and patients.

Intended learning outcomes

It is the first and last bullet points of paragraph 72 (above) that are the particular concern of this chapter – adhering to health and safety legislation and ensuring a safe and efficient working environment. The specified learning outcome that relates to Health and Safety is recorded in paragraph 111 (GDC 2002) 'be familiar with the legal and ethical obligations of registered dental practitioners'.

Ethical and legal obligations

It is incumbent on the practitioner to reduce the risks of untoward incidents. The extent to which this is practical will depend on the interaction between the likelihood of such an incident, the potential consequences and the cost of prevention.

The legal framework underpinning this is the Health and Safety at Work Act (1974). This was enabling legislation that allowed the introduction of specific Regulations (see later) and modifies previous Acts.

Section 2 of the act placed certain responsibilities on all employers. They must, as far as is reasonably practicable:

- Ensure the health, safety and welfare at work of all employees.

- Provide and maintain plant and systems of work that are safe and without risk to health.

- Make arrangements to ensure the safe use, storage, handling and transport of articles and substances.

- Provide instruction and training which ensures the health and safety at work of employees.
- Maintain the workplace and its access in a safe condition.
- Provide a written statement of health and safety policy.
- These requirements also extend to others who may be affected by the business, e.g. patients.

  Various other regulations impact on dental practice:

- Ionising Radiation Medical Activity Regulation (2000) – see Chapter 1.11
- The Control of Substances Hazardous to Health Regulations (1988)
- The Electricity at Work Regulations (1988)
- The Pressure Systems And Transportable Gas Containers Regulations (1989)
- Health and Safety (First Aid) Regulations (1981)

  Further regulations followed in 1992.

- The Management of Health and Safety at Work Regulations (the Framework Regulations)
- The Personal Protective Equipment at Work Regulations
- The Provision and Use of Work Equipment Regulations
- The Health and Safety (Display Screen Equipment) Regulations
- The Manual Handling Operations Regulations
- The Workplace (Health Safety and Welfare) Regulations

  Health and safety can be considered under three headings: people, premises and substances.

People

- Welfare of employees:
  - Safe systems of work
  - Competent and suitable fellow employees
  - Employers own actions
- Accidents and RIDDOR:
  - Notification and recording of accidents
  - Provision of First Aid
- Protective clothing etc.:
  - Provision
  - Replacement

- Ensuring use
- Vaccinations:
  - Hepatitis B

Premises

- Workplace safety:
  - Effective maintenance
  - Adequate ventilation
  - Reasonable temperature
  - Appropriate lighting
  - Cleanliness
  - Suitable seating and workstations
- Traffic routes safe
- Window and door glazing of safety type
- Windows etc. operated and cleaned safely
- Safe doors
- Adequate toilets and washbasins
- Access to drinking water
- Changing and rest facilities
- Electricity safety
- Fire precautions
- Waste disposal:
  - Non-clinical waste
  - Clinical waste
- Water/effluent pollution
- Radiation:
  - X-rays,
  - lasers
- Autoclaves and pressure vessels:
  - Designed for safe use and inspection
  - Appropriate instructions and labels

- Properly installed
- Properly operated
- Periodically inspected
- Correctly maintained and recorded.

Substances

- COSHH assessments:
  - Maximum Exposure Limits (MELS)
  - Ocupational Exposure Standards (OES)
- Mercury:
  - Safe handling
  - Safe disposal

Table 1.4.1 Health and safety checklist when starting work in an unfamiliar dental environment

Fire	Where are the fire extinguishers, exit and assembly area?
Electrical apparatus	Is there a record of current safety certification?
Compressor	Is there a record of current safety certification?
Autoclave	Is there a record of current safety certification, and efficiency?
X-ray equipment	Is there a record of current safety certification, and efficiency?
Personal safety	Are there safety glasses, protective clothing and suitable gloves?
Clinical waste	Is there a appropriate and certified method of disposal?
Mercury	Is there mercury spillage kit? Is there appropriate disposal of waste amalgam?
Working environment	Adequately lit? No obstructions to free movement, suitable methods for cleaning potentially contaminated clinical surfaces etc.
First Aid equipment	Where are the First Aid box, emergency drugs, oxygen cylinder?
Accident reporting	System in place?
Staff	Adequately trained for the duties expected of them, including CPR?
	Appropriate current Hepatitis B immune status?

References and further reading

GDC (2002) *The First Five Years: a framework for undergraduate dental education*, 2nd edn. London, The General Dental Council.

Illey R. and Lambden P. (2002) *A Toolkit for Dental Risk Management*. Abingdon, Radcliffe Medical Press Ltd.

Mathews J. R. (1995) *Risk Management in Dentistry*. Oxford, Wright.

QAA (2002) *Dentistry: academic standards*. Subject benchmark statements. Gloucester, Quality Assurance Agency for Higher Education.

RIDDOR (1995) Available at: www.healthandsafetysmart.co.uk/riddor/htm

Acts of Parliament and Regulations

Health and Safety (First Aid) Regulations (1981)

The Control of Substances Hazardous to Health Regulations (1988)

The Electricity at Work Regulations (1988)

The Pressure Systems and Transportable Gas Containers Regulations (1989)

The Management of Health and Safety at Work Regulations (the Framework Regulations) (1992)

The Personal Protective Equipment at Work Regulations (1992)

The Provision and Use of Work Equipment Regulations (1992)

The Health and Safety (Display Screen Equipment) Regulations (1992)

The Manual Handling Operations Regulations (1992)

The Workplace (Health Safety and Welfare) Regulations (1992)

Ionizing Radiation Medical Activity Regulation (2000)

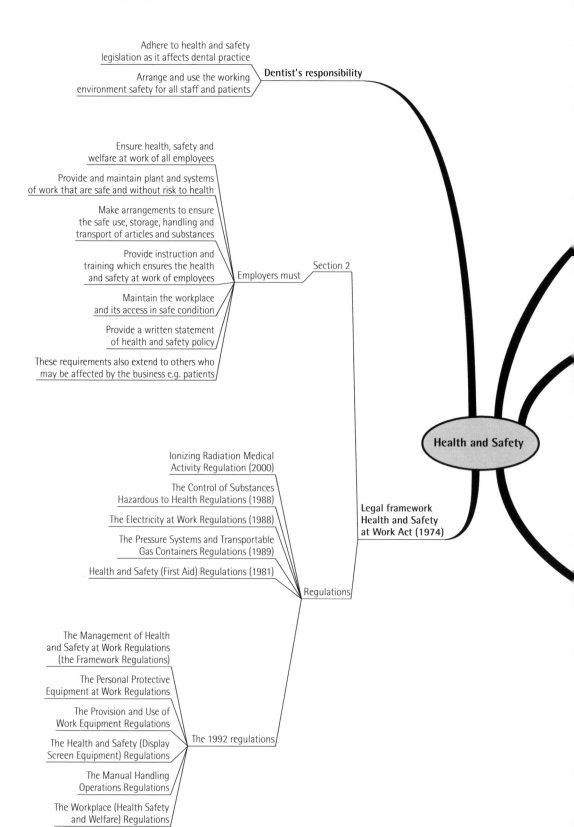

Adhere to health and safety legislation as it affects dental practice

Arrange and use the working environment safety for all staff and patients

Dentist's responsibility

Ensure health, safety and welfare at work of all employees

Provide and maintain plant and systems of work that are safe and without risk to health

Make arrangements to ensure the safe use, storage, handling and transport of articles and substances

Provide instruction and training which ensures the health and safety at work of employees

Maintain the workplace and its access in safe condition

Provide a written statement of health and safety policy

These requirements also extend to others who may be affected by the business e.g. patients

Employers must

Section 2

Ionizing Radiation Medical Activity Regulation (2000)

The Control of Substances Hazardous to Health Regulations (1988)

The Electricity at Work Regulations (1988)

The Pressure Systems and Transportable Gas Containers Regulations (1989)

Health and Safety (First Aid) Regulations (1981)

Regulations

Legal framework Health and Safety at Work Act (1974)

Health and Safety

The Management of Health and Safety at Work Regulations (the Framework Regulations)

The Personal Protective Equipment at Work Regulations

The Provision and Use of Work Equipment Regulations

The Health and Safety (Display Screen Equipment) Regulations

The Manual Handling Operations Regulations

The Workplace (Health Safety and Welfare) Regulations

The 1992 regulations

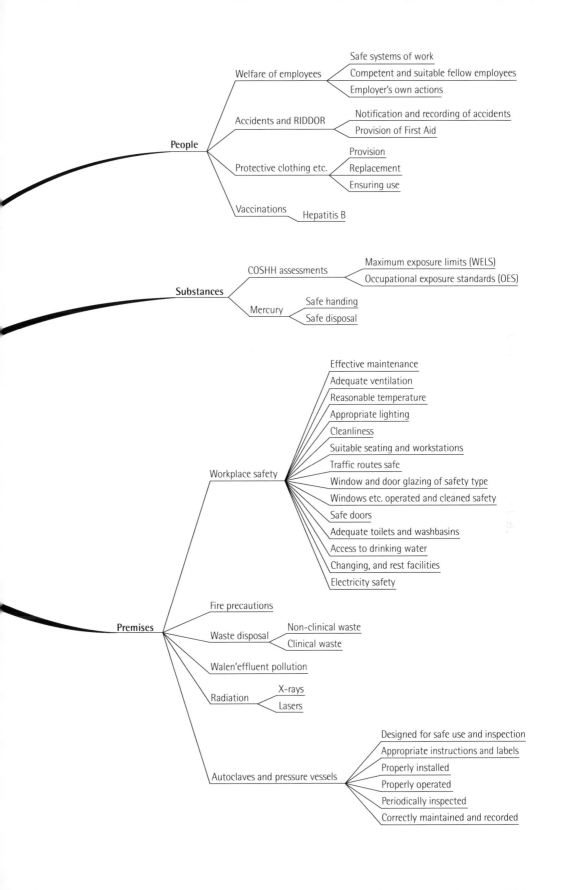

People
- Welfare of employees
  - Safe systems of work
  - Competent and suitable fellow employees
  - Employer's own actions
- Accidents and RIDDOR
  - Notification and recording of accidents
  - Provision of First Aid
- Protective clothing etc.
  - Provision
  - Replacement
  - Ensuring use
- Vaccinations
  - Hepatitis B

Substances
- COSHH assessments
  - Maximum exposure limits (WELS)
  - Occupational exposure standards (OES)
- Mercury
  - Safe handing
  - Safe disposal

Premises
- Workplace safety
  - Effective maintenance
  - Adequate ventilation
  - Reasonable temperature
  - Appropriate lighting
  - Cleanliness
  - Suitable seating and workstations
  - Traffic routes safe
  - Window and door glazing of safety type
  - Windows etc. operated and cleaned safety
  - Safe doors
  - Adequate toilets and washbasins
  - Access to drinking water
  - Changing, and rest facilities
  - Electricity safety
- Fire precautions
- Waste disposal
  - Non-clinical waste
  - Clinical waste
- Walen'effluent pollution
- Radiation
  - X-rays
  - Lasers
- Autoclaves and pressure vessels
  - Designed for safe use and inspection
  - Appropriate instructions and labels
  - Properly installed
  - Properly operated
  - Periodically inspected
  - Correctly maintained and recorded

1.5 Infection control in dentistry

Mike Martin

Key points

- Under their duty of care obligation, dentists must take precautions to implement infection control procedures, and failure to do so leaves them open to serious professional misconduct.

- All dental staff must be adequately trained in the practice procedures and routines which should be in place for sterilization and infection control, and in particular the concept of 'universal precautions'.

- Graduating dentists should be aware of the implications of infection control in dentistry in relation to the micro-organisms (including prions) that potentially could cause infection in dentistry, and of patients at risk.

- There are regulations covering the disposal of non-infected waste, clinical waste and sharps, and for transport of clinical materials through the postal system.

- Any student who knows or has reason to believe that he or she is the carrier of a transmissible blood-borne virus has the responsibility to declare that fact to the dental dean or equivalent person.

Introduction

The GDC *The First Five Years* (2002) document refers to medical emergencies in the undergraduate curriculum in the following paragraphs:

> Health and safety and infection control
>
> **Paragraph 72** With the introduction to clinical dentistry, even though working under close supervision, the student takes responsibility for the safety of patients. Wider aspects of this include the safety of staff and fellow students. Therefore topics which must be discussed at this stage include infection control, substances hazardous to health, fire regulations and safety problems associated with dental equipment, including dental radiographic equipment. A modern approach to health and safety in the workplace should be an essential component of this part of the curriculum. Students must be able to:

◆ adhere to health and safety legislation as it affects dental practice;

◆ implement and perform satisfactory infection control and prevent physical, chemical and microbiological contamination in the practise of dentistry;

◆ arrange and use the working practice environment in the most safe and efficient manner for all patients and staff.

Transmissible diseases

Paragraph 73 Students should be advised that if they may be infected with transmissible diseases that could be a biohazard to patients or colleagues during the dental programme they must obtain medical advice and, if found to be infected, must receive regular medical supervision. Students must act upon any medical advice they receive, which might include the necessity to cease carrying out invasive dental procedures and therefore withdraw from the dental programme. This rule conforms to *Guidance on Professional and Personal Conduct* issued to all dentists by the GDC in *Maintaining Standards*. Any student who knows or has reason to believe that he or she is the carrier of a transmissible blood-borne virus has the responsibility to declare that fact to the dental dean or equivalent person.

Paragraph 95 The course in oral pathology and oral microbiology should integrate with pathology and medical microbiology.

Infection control is also referred to in the Subject Benchmark Statements for Dentistry (QAA 2002) as follows:

Under 'The nature and extent of programmes in dentistry', paragraph 1.8 'Graduating dentists must appreciate the need to deliver dental care in a safe environment for both patients and staff in compliance with health and safety regulations. They must be familiar with the principles and practice of infection control.'

Under 'Subject knowledge and understanding', paragraph 2.7 states that 'graduating dentists should demonstrate knowledge and understanding of sources of infection and the means available for infection control'.

Under 'Working environment', paragraph 3.23 states that graduating dentists should implement and perform satisfactory infection control and prevent physical, chemical or microbiological contamination in the practise of dentistry. They should arrange and use the working practice environment in the most safe and efficient manner for all staff and patients.

For the understanding of infection control in dentistry based on the *The First Five Years* document, the dentist at graduation will need to have a sound working knowledge of the following subjects:

1. Which micro-organisms can potentially cause cross-infection in dentistry.

2. History taking with reference to infection control.

3. The concept of universal precautions.

Table 1.5.1 Intended learning outcomes for infection control in dentistry

Be competent at	Have knowledge of	Be familiar with
Implementing and performing satisfactory infection control to prevent microbiological contamination in the practice of dentistry	Sources of infection and the means available for infection control	The principles and practice of infection control
Maintaining an aseptic technique throughout surgical procedures	The causes and effects of oral diseases needed for their prevention, diagnosis and management	
Knowing when and how to prescribe appropriate anti microbial therapy in the management of plaque-related disease	The scientific principles of sterilization, disinfection and antisepsis	
	The role of laboratory investigations in diagnosis of infectious disease	

4. Personal protection.

5. Surgery design and infection control.

6. Disinfection.

7. Sterilization.

8. Disposal of clinical waste.

9. Clinical materials and the postal system.

Micro-organisms that potentially could cause cross-infection in dentistry

Standards

The student should understand that all the methods used for the prevention of cross-infection in dentistry are based on knowledge of the way micro-organisms cause infection (Marsh and Martin 1999). This knowledge is used to prevent contamination with micro-organisms and subsequent infection. The micro-organisms of interest are:

The blood-borne viruses

- Hepatitis B, C, D, G, and TTV

- Human immunodeficiency virus (HIV)
- Herpes 1, 2, 3, 4, 5
- Respiratory viruses.

Bacteria

- Mycobacterium spp. especially tuberculosis
- Methicillin resistant *Staphylococcus aureus* (MRSA)

Fungi

- *Candida spp.*
- *Aspergillus spp.*

Prions

- Transmissible spongiform encephalopathies (vCJD)

In February 2003, the British Dental Association (BDA) produced a revised infection control booklet (BDA 2003) and in July 2003 dealt specifically with the acquired human prion diseases including sporadic, iatrogenic and variant CJD (Department of Health 2003).

Underpinning knowledge

For each of the above infectious agents the student should:

- Be aware of those groups of people who are at risk.
- Understand the life cycle of the agent.
- Where it is found and how it is commonly transmitted.
- What can be used to destroy it (e.g. autoclaving or disinfection).
- If there is a carriage state, understand the consequences for the operator and the patient.
- The long-term effects of infection (e.g. the relation between hepatitis C and cancer of the liver).

Medical history and infection control

Whilst medical histories can be helpful in eliciting the presence of infectious disease, they may not always be accurate. This is because patients may be 'economical with the truth' or they may not know they have a disease.

In addition to all the standard questions in the medical history (Chapter 1.1) the following should be added:

Do you suffer fomr or have you have had any of the following:

- Hepatitis or jaundice?
- Tuberculosis?

◆ Have any of your close relatives (parent, child, grandparent or grandchild) ever suffered from Creutzfeld–Jakob disease?

◆ Are you taking any antibiotics?

The concept of universal precautions

The student should understand that in order to prevent infection being transferred, all patients should be treated as at risk of being infected and so a common routine for infection control procedures is to be used (General Dental Council 1997). This routine is called universal precautions (see **Checklist 6**).

Personal protection

Personal protection encompasses the following areas of which the student should understand:

1. Immunization
2. Hand protection
3. Masks
4. Eye protection
5. Surgery clothing
6. Innoculation injuries
7. Aerosol and blood splatter
8. Training.

Immunization

The student should understand and have knowledge of the immunizations that are used for the following diseases:

◆ Diptheria
◆ Hepatitis B
◆ Pertussis
◆ Poliomyelitis
◆ Rubella
◆ Tetanus
◆ Tuberculosis.

The route of administration and length of protection is also important.

Hand protection

The care and maintenance of the hands is important in infection control.

Knowledge of the transient and persistent microbial flora is important. The use of a systematic hand wash technique, e.g. the six step procedure (Ayliffe 1975), ensures that hands are cleaned and therefore disinfected during washing.

The student should appreciate the difference between the three types of handwash. These are:

- Social – used in everday life, not systematic;
- Hygienic – systematic, used between patients;
- Surgical – systematic, used to prepare hands prior to invasive operations.

Masks
The use of masks prevents physical splatter of material onto the face. Masks are not a protection against micro-organisms as most are permeable.

Eye protection
The danger of infection or physical damage to the eyes must be clearly understood.

Eye protection is mandatory for both the operator and nurse if damage is to be avoided.

Surgery clothing
This protects the operator and assistants from contamination and during operating procedures it is heavily contaminated. Clothing has to be capable of being washed at temperatures greater than 65°C; this temperature reduces the microbial load below infective doses.

Inoculation injuries (sharps injuries, needlestick injuries)
These are accidents in which the skin may or may not be penetrated. The student should understand the following:

- The principle of assessment of sharp injuries (epithelial penetration or not).
- The first aid associated with these type of injuries (wash with no scrubbing), cover with adhesive dressing.
- Has the wound penetrated the skin?
- If no penetration take no further action.
- If yes consider hepatitis B status and revaccination.
- Is the donor patient carrying HIV? If yes, consider post-exposure prophylaxis with antiretroviral drugs.
- Audit to prevent the injury happening again.

Aerosol and splatter
There should be an understanding of the dangers to the eyes and broken skin of splatter, particularly in relation to the eyes. Aerosols and their generations should be understood in relation to tuberculosis.

Training
The responsibility for infection control lies with the operating dentist, who must ensure that risks are understood.

Surgery design

Surgery design is paramount importance for effective infection control.

♦ The design of the surgery should incorporate the establishment of operating zones for dentist and dental nurse.

♦ The decontamination zone should contain dirty areas for receiving the instruments and all equipment for decontamination. Clean areas should contain an autoclave and space for aseptic storage.

Disinfection

The term is defined as the removal of some pathogens but not necessarily spores. There are four areas of use for disinfection:

1. Surface disinfection. This relies mainly on cleaning and the disinfectant should contain a detergent or surfactant in addition to the agent active against the microbes.

2. Drains, spittoons and sinks. A cidal disinfectant is necessary to kill the micro-organisms and a detergent to remove the adherent films forming on the tubing (biofilm).

3. Impressions and appliances must be disinfected before leaving the surgery.

4. Dental unit water supplies must be disinfected regularly to prevent the build-up of biofilm and the subsequent contamination of the water supply.

Sterilization

This is the killing of all living micro-organisms and prions. There are three key processes:

1. Decontamination of the instruments by manual cleaning, ultrasonics, enzymes or washer/disinfectors.

2. Sterilization by autoclaving.

3. Aseptic storage.

Disposal of clinical waste

By definition clinical waste is material generated during dental procedures, which has been in contact with blood, saliva and oral tissues. This material needs incineration or burial in a deep fill site by a specialist company. Medicines including part-full used local anaesthetic cartridges need disposal separately. Sharps need placement in a rigid box. All waste must be disposed of by specialist companies licensed for this operation.

Clinical materials and the postal system

Students should understand how to send either biopsy material or microbiological samples through the postal system. The need for 'pathological specimens handle with care' labels and leak-proof containers must be emphasized.

Checklist 6 **Universal precautions**

Setting up a dental unit for patient treatment			
SCOT plus mini-viva			
Student			
Observe			
Task	**Yes**	**No**	**N/A**
Student not wearing wrist jewellery, watches or sharp rings			
Wet hands before applying disinfectant soap (Hibiscrub or similar)			
Wash hands, using approved technique			
Turn off tap with wrist/elbow			
Dispose of towel in non-infected waste			
Glove up			
Wipe designated work surfaces with a vigorous scrubbing action			
Wipe headrest and armrest			
Dispose of wipe in infected waste			
Dry the above with paper towels			
Flush all water lines for 30 seconds			
Disinfect designated work surfaces with 70% alcohol wipes			
Disinfect headrest and armrest with 70% alcohol wipes			
Dispose of alcohol wipes in infected waste			
Change gloves, washing hands if contaminated (i.e. glove perforated) or using an alcohol-based disinfectant hand rub if not contaminated			
Place impervious sheet (Traymaid or similar) on bracket table			
Drop mirror, probe tweezers, cotton wool rolls, 3 in 1 tip onto bracket table			
Set up aspirator tips			
Fit barrier sleeves, as appropriate, to difficult to clean surfaces			

Checklist 6 **Universal precautions** – *continued*

Setting up a dental unit for patient treatment			
SCOT plus mini-viva			
Student			
Observe			

Task	Yes	No	N/A
Mini viva			
Student can describe the rationale for the sequence:			
Vigorous cleaning with detergent wipe dry thoroughly			
Disinfect with 70% alcohol			
Student can describe procedures to follow if requiring an item from a drawer/cupboard when assistance unavailable			
Student can demonstrate knowledge of infection control procedure for work passing between clinic and laboratory			
Date completed .... Staff			

Enough absorbent material has to be wrapped around the specimen to ensure that it is absorbed if the container it is placed in breaks.

References and further reading

British Dental Association (2003) *The Decontamination of Surgical Instruments in the NHS in England Update Report*. London, Department of Health. Gateway reference 4625, available at www.dh.gov.uk/assetROOT/04/11/35/44/04113544.pdf

Department of Health (July 2003) *Risk Assessment for vCJD and Dentistry*. Available at www.dh.gov.uk/PolicyAndGuidance/HealthAndSocialCareTopics/CJD

Ayliffe G. A., Bridges K., Lilly H. A., Lowbury E. J., Varney J. and Wilkins M. D. (1975) Comparison of two methods for assessing the removal of total organisms and pathogens from the skin. *J Hyg (Lond)* 75(2), 259–74,

GDC (2002) *The First Five Years: a framework for undergraduate dental education*, 2nd edn. London, The General Dental Council.

General Dental Council (1997) *Maintaining Standards*. Cross infection, paragraph 4.1, and Disposal of clinical waste, paragraph 6.4. London, The General Dental Council.

Lilley, R. and Lambden P. (2002) *The Tool Kit for Dental Risk Management*. Abingdon, Radcliffe Medical.

Marsh P. D. and Martin M. V. (1999) *Oral Microbiology*, 4th edn, Chapter 14, pp. 178–84. Wright, Edinburgh.

QAA (2002) *Dentistry: academic standards*. Subject benchmark statements. Gloucester; Quality Assurance Agency for Higher Education.

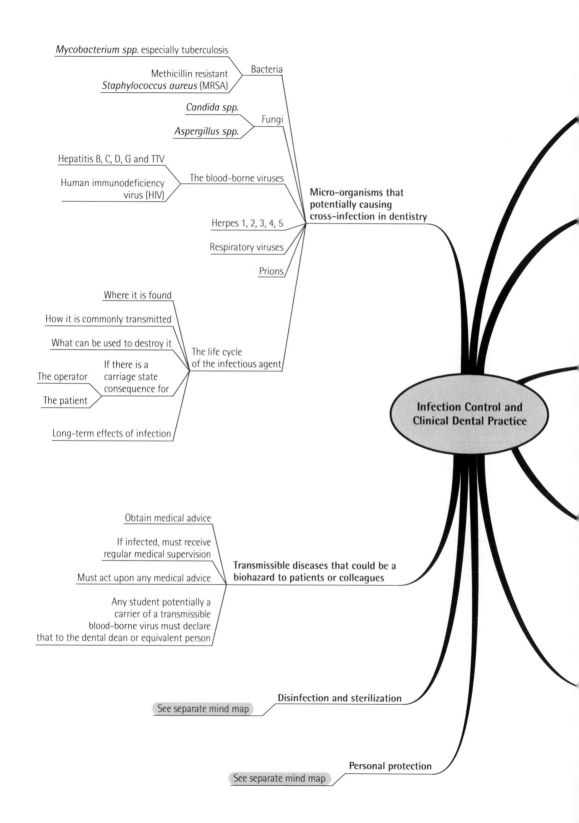

Mycobacterium spp. especially tuberculosis

Methicillin resistant
Staphylococcus aureus (MRSA)

Bacteria

Candida spp.

Aspergillus spp.

Fungi

Hepatitis B, C, D, G and TTV

Human immunodeficiency
virus (HIV)

The blood-borne viruses

Herpes 1, 2, 3, 4, 5

Respiratory viruses

Prions

Micro-organisms that
potentially causing
cross-infection in dentistry

Where it is found

How it is commonly transmitted

What can be used to destroy it

The operator

If there is a
carriage state
consequence for

The patient

The life cycle
of the infectious agent

Long-term effects of infection

Infection Control and
Clinical Dental Practice

Obtain medical advice

If infected, must receive
regular medical supervision

Must act upon any medical advice

Any student potentially a
carrier of a transmissible
blood-borne virus must declare
that to the dental dean or equivalent person

Transmissible diseases that could be a
biohazard to patients or colleagues

Disinfection and sterilization

See separate mind map

Personal protection

See separate mind map

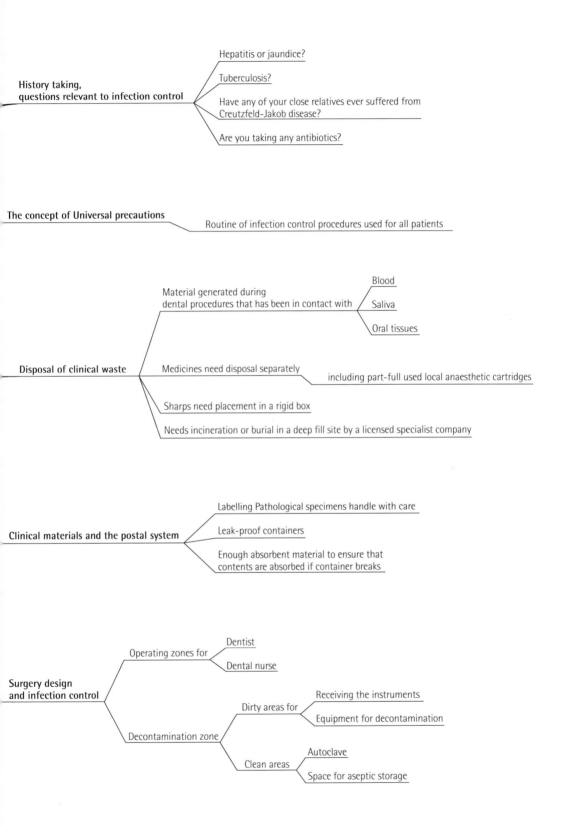

History taking,
questions relevant to infection control
- Hepatitis or jaundice?
- Tuberculosis?
- Have any of your close relatives ever suffered from Creutzfeld-Jakob disease?
- Are you taking any antibiotics?

The concept of Universal precautions
- Routine of infection control procedures used for all patients

Disposal of clinical waste
- Material generated during dental procedures that has been in contact with
  - Blood
  - Saliva
  - Oral tissues
- Medicines need disposal separately — including part-full used local anaesthetic cartridges
- Sharps need placement in a rigid box
- Needs incineration or burial in a deep fill site by a licensed specialist company

Clinical materials and the postal system
- Labelling Pathological specimens handle with care
- Leak-proof containers
- Enough absorbent material to ensure that contents are absorbed if container breaks

Surgery design and infection control
- Operating zones for
  - Dentist
  - Dental nurse
- Decontamination zone
  - Dirty areas for
    - Receiving the instruments
    - Equipment for decontamination
  - Clean areas
    - Autoclave
    - Space for aseptic storage

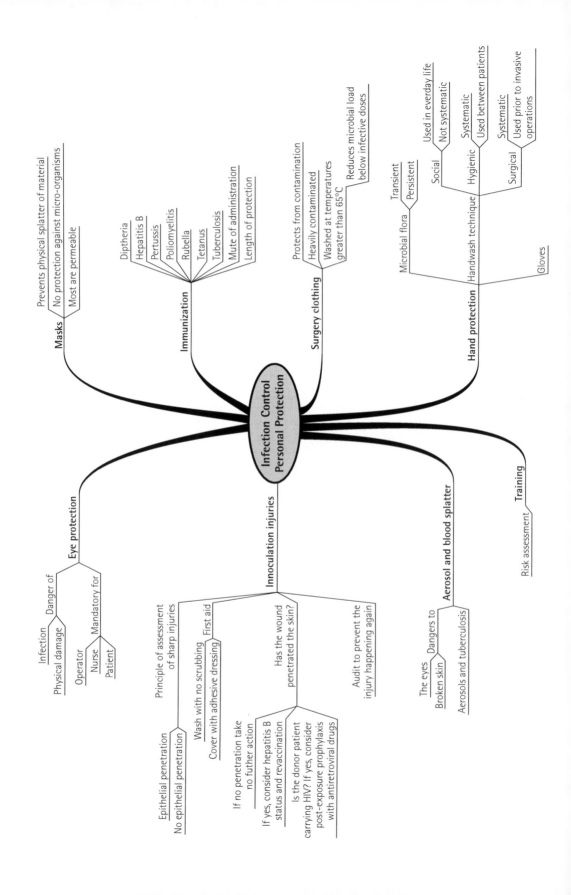

Infection Control Personal Protection

Masks
- Prevents physical splatter of material
- No protection against micro-organisms
- Most are permeable

Immunization
- Diptheria
- Hepatitis B
- Pertussis
- Poliomyelitis
- Rubella
- Tetanus
- Tuberculosis
- Mute of administration
- Length of protection

Surgery clothing
- Protects from contamination
- Heavily contaminated
- Washed at temperatures greater than 65°C
- Reduces microbial load below infective doses

Hand protection
- Microbial flora
  - Transient
  - Persistent
- Handwash technique
  - Social
    - Used in everday life
    - Not systematic
  - Hygienic
    - Systematic
    - Used between patients
  - Surgical
    - Systematic
    - Used prior to invasive operations
- Gloves

Eye protection
- Danger of
  - Infection
  - Physical damage
- Mandatory for
  - Operator
  - Nurse
  - Patient

Innoculation injuries
- Principle of assessment of sharp injuries
  - Epithelial penetration
  - No epithelia penetration
- First aid
  - Wash with no scrubbing
  - Cover with adhesive dressing
- Has the wound penetrated the skin?
  - If no penetration take no futher action
  - If yes, consider hepatitis B status and revaccination
  - Is the donor patient carrying HIV? If yes, consider post-exposure prophylaxis with antiretroviral drugs
- Audit to prevent the injury happening again

Aerosol and blood splatter
- Dangers to
  - The eyes
  - Broken skin
- Aerosols and tuberculosis

Training
- Risk assessment

1.6 Dental public health

Cynthia Pine and Rebecca Harris

Key points

- Graduating dentists should know the prevalence of oral disease in the UK adult and child populations, and understand the health care system in which they will work.

- It is incumbent on the dentist to evaluate social, cultural, psychological, and environmental factors which contribute to general and oral health.

- There is an increasing recognition of the role of the dental professional in and responsibility for improving the general and oral health of the community through treatment strategy, education and service.

- With the increasing amount of information and techniques available to dentists, treatment options, and public access to information on the internet, the dentist must understand the broad principles of scientific research and evaluation of evidence and provide evidence-based advice.

- Graduating dentists should understand the oral health needs of different sections of the community, including those with special needs (see Chapter 2.2).

Introduction and background

Dental public health (also known as 'community oral health' and 'community dentistry') is the branch of dentistry that aims to prevent oral disease and maintain oral health by focusing on societal influences and working with communities as opposed to individual patients. By studying dental public health the dental undergraduate will develop an understanding of how the nature of the community, access to material goods and services, and broad cultural composition will impact on disease experience, type of dental services people prefer, their likely attendance and ability to maintain their own dental health (Pine and Harris 2006). The study of dental public health therefore requires an understanding of the relevant aspects of:

- sociology
- psychology

- population health science including epidemiology and statistics
- health economics
- evidence-based practice
- health promotion and
- health service organization.

In the United Kingdom, dental public health is a recognized speciality of dentistry. At the undergraduate level the role of the dentist as a professional within society with a responsibility in shaping future dental services and responding to demographic shifts, broader health needs and societal change is emphasized (Bradnock and Morris 2000).

The teaching of dental public health should occur throughout the undergraduate course. This will help undergraduates to develop and maintain an appreciation of how the environment in which people live impacts directly on the prevalence of diseases and conditions, beliefs, attitudes and behaviours and the ability of clinicians to intervene successfully and holistically to improve oral health. This is summarized in paragraphs 84 and 85 of *The First Five Years* (GDC 2002) as follows:

DENTAL PUBLIC HEALTH

Paragraph 84 In addition to teaching directed towards the treatment of individual patients, students should be imbued with the concept of the profession's wider responsibilities towards the community as a whole. Teaching in dental public health should emphasise the sociological aspects of healthcare, including the reasons for the widely varying oral and dental needs of different sections and age groups within the population. Knowledge of the social, behavioural, environmental and economic influences on oral and dental health is important, as is an understanding of epidemiological techniques used to determine such effects. The curriculum should include behavioural and epidemiological science relevant to dentistry, the interpretation of data, and the aetiology and natural history of diseases. It should also include an understanding of the social, cultural and environmental factors which contribute to health or illness, the capacity of healthcare professionals to influence these, the principal methods and limitations of disease prevention and health promotion, and the contribution of research methods in dentistry. Students should understand basic statistical and epidemiological concepts and the complexity of service delivery. The understanding should include:

- the different methods of payment and employment of dentists;
- the role of different professional groups;
- equity of service provision and access to care and treatment for people with special needs.

Paragraph 85 Dental students should learn that health promotion involves helping individuals and communities to benefit from increased control over their own health with the intention of improving it. Although many groups and organisations in addition to those composed of healthcare professionals are involved, doctors and dentists can play an important role. Dental students should understand the principles of health promotion and apply them when in contact with patients and at other times, particularly in matters of tooth-brushing with fluoridated dentifrices, diet and nutrition, tobacco avoidance and public health measures such as fluoridation.

The QAA Benchmark Statement for Dentistry also includes dental public health in its description of the nature and characteristics of an undergraduate programme in dentistry. There is a specific section concerned with dental public health in this document, although some aspects of the underpinning knowledge and understanding which are identified as requiring an integration of material from different parts of the undergraduate course will also be relevant to dental public health teaching programmes.

Dental public health

Graduating dentists should understand the health care system in which they will work, and should be able to:

- evaluate social and economic trends and their impact on oral health care.
- recognise their role in and responsibility for improving the general and oral health of the community through treatment strategy, education and service.
- describe and understand the prevalence of oral disease in the UK adult and child populations.

Through integrated learning graduates should be able to demonstrate knowledge and understanding in relation to:

- patients' responses to dental care and how these may be affected by experience and psychological, social and cultural influences.
- the principles and importance of health promotion, health education and prevention in relation to dental disease, and how these principles are applied.
- the system of delivery of health care in the UK with special reference to oral health care.
- the oral health needs of different sections of the community, such as those with special needs.
- the broad principles of scientific research and evaluation of evidence that are necessary for an evidenced-based approach to dentistry (QAA 2002).

74 DENTAL PUBLIC HEALTH

Table 1.6.1 Intended learning outcomes for dental public health and epidemiology

Have knowledge of	Be familiar with
The organization and provision of health care in the community and in hospital	The principles of recording oral conditions and evaluating data
	The prevalence of certain dental conditions in the UK
	The social, cultural and environmental factors which contribute to health or illness
	The principles of health promotion and disease prevention
	The importance of community-based preventive measures

Table 1.6.1 sets out the dental public health learning outcomes listed in *The First Five Years*. Four learning outcomes are listed in paragraph 111 as specifically dental public health learning outcomes, whereas two listed as generic learning outcomes in paragraph 18. All four of the dental public health learning outcomes are identified as areas where the student should 'be familiar with'. Dental graduates are not expected to competent in dental public health since this is a more specialist skill. They are expected to be familiar with, i.e. have developed a basic understanding of these topics, so that they have an awareness of the relevance of the broader context of public health in the provision of dental care.

The order as listed in Table 1.6.1 is preferred as it allows those organizing dental public health courses to build on common sequencing within many dental courses and to complement clinical instruction. It is essential that dental public health is not seen as a topic only for the final year or irrelevant to patient care. The principles should be introduced from the first year and incorporated into clinical courses from the outset using practical examples to make the subject relevant and central to the developing clinician.

Starting off by introducing indices

Students are often introduced to clinical dentistry by examination of colleagues within their own class. This approach allows a number of topics to be introduced in one exercise, for example: cross-infection control, ergonomics, oral examination, correct handling of simple dental instruments and methods to record the dental conditions observed. From this simple data, students can learn how to compose common dental and oral indices. Using this class data can provide an introduction to methods of drawing data together, calculation of mean indices and introducing the concepts of local and national surveys to look at normative need.

Standardizing measurement of disease

As students learn the principles of undertaking and recording an individual's history and examination, there is an opportunity to introduce the concept of how clinicians naturally vary in measuring the severity of oral disease and disorders. This supports a consideration of why there is a need to standardize methods when undertaking surveys to estimate the health status of groups of people to determine the prevalence of certain dental conditions in the UK.

Impact of poor oral health

Experience of working with patients will highlight graphically why a simple record of disease status is insufficient. In order to draw up appropriate treatment plans, under-graduates will need to consider how the condition is impacting on their patients in terms of pain, limited function, loss of sleep, psychological impairment. They will become familiar with recording these impacts for individuals and public health dentists can use this understanding to take the topic into the population perspective. For example, oral health impacts will have social and economic consequences for society at large in terms of lost time from school and work.

Social, cultural and environmental impacts

Providing clinical care for patients of different ages and from different ethnic groups will provide real-life examples of variations of oral health prevalence and expectations of care. Public health dentists can use this common experience to provide a forum for discussion as to why disease prevalence varies, for example, with age, gender, ethnic group, and geographically. It gives a framework for considering the social, cultural, and environmental impacts on health.

Promoting health

Individual advice and counselling to support behaviour change in the use of dietary sugar, tobacco and oral hygiene behaviour will be a core part of the curriculum. However, this needs to be grounded in an understanding of the likely patterns of behaviour and access to material goods and services patients have within their own community. This provides an opportunity to present the concepts of general health promotion and the benefits of taking a common risk factor approach within community based preventive programmes. The key role of professionals complementary to dentistry (DCPs) in delivering prevention both chair-side and within community programmes can form part of the teaching.

Community-based outreach programmes

Dental undergraduates are increasingly able to undertake clinical placements in primary dental settings outside of the dental hospital. This provides excellent opportunities to make dental public health a very real subject for students. It provides extended possibilities for team training and multi-professional placements. A number of projects can be organized that support the development of understanding of the discipline. For example, students may identify as case studies, two or three of their patients seen within primary care and document their history (including social and diet history), examination and treatment plan, together with information on the community setting within which the patient lives and the configuration of local services, to demonstrate how these impact on the uptake and outcome of treatment (Harris *et al.* 2003). This project work can be complemented by formal teaching on the changing structure of dental services in the UK, including how local need will inform commissioning and service provision. The primary care settings will also provide examples of how payment of both the service provider and that required from patients may lead to the emergence of varying patterns of care, provision and uptake.

Learning outcome 1: be familiar with the principles of recording oral conditions and evaluating data

This learning outcome encompasses two distinct aspects, and the standards are therefore listed separately. Evaluation of data is the principle component skill of effective critical appraisal of original scientific papers. Therefore this framework is the one chosen to assess familiarity with this competency.

Standards
Of the principles of recording oral conditions
  The student should:

◆ Be able to define the components of common indices used to measure disease experience, e.g. the DMFT (decayed, missing, filled teeth) index.

◆ Understand that individual clinical assessment is variable and how a standardization process improves the accuracy of measurement of disease experience of a group.

◆ Have knowledge of methods to combine data from oral examinations to produce an average for a group and understand how variation is estimated, e.g. mean DMFT, standard deviation and confidence intervals.

◆ Be able to describe the aims of a screening programme and how screening differs from epidemiology.

Standards
Of the principles of evaluating data.
  The student should:

◆ Be able to examine an original scientific paper describing a survey, clinical study or clinical trial and using a framework like the one below give an assessment of whether the discussion and conclusions are consistent with the data given in the results.

Critical appraisal framework

◆ Why was the study done and what clinical question is being addressed?

◆ What type of study was done?

- Was the study design appropriate to the research question?
- Was the data collected accurately, with possible sources of bias in sampling and measurement addressed?
- Were appropriate statistical tests used in the analysis?
- Do the conclusions drawn by the authors reflect the results?
- What are the implications of the findings?

Checklist 7 For surveys of dental health: recording, compiling and evaluating data on oral conditions

	YES	NO
List the properties of an ideal index		
Describe the components of dental indices e.g. DMFT, basic periodontal examination (BPE), index of orthodontic treatment need (IOTN) and compare these to properties of an ideal index		
Illustrate how to record and calculate common dental indices		
Calculate common statistical parameters from dental indices to measure average occurrence, variation, and understand what simple statistical tests would be appropriate to detect difference between groups		
Examine relevant web pages showing the mapping of composite data on oral conditions using geographical information systems		

Assessment methods

- Practical exercise, e.g. draw up database from dental examinations within class/compare subgroups, e.g. men and women
- OSCE station showing six dental charts, calculate mean DMFT and standard deviation.

Learning outcome 2: be familiar with the prevalence of certain dental conditions in the UK

The student should:

- Be able to define the stages in undertaking a descriptive epidemiological survey.
- Appreciate the principal factors that reduce the quality of survey findings and validity of results leading to biased estimates.
- Know the sequence and key results of national surveys of child and adult dental health in the UK.

- Have the skill to search relevant web sites to find results of national and local surveys.
- Be able to describe major trends in dental and oral health in the UK over time, for adults and children and for different socio-economic groups.

Checklist 8 **For surveys of dental health: study design**

	YES	NO
Describe the principles of study design for epidemiological surveys, case control studies, and clinical trials		
List the essential stages in conducting a cross-sectional epidemiological survey		
Give examples of potential sources of bias in epidemiological surveys and methods to minimise them		
Be able to calculate common statistical parameters to measure average occurrence, variation, and understand what simple statistical tests would be appropriate to detect difference between groups		

Assessment methods

Draw up database from dental examination within the whole class/critical review a paper of a descriptive epidemiological study.

Checklist 9 **For surveys of dental health: national and local UK surveys**

	YES	NO
Give an explanation of how the national surveys of dental health of UK are conducted		
List the years in which child and adult dental health have been surveyed in the UK and describe the change in key parameters, e.g.:		
• level of edentulousness in UK adults		
• changes in mean DMFT in children		
Give examples of differences in dental health of men and women, and of those from different socio-economic groups as measured in national surveys		
Describe the most common barriers to dental attendance		
List the prevalence of self-reported oral hygiene practices		
Give examples by accessing the relevant web site of local variation in dental health of children as recorded by BASCD co-ordinated surveys		

Assessment methods

Web-based search for survey data, students to compile short report of dental health in home area using available data from British Association for the Study of Community Dentistry (BASCD) co-ordinated surveys.

Learning outcome 3: be familiar with social, cultural and environmental factors that contribute to health or illness

The student should:

♦ Be able to define poverty and discuss how access is restricted to material goods and services.

♦ Be able to give a holistic definition of health and describe the difference between normative, felt and expressed need.

♦ Be able to describe oral health-related behaviours that are associated with health and illness and appreciate how these behaviours vary by social and cultural group.

♦ Consider how differences between cultural groups may simply reflect reduced access to preventive health messages, to health services or different health-related habits rather than any inherent variation in disease susceptibility.

♦ Be aware that it is incorrect to assign to an individual characteristics which may describe behaviour of population groups, i.e. avoiding stereotyping.

Checklist 10 For social, cultural and environmental factors that contribute to health or illness

	YES	NO
Describe commonly used classifications of socio-economic status and their limitations		
Give examples of inequalities in oral health		
Give examples of cultural barriers to care		
Discuss reasons for varying dental needs of sections of the population		

Assessment methods

Students to compile case studies of patients during their community outreach placement and discuss how the patients' treatment goals may be influenced by the community setting within which the patient lives.

Learning outcome 4: understand the principles of health promotion and disease prevention

The student should:

◆ Have an understanding of the principles of health promotion as set out in the WHO's Ottawa Charter.

◆ Be able to distinguish between oral health education and oral health promotion.

◆ Be able to define the differences between knowledge, attitudes and beliefs and health-related behaviour.

◆ Be aware of the relative size and influence of advertising of foods and drinks containing high fat, salt, and sugar in contrast to fruits, vegetables and health promotion messages.

◆ Understand that there are cross-departmental government initiatives to promote health and development, e.g. Sure Start.

◆ Describe population approaches to smoking cessation including effect of fiscal measures, changes in advertising and smoking in the workplace on society's attitudes to smoking and prevalence rates.

Checklist 11 Understanding the principles of health promotion and disease prevention

	YES	NO
Outline a range of public health approaches to oral cancer prevention		
Identify opportunities for prevention of oral cancer within the clinical environment		
Within the dental surgery (West *et al.* 2000):		
• ASK a patient about whether they smoke, and if they smoke whether they are interested in stopping. If interested in stopping		
• ADVISE with clear personalized advice and		
• ASSIST by giving self-help literature and helpline number and helping them set a date to quit		
• ARRANGE a follow-up visit within 1–2 weeks after quitting		

Assessment methods

Write a summary of opportunities for the prevention of cancer in a clinical environment and also actions which may be taken by health promoters at a community and
national level.

Learning outcome 5: be familiar with the importance of community-based preventive measures

The student should:

- Differentiate between primary, secondary and tertiary prevention and give examples of individual and population or community-based measures.

- Be able to describe the most common community-based preventive measures and compare advantages and disadvantages.

- Be able to compare and contrast the different community vehicles for the delivery of fluoride.

Checklist 12 **For the importance of community-based preventive measures**

	YES	NO
State the level of fluoride in the water locally and in community outreach area		
Describe any community-based preventive programmes operating locally and in community outreach area e.g. fruit in schools programme, fissure sealants, tooth-brushing programmes		
Discuss systematic review on the effectiveness and safety of water fluoridation		

Assessment methods

A case scenario is given whereby a patient asks his dentist his opinion relating to a
proposal for a water fluoridation programme in the local (low socio-economic) area.
Student to reply to the query.

Learning outcome 6: have knowledge of the organization and provision of health care in the community and in hospital

The student should:

* Understand the differences between primary, secondary and tertiary care.

* Have knowledge of different forms of contracting for dental services, e.g. fee-for-item of service, capitation and of patient co-payments.

* Understand the role of the health authorities in commissioning and performance monitoring dental services, e.g. Primary Care Trusts and Strategic Health Authorities.

* Develop an understanding of the role of members of the primary medical care team in community settings, e.g. the roles of health visitors and community pharmacists.

* Be able to define access to oral health care and discuss how access may be limited for certain groups.

Checklist 13 **For the organization and provision of health care in the community and in hospital**

	YES	NO
Meet and discuss the role of at least three different members of the primary health care team		
Describe different methods of payment and employment of dentists in the UK		
Describe the role and permitted duties of all members of the primary dental care team		

Assessment methods
OSCE station matching roles/permitted duties of members of primary health care team and primary dental care team.

References and further reading

Bradnock G. and Morris J. (2000) The academic discipline of dental public health. *Community Dental Health* 17, 65–7.

GDC (2002) *The First Five Years: a framework for undergraduate dental education*, 2nd edn. London, The General Dental Council.

Harris R. V., Dailey Y. and Lennon M. A. (2003) Recording and understanding social histories by dental undergraduates in a community-based clinical programme. *European Journal of Dental Education* 7, 34–40.

Pine C. M. and Harris R. V. (eds) (2006) *Community Oral Health*, 2nd edn. Berlin, Quintessence.

QAA (2002) *Dentistry: academic standards*. Subject benchmark statements. Gloucester, Quality Assurance Agency for Higher Education.

West R., McNeil A. and Raw M. (2000) Smoking cessation guidelines for health professionals: an update. *Thorax* 55, 987–99.

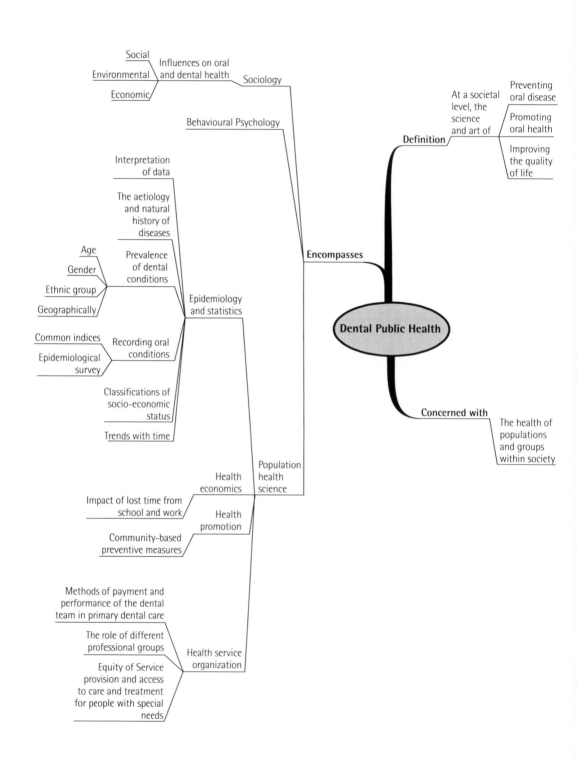

Social
Environmental
Economic
Influences on oral
and dental health
Sociology

Behavioural Psychology

Interpretation
of data

The aetiology
and natural
history of
diseases

Age
Gender
Ethnic group
Geographically
Prevalence
of dental
conditions

Common indices
Epidemiological
survey
Recording oral
conditions

Epidemiology
and statistics

Classifications of
socio-economic
status

Trends with time

Health
economics
Population
health
science

Impact of lost time from
school and work
Health
promotion

Community-based
preventive measures

Methods of payment and
performance of the dental
team in primary dental care

The role of different
professional groups
Health service
organization

Equity of Service
provision and access
to care and treatment
for people with special
needs

Encompasses

Dental Public Health

Definition
At a societal
level, the
science
and art of
Preventing
oral disease

Promoting
oral health

Improving
the quality
of life

Concerned with
The health of
populations
and groups
within society

1.7 Medical emergencies including therapeutics

Farida Fortune

Key points

♦ It is imperative that the dental graduate should be able to diagnose and deal appropriately with all types of medical emergencies.

♦ The dental graduate must be able to recognize cardiac arrest and be able to perform cardiopulmonary resuscitation.

♦ Medical emergencies may be avoidable with underpinning knowledge of the main medical disorders and medications that may place a patient at risk.

♦ Sound knowledge of medical conditions and medications that impinge on dental treatment is essential.

♦ Introduction to medical emergencies should take place in the first year of dental undergraduate training and students throughout their clinical training should be exposed to the diagnosis of and handling of all types of medical emergency.

Introduction

The importance of medical emergencies within the dental setting cannot be overestimated. They may range from commonly encountered vasovagal and hyperventilation episodes to life threatening events.

The GDC *The First Five Years* (2002) document refers to medical emergencies in the undergraduate curriculum:

> **Paragraph 60** The GDC expects that all students will undertake an attachment to the accident and emergency department of a teaching or general hospital. During this attachment the student must not be diverted to dental emergencies but should gain experience of the treatment of acutely ill patients by observing the procedures of triage, prioritisation in terms of airway, breathing, circulation and resuscitation. It is also intended they will develop their interpersonal skills by observing interactions of doctors and other healthcare professionals with acutely ill patients.

Paragraph 61 The GDC considers that at an early stage in the dental programme students must be given instruction in first aid, including the principles of cardiopulmonary resuscitation and its practise under realistic conditions. It is necessary for this practise to be repeated on an annual basis throughout the programme. Students should learn how to recognise and take appropriate action in situations such as:

- Anaphylactic reaction, hypoglycaemia, upper respiratory obstruction, cardiac arrest, fits, vasovagal attack, inhalation or ingestion of foreign bodies and haemorrhage.

Paragraph 62 Dental students must be aware of the relevant information concerning medical emergencies in the GDC's document *Maintaining Standards: Guidance to Dentists on Professional and Personal Conduct* or its successors. It is essential that all premises where dental treatment takes place have available and in working order: portable suction apparatus to clear the oropharynx, oral airways to maintain the natural airway, equipment with appropriate attachments to provide intermittent positive pressure ventilation of the lungs and a portable source of oxygen together with emergency drugs. Graduates should be able to use this equipment and administer drugs effectively.

Medical emergencies are also referred to in the Subject Benchmark Statements for Dentistry (QAA 2002) as follows:

Paragraph 2.8 Graduates should be able to demonstrate knowledge and understanding of medical emergencies that may occur in the dental surgery and their prevention and management, including basic life support and resuscitation.

Paragraph 3.12 Identify and manage dental emergencies and appropriately refer those that are beyond the scope of management by a primary care dentist.

Paragraph 3.24 Provide basic life support for medical emergencies.

Causes of collapse

Learners should have knowledge of:

- Hypersensitivity reactions in a clinical setting.
- Causes of collapse with special reference to:
  - Anaphylactic reaction
  - Diabetic collapse especially hypoglycaemia
  - Myocardial infarction

Table 1.7.1 Intended learning outcomes for medical emergencies

Be competent at	Have knowledge of	Be familiar with
Carrying out resuscitation techniques and immediate management of cardiac arrest	Diagnosing medical emergencies and delivering suitable emergency drugs, where appropriate, using intravenous techniques	Treatment of acutely ill patients by observing the procedures of triage, prioritization in terms of airway, breathing, circulation
Immediate management of anaphylactic reaction, upper respiratory obstruction, collapse, vasovagal attack, haemorrhage, inhalation or ingestion of foreign bodies and diabetic coma		

- Cardiac arrest
- Respiratory arrest
- Respiratory obstruction due to foreign body or reversible obstruction in an acute asthmatic attack
- Addisonian collapse
- Epileptic fit
- Cerebrovascular accident
- Vasovagal attack
- Haemorrhage.

Several skills are entrenched in the above statement:

- The ability to recognize when a patient's condition is deteriorating or that a patient is becoming very unwell;
- When a patient becomes unwell recognize whether the patient has a life-threatening event resulting in a medical emergency;
- Identify and assess the signs and symptoms of all types of medical emergency, or pending emergency.

The ASA (American Society of Anesthesiologists) Physical Status Classification (Table 1.7.2) is a useful tool in routine outpatient and inpatient dental care to assess all patients, and helps to assess risk of an untoward incident occurring during a patient treatment visit. The higher the number in the classification the more likely a patient is of having an untoward event.

Table 1.7.2 ASA Physical Status classification

I	Healthy patient
II	Patient with mild, controlled, functionally non-limiting systemic disease. Examples are well-controlled diabetes, hypertension and epilepsy. A pregnant woman also falls into this category
III	Patient with severe or poorly controlled systemic disease that is functionally limiting, e.g. poorly controlled diabetes, hypertension, epilepsy, and angina
IV	Patient with severe systemic disease that is a constant threat to life, e.g. recent cardiac event or surgery. These patients are usually inpatients who tend only to need emergency dental treatment
V	Moribund patient not expected to survive 24 hours with or without surgery

To elicit vital signs

The dentist should be competent at eliciting vital signs without which the diagnosis of medical emergencies becomes unachievable.

Vital signs:

♦ Pulse, radial, brachial, carotid rate and rhythm

♦ Blood pressure

♦ Respiratory rate

♦ Pupil size, although not a vital sign should be included as it gives invaluable evidence of the state of brain functioning during an emergency.

♦ Temperature.

The knowledge and skill of 'delivering suitable emergency drugs' and 'where appropriate by intravenous route' requires a higher level of learning outcome.

Underpinning knowledge includes

♦ surface anatomy of the upper limb with particular reference to the venous and arterial circulation, and knowledge of skin subcutaneous and muscle layers.

♦ Risk assessment and establishing the need to deliver an intramuscular or intravenous injection is essential.

Perform cardiopulmonary resuscitation

Competent at carrying out resuscitation techniques and immediate management of cardiac arrest, anaphylactic reaction, upper respiratory obstruction, collapse, vasovagal attack, haemorrhage, inhalation or ingestion of foreign bodies and diabetic coma.

(GDC 2002)

To become competent numerous skills are required. Cardiopulmonary resuscitation (CPR) should be taught each year at all dental schools. However, the skill is taught in isolation on manikins. Dental graduates are able to reproduce the practical procedure consistently, when a manikin is used. However, there is no evidence that practitioners are able to transfer this skill effectively in the live situation (AHA Evidence Evaluation Conference 1999).

Although very serious, cardiac arrest is not the most common medical emergency that occurs in the dental surgery.

- The skills to be competent for all stated emergencies should be part of the learners experience and reinforced at several levels during training in order to continue to maintain their skills by repeated CPD reinforcement.

- The most appropriate way to become competent is to combine realistic role-playing with exposure to general medical emergencies in accident and emergency departments.

In an emergency in a dental surgery the dental learner should be able to recognize, identify, and assess and manage the signs and symptoms of any emergency mentioned above.

For all emergencies the learner should be able to carry out an initial assessment: the initial assessment includes the ability to:

- Recognize there is a problem

- Stop dental treatment

- Assess consciousness

- Position the patient

- Assess the airway

- Assess breathing

- Assess circulation

- Apply basic life support – ABC – if necessary

- Assess level of consciousness AVPU (**A**lert, **V**erbal response, **P**ain response, or **U**nresponsive).

The above should result in the learner being able to either initiate further management or call for outside assistance.

Further management will include the ability to:

- Administer oxygen

- Monitor vital signs (pulse rate and rhythm, blood pressure, respiratory rate)

- Make a differential diagnosis

- Be able to initiate treatment for the above list of emergencies

- Where a patient remains unconscious apply basic life support until assistance arrives.

Competency of being able to use appropriate intravenous techniques is not a requirement of the dental graduate, but knowledge is and requires:

♦ Awareness of cross-infection control in relation to medical emergencies

♦ Practical skill of intramuscular injection

♦ Knowledge of placing a venous cannula, venesection and venous delivery.

The most appropriate setting to achieve this is during the human disease course, first on a manikin with reinforcement and observation or practising of this skill during oral medicine and oral surgery outpatient clinics.

Pharmacology and therapeutics

Modern drugs, polypharmacy and changes in lifestyle may have a significant impact on dental care of a patient, and the dental graduate should be able to access and interpret information on pharmacology and therapeutics.

Knowledge

1. The course should ensure that learners have knowledge of and understanding of the pharmacology of common drugs:

    ♦ The principles of absorption, distribution and elimination of drugs in the body

    ♦ The characteristics of drug interactions

    ♦ The pharmacology and mechanism of action of drugs used in infection, inflammation, and pain management

    ♦ The pharmacology of drugs used in the management of cardiovascular, respiratory, endocrine, and central nervous system disorders

    ♦ Local anaesthetics, drugs used in sedation and general anaesthetics

    ♦ Antibiotics, antiviral, and antifungal drugs

    ♦ Haemostatics and anticoagulants

    ♦ Drugs of abuse.

2. The effect of non-dental medication on the management and proposed dental treatment planning. Have knowledge of:

    ♦ The indications and contraindication for drug use

    ♦ Drug dosage

    ♦ Routes of administration

    ♦ Drug action and reaction to dental problems

    ♦ Adverse drug reactions.

3. Have knowledge of all therapeutic agents used in clinical dentistry:
   - describe drugs used in routine clinical dentistry
   - have knowledge of the way these agents are chosen, prescribed and administered
   - discuss adverse reactions to the above therapeutic agents.
4. The essentials of the design of clinical trials. Have knowledge of:
   - Single and double blind aspects
   - Statistical method.

Skill

- Write a prescription using the *Dental National Formulary* (DNF) which is legible and legal
- Prescribe and administer an appropriate drug for given situations in the dental setting
- Use different sources of drug information both the *DNF* and *British National Formulary* (BNF), data sheets, and local Poison and Drug Information Units
- Recognize and administer using appropriate dosage, and correct route agents used in the treatment of medical emergencies that may occur in dental practice.

Checklist 14 **Management of the collapsed dental patient**

	YES	NO
Stop dental treatment		
Assess consciousness		
Alert?		
Verbal response?		
Pain response		
Unresponsive		
Position patient		
Assess airway		
Assess breathing		
Assess circulation:		
• pulse rate, rhythm and magnitude		
Apply basic life support as necessary*		
Get assistance as needed		

* See **Checklist 15**.

Checklist 15 **Sequence of actions for adult CPR (UK Resuscitation Council)**

	YES	NO
Ensure safety of rescuer and victim		
Check the victim and see if he responds:		
If he does not respond:		
• Shout for help		
• Turn the victim on to his back and then open the airway:		
Keeping the airway open, look, listen and feel for breathing (more than an occasional gasp or weak attempts at breathing):		
• Look for chest movement		
• Listen at the victim's mouth for breath sounds		
• Feel for air on your cheek		
If the victim is not breathing and you are alone – summon help, and if there are occasional gasps or weak attempts at breathing:		
• **Give 2 slow, effective** rescue breaths, each of which makes the chest rise and fall:		
• Ensure head tilt and chin lift		
• Pinch the soft part of his nose closed with the index finger and thumb of your hand on his forehead		
• Open his mouth a little, but maintain chin lift		
• Take a deep breath to fill your lungs with oxygen, and place your lips around his mouth, making sure that you have a good seal		
• Blow steadily into his mouth whilst watching his chest; take about 2 seconds to make his chest rise as in normal breathing		
• Maintaining head tilt and chin lift, take your mouth away from the victim and watch for his chest to fall as air comes out		
Assess the victim for signs of a circulation:		
• Look, listen and feel for normal breathing, coughing or movement by the victim and check the carotid pulse		

Checklist 15 **Sequence of actions for adult CPR (UK Resuscitation Council)** – *continued*

	YES	NO
If there are no signs of a circulation, or you are at all unsure, start chest compressions:		
Combine rescue breathing and chest compression:		
• After 30 compressions tilt the head, lift the chin, and give 2 effective breaths		
Continue resuscitation until:		
• Qualified help arrives and takes over;		
• The victim shows signs of life;		
• You become exhausted		

References and further reading

Fortune F. (2004) *Human disease for dentistry.* Oxford, Oxford University Press.

Resuscitation Council (UK) (2005) New international consensus on cardiopulmonary resuscitation. *British Medical Journal* 331, 1281–2.

GDC (2002) *The First Five Years: a framework for undergraduate dental education,* 2nd edn. London, The General Dental Council.

QAA (2002) *Dentistry: academic standards.* Subject benchmark statements. Gloucester, Quality Assurance Agency for Higher Education.

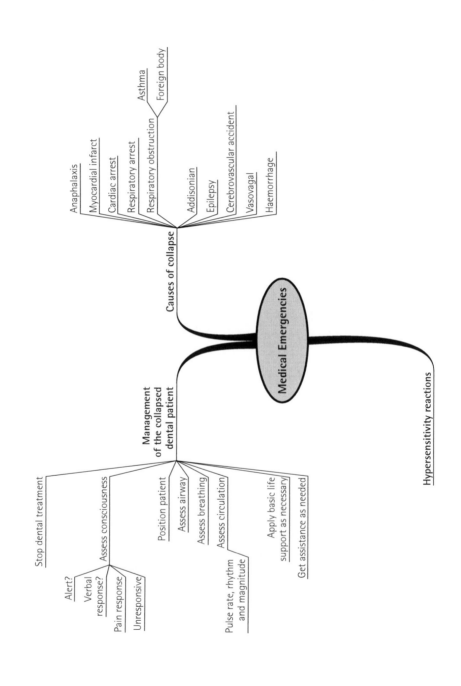

Medical Emergencies

Causes of collapse
- Anaphalaxis
- Myocardial infarct
- Cardiac arrest
- Respiratory arrest
- Respiratory obstruction
  - Asthma
  - Foreign body
- Addisonian
- Epilepsy
- Cerebrovascular accident
- Vasovagal
- Haemorrhage

Management of the collapsed dental patient
- Stop dental treatment
- Assess consciousness
  - Alert?
  - Verbal response?
  - Pain response
  - Unresponsive
- Position patient
- Assess airway
- Assess breathing
- Assess circulation
  - Pulse rate, rhythm and magnitude
- Apply basic life support as necessary
- Get assistance as needed

Hypersensitivity reactions

1.8 Human disease

Farida Fortune

Key points

- Human disease and therapeutics requires integrated learning between basic sciences and the clinical dental specialties.

- At the completion of training the dental graduate should have a broad knowledge, understanding, and clinical skills derived from the human disease curriculum throughout the undergraduate curriculum.

- Communication skills are an integral part of the examination of the clothed patient, obtaining and assess the medical history and discussion of the findings with the patient and other professionals.

- Human disease and therapeutics provides the ideal learning opportunity for undergraduates to appreciate that clinical care should be based on a team approach.

- The dental graduate must be able to select and interpret findings from an ever-increasing round of other investigations in order to understand the pathogenesis and diagnosis of the oral condition.

- Recognition of the systemic manifestations of oral disease and the implications systemic disease and its treatment on the management of oral health are important skills for the dentist.

- It is important for dentists to be able to manage dental and orofacial pain by intervention and prescription within limits of competence, recognize personal limitations in providing care and refer appropriately.

Introduction

In the context of undergraduate dental education, the study of human disease encompasses the aspects of medicine and surgery as they pertain to the practice of dentistry.

The GDC document *The First Five Years* (GDC 2002) states that:

> The practice of dentistry has always been characterised both by its closeness to the practice of medicine and its distinctiveness from it. Thus, whilst it is universally acknowledged that those dentists subscribe to the core values of a doctor, certain features of the practice of dentistry ensured that the identity of a separate profession has maintained.

The focus of teaching and learning in this subject area is evolving as the curriculum content becomes focused on those aspects of human disease that impact on the provision of dental care and not just general medicine and surgery courses lacking appropriate emphasis on the applicability of content to the needs of future dentists.

The First Five Years gave clear indication that responsibility and authority for co-ordination resides within the dental school.

> The course should be co-ordinated by a member of staff of the dental school, who should liaise with NHS Trusts and the appropriate university department, which are required to provide the appropriate facilities and teaching support.

> **(GDC 2002)**

There is a change in emphasis within the health care services epitomized by the following quotations: 'patients always come first' and 'patients are in the driving seat able to make informed choices about their care' (A. Milburn MP, New Health Network, 15 January 2002).

Statements like these should drive the learning experience of dental students and practitioners. To ensure high-quality learning, learning objectives need to be made clear to dental graduates and competencies defined. The aim is to make the learning experience in human disease constructive and contextual, will allow dental students to develop the ability to adapt to constant and rapid changes in knowledge.

In specific reference to various parts of the human disease and therapeutics undergraduate curriculum, *The First Five Years* (GDC 2002) document states:

> **Paragraph 11** The GDC remains concerned to ensure that dentists continue to play an important role in society not only through the care of individual patients but also by contributing to the health and well-being of the general public. The practise of dentistry demands that practitioners demand a wide variety of responsibilities ranging from health promotion through to illness prevention, diagnosis and treatment.
>
> **Paragraph 19** The dental graduate must be able to: obtain and record a comprehensive history, perform an appropriate physical examination, interpret the findings and organise appropriate further investigations.

Paragraph 54 The course in human disease provides dental students with an insight into the manifestations of human diseases and disorders and the diagnostic services used in their investigation and treatment. In addition to providing an excellent basis for studies of clinical dental subjects, the course allows the dentist to communicate effectively thereafter with physicians and surgeons about patients in their joint care. Integration of the teaching of medicine, surgery and allied subjects under the general heading of human disease could help decongest the undergraduate curriculum and emphasise the importance of biomedical sciences in clinical diagnosis and management.

Paragraph 56 Sufficient instruction in human disease should be given to enable the student to understand its manifestations insofar as they may be relevant to the practise of dentistry. Relevant topics include maintenance of the well-being of patients, the recognition of physical and mental illness dealing with emergencies and communicating effectively with patients, their relatives and medical practitioners about professional matters. Courses require careful structuring and should involve clinical teaching on patients. This may be carried out in in-patient and out-patient medical and surgical departments or in specialist clinics situated in teaching or district general hospitals or in a relevant teaching environment within a dental setting or a primary care trust. The course should be co-ordinated by a member of staff of the dental school, who should liaise with NHS Trusts and the appropriate university department, which are required to provide the appropriate facilities and teaching support.

Paragraph 57 Students should acquire the skills necessary to elicit an appropriate medical history, with particular reference to cardio-respiratory diseases, haemorrhagic disorders, allergies and drug therapy. They must be able to observe and interpret physical signs in the clothed patient and know how to give intra-muscular, subcutaneous and intravenous injections.

Paragraph 58 The variety and complexity of drugs used in medical and dental treatment including those used in the control of pain and anxiety, add to the importance of pharmacology and therapeutics in the curriculum. Instruction should be given in prescription writing and the legislation concerning the supply of drugs and medicines. There are considerable advantages in teaching these subjects in courses specifically designed for dental students by teachers who have an interest in clinical, oral and dental problems. The teaching of therapeutics is best done at a point in the undergraduate curriculum when students have experience in the examination and treatment of patients.

Human disease and therapeutics is also referred to in the Subject Benchmark Statements for Dentistry (QAA 2002) as follows:

Paragraph 1.1 Dentistry is based on sound scientific and technical principles with the clinical aspects of dentistry underpinned by knowledge and understanding of the biological and clinical medical sciences.

Paragraph 2.2 Graduates should be able to demonstrate knowledge and understanding of the integration of body systems, normal homeostasis and mechanisms of responses to and including trauma and disease.

Paragraph 2.4 Graduates should be able to demonstrate knowledge and understanding of human diseases and pathogenic process including genetic disorders and the manifestation of those diseases which are particularly relevant to the practise of dentistry.

Paragraph 3.8 Assess and appraise contemporary information on the significance and effective drugs and other medicaments, taken by the patient, on dental management, and:

Perform a physical and oral examination to include head and neck, hard and soft tissues, vital signs and recognise disease states and abnormalities including detrimental oral habits.

Paragraph 3.21 Recommend and prescribe appropriately pharmaco-therapeutic agents, monitor their effectiveness and safety and be aware of drug interactions.

Paragraph 3.24 Medical conditions and emergencies. Evaluation of patients for fitness to undergo routine dental care, modify treatment plans to take account of general medical status and recognise those patients who are beyond the scope of their management.

Intended learning outcomes: knowledge, skills and attitudes

Human disease should combine the learning opportunities and experiences of the biomedical sciences into clinical practice. This will ensure a seamless learning experience where the application of the scientific principle underpins the understanding of disease process. It will encourage both undergraduates and postgraduates to develop and apply logic and judgement when proffering clinical care and in so doing provide a safe and effective clinical dental environment for patients. Human disease introduces dental students to principles of safe clinical and medical emergency practice together with basic medical science at the beginning of the curriculum. The dental student is able to develop clinical skills with an increasingly broad knowledge base and its applied and underlying scientific principles resulting in the consolidation of core competencies in the final year. These can then be taken into vocational dental practice and form the basis of life-long learning.

Human disease also provides the ideal learning opportunity for undergraduates to appreciate that clinical care should be based on a team approach. That core activities such as the management of medical emergencies can only be effectively delivered in an inter-professional team in the working environment.

During the course key personal issues of professionalism, attitudes and behaviour may be addressed. Broader issues such as communication, consent, disabilities, and health and safety are an essential part of the learning experience

The use of a clinical diary on the medical problems of current dental patients during the clinical years helps foster reflective learning.

Knowledge and understanding

♦ Understanding of basic and clinical sciences and underlying principles

Table 1.8.1 Intended learning outcomes for human disease and therapeutics

Be competent at	Have knowledge of	Be familiar with
Eliciting and recording accurately the patient's history	Scientific principles of sterilization, disinfection and antisepsis	The pathological features and dental relevance of common disorders of the major organ systems
Performing an appropriate and relevant examination of the clothed patient	Pharmacological properties of those drugs used in general practice including their unwanted effects	The role of therapeutics in the management of patients requiring dental treatment
Interpreting the findings in a reflective manner		The general aspects of medicine and surgery
Communicating effectively with patients, their relatives and carers, the dental team, colleagues and other health professionals		The main medical disorders that may impinge on dental treatment
Obtaining informed consent for examination and treatment		The place of dentistry in the provision of health care and the roles of other health care workers
		The complex interactions between oral health, nutrition, general health, drugs and diseases that can have an impact on dental care and disease.

Integration of the teaching of medicine surgery and allied subjects under the general heading of human disease could decongest the undergraduate curriculum and emphasize the importance of biomedical sciences in clinical diagnosis and management.

General Dental Council (2002)

Although it is increasingly becoming apparent that the dental undergraduate syllabus needs decongesting, this should not be at the expense of providing sufficient time to enable teachers and learners to explore innovatively the interaction between scientific principles applied to clinical method. Didactic teaching may be used early on in the curriculum during the human disease course.

The dental graduate must know and understand:

+ The science and scientific method of the basic medical sciences and its application to clinical human disease

+ Communication with particular reference to special groups such as children, the aged, patients with physical (hearing-impaired and blind), learning and mental disabilities. Integrating behavioural sciences with human disease fosters early understanding of these issues (Chapter 2.2)

+ Principles of health promotion and disease prevention (Chapter 1.6)

+ Broader issues such as law, ethics and health and safety regulations in relation to human disease impact on the work environment (Chapter 1.2)

Attitudes

+ Clinical attachments at district general hospitals, accident and emergency departments and outpatient clinics require professional behaviour and attitudes of the highest standard. This may be the first time dental students are outside the 'safe environment' of the dental school and working and learning alongside health professionals practicing in close proximity to dentistry. They are initially intimidated by the environment but soon find their behaviour and attitudes, and in many cases their knowledge base compares favourably to medical students. Feedback from 'away attachments' indicates an increase in confidence at the end of the period (Mofidi *et al.* 2003).

In dentistry at both an undergraduate and postgraduate level the teaching of attitudes and professionalism has not been formalized and is arrived at through the *ad hoc* apprentice and mentoring method. It is interesting to note that both are frequently assessed at dental school by very subjective criteria.

Skills

+ Human disease provides an opportunity for the learner to be able to spend time developing one of the most essential skills needed by the dentist. This is the ability to both elicit and record accurately the patient's history, and perform an appropriate and relevant examination and thereafter to interpret the findings in a reflective manner.

◆ The human disease curriculum should provide a sound basis for the understanding of the impact of systemic disease on the dental management, and the manifestations of systemic disease on oral cavity pathology when seen in oral medicine and oral surgery.

Effective communication with patients, their relatives and carers, the dental team, colleagues and other health professionals may be developed during the core course and during year 1 and 2 during the communication skills courses which are now embedded within the dental curriculum. During this time they may acquire specific skills pertinent to human disease.

What the dentist should be able to do

The medical history

Although a separate entity in the syllabus, communication forms an integral part of human disease. Without communication skills learners will be unable to elicit a competent history and unable to make an assessment of the patient's treatment needs. They will also be unable to communicate effectively with the patient or their family, the dental team, colleagues and other health professionals.

Emphasis early in the curriculum and integration with human disease and dental clinical practice is essential and cannot be over-emphasized (see Chapter 1.3).

The GDC (2002) notes that the dentist should be competent at obtaining a relevant medical history.

Dental students have already started clinical work before starting the human disease course but despite this they find the history taking intimidating.

The aim of history taking is to characterize the history, attributes (medical and psychosocial) and context of the problem. Although the sequence given below is a logical guide, it is unusual for patients to present information in this order.

The interview should be patient-centred. This aims to understand the complaint in terms of:

◆ The disease framework

◆ Medical and psychosocial terms

◆ The dentist's agenda

◆ The patient's perspective.

A model of the patient-centred interview is given below. This is *The Calgary–Cambridge Guide: A Guide To The Medical Interview.*

The Calgary–Cambridge Guide

The *Guide* identifies a number of specific skills (behaviours) which a doctor or dentist uses to achieve the five steps in an interview.

The provision of a structure to the interview and the building of the relationship with the patient.

Table 1.8.2 The patient-centred clinical interview: The Cambridge–Calgary Guide
Providing structure:

	1. Initiating the session	Building the relationship:
• Summary		
• Signposting	• Preparation	• Non-verbal behaviour
• Sequencing	• Establishing initial rapport	• Developing rapport
• Timing		• Involving the patient
	• Identifying the reason(s) for the consultation	
	2. Gathering information	
	• Exploration of the patient's problem to discover:	
	(i) the bio-medical perspective (disease)	
	(ii) essential background history	
	(iii) the patient's perspective (illness)	
	3. Physical examination	
	4. Explanation and planning	
	• providing the correct amount and type of information	
	• aiding accurate recall and understanding	
	• achieving a shared understanding: incorporating the	
	• patient's illness framework	
	• planning: shared decision-making	
	5. Closing the session	

The skill of history taking (see also Chapter 1.1) should be reinforced at every opportunity during both undergraduate and postgraduate training. The predominance of diagnostic and treatment decisions are made after eliciting the history with very little change after the examination and investigations. The current vogue for printed medical histories in both dental schools and general dental practice surgeries deprives the learner of effective communication with the patient and loss of the opportunity of engaging patients to reflect on lifestyle and behaviour which compromises their health.

A checklist on history taking is provided in Chapter 1.1. Guidance on aspects to consider in the context of human disease including the following.

All histories must start with the patient's age and sex.

The history should follow the format given below.

History of presenting complaint

Past medical history

- Medical history: ask specifically about endocarditis, rheumatic fever, tuberculosis, jaundice, diabetes and hypertension
- Record any serious illness, hospital admissions, accidents, childhood illnesses and complications
- Gynaecological and obstetric history. Consequences of these form an important cause of oral pathology in women

Review of systems

This should cover symptoms which are not covered in the presenting complaint.

Medication and allergies

- Enquire about all recent prescribed drugs and self-medication
- Allergies should include details of all adverse reactions to drugs, foods and inhalants and environmental antigens.

Family history

- Record any familial illnesses
- Record state of health of immediate relatives
- Parents
- Siblings
- Husband/wife/partner
- Both age and cause of death.

Social history

- Living environment including nature of housing who and how many resident
- Pets
- Nutrition, including diet, mealtime patterns and snacking, dietary beliefs
- Smoking (tobacco-smoking years)
- Cultural use of drugs such as qaat, paan
- Alcohol intake (units per week of beer/wine/spirits)

♦ Occupation

♦ Stress

♦ Travel abroad if indicated.

(See **Checklist 16**.)

Patient examination

♦ The dentist is required to be able to examine the clothed patient.

♦ Explain actions while the patient is being examined.

♦ Ensure the patient is comfortable and at ease.

General examination

♦ Observation of the patient is important.

♦ Learners do not realize that they need to learn to look at the patient and find this the most difficult part of the examination.

♦ Learners feel that examining means palpation and eliciting signs.

♦ Note whether the patient looks well or unwell, anxious, distressed or unconcerned, alert or drowsy, obese, thin or cachexic, short or tall.

♦ Reinforcement at frequent intervals is necessary as the learner often sits behind the patient without observing facial characteristics and expressions.

Specific areas in which to develop competence in examining
Examination of:

The hands

♦ Inspection, size of hands and digits, joint abnormalities and deformities

♦ Nail colour, curvature, presence of spots, nail bed vessels, splinter haemorrhages

♦ Skin colour on palmar and dorsal aspect

♦ Markings to indicate specific underlying diseases

♦ Temperature of extremities

♦ The pulse is always taken during the examination.

Temperature pulse (radial and carotid) and blood pressure
Lymph nodes of the head and neck area
With special reference to the cervical nodes. Note the size and location of any palpable nodes their consistency whether they were hard, firm, rubbery or soft, tender, mobile or fixed to underlying tissue (see **Checklist 17**).

Patient investigations

The dentist should be able to:

- Interpret basic haematological and biochemical investigations to decide if and how they may impact on the patient's dental management.

- Decide whether a patient requires urgent or routine referral to a medical practitioner.

- Understand reports of complex imaging techniques for their patient who might be under a specialist carer, e.g. a radiologist or oncologist for cancer or trauma care.

Patient management

The management of a patient in human disease refers to the impact of systemic disease on the dental management as well as the management of the acute emergency. All aspects of management are important;

- the dental and medical history

- the examination of the clothed patient

- the relevant investigations

- treatment and

- implications for the patient's medical care.

This gives the dentist the understanding of the complaint as well as its context.

Fig. 1.8.1

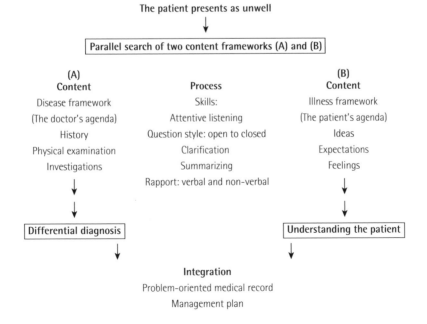

The patient presents as unwell
↓
Parallel search of two content frameworks (A) and (B)

(A) Content	Process	(B) Content
Disease framework	Skills:	Illness framework
(The doctor's agenda)	Attentive listening	(The patient's agenda)
History	Question style: open to closed	Ideas
Physical examination	Clarification	Expectations
Investigations	Summarizing	Feelings
	Rapport: verbal and non-verbal	

Differential diagnosis

Understanding the patient

Integration
Problem-oriented medical record
Management plan

Checklist 16 **History of present complaint**

	YES	NO
What is the complaint?		
Writes down the problem in the patient's own words in a clear logical sequence		
Avoids the use of the patient's or their friends' and relatives' diagnosis		
History of presenting complaint		
Listens to patient's description in their own words		
Finds out when the patient was last fit and well		
Records the timing (date) of onset of symptoms		
Enquires about elaboration of symptoms		
Site		
Onset		
Character		
Radiation		
Alleviation		
Time		
Exacerbation		
Severity		
Associated manifestations e.g. nausea, aura etc.		
Enquires about the reasons for the problem arising		
Uses open questions for:		
• What and how has the patient responded to the complaint?		
• Are there social, psychological or physical difficulties associated with the onset of the complaint?		
• Does the complaint interfere with daily activities?		
• What are the patient's views and worries?		
• What are the consequences of the complaint for the patient?		
• What are the problems in the context of the patient's dental health?		
• Are there any problems which may affect your own or your health professional colleagues' health?		

Within the above domain contents, taking the history challenges the learner's interpersonal skills and the ability to cross social, ethnic, age, disability boundaries in making the initial assessment is both an art and science which should be a large part of the learning experience.

Knowledge and understanding of pharmotherapeutic principles of drug kinetics and interaction must be incorporated into both the basic medical sciences and the clinical environment if therapeutic mishaps, with consequent patient morbidity, are to be avoided (see Chapter 1.7).

Checklist 17 **Lymph node and thyroid examination**

	YES	NO
Palpates lymph nodes from behind		
Supraclavicular (triangle between sternomastoid and the sternum), anterior and posterior triangles		
Auricular area preauricular (in front of the ear and postauricular behind the ear)		
Submandibular (under the jaw on the side and submental areas under the jaw in the midline)		
Occipital (at the base of the skull)		
Jugulo-digastric (at the angle of the jaw at the level of hyoid)		
Superficial or anterior cervical lies along sternocleidomastoid		
Posterior cervical lies behind the sternomastoid muscle		
The deep cervical chain lies below the sternomastoid and must be palpated by lifting the muscle		
Lift the edge of the sternomastoid muscle		
Make sure there is no stretch on the muscle; move the muscle backward and palpate for the deep nodes underneath		
Thyroid gland (the normal gland cannot be felt or seen, and an enlarged thyroid or goitre is inspected from the front and palpated from behind)		
Auscultation for bruits		
Inspect/palpate surrounding area for lymph nodes		
Associated signs of specific thyroid abnormalities		
Mass/lump: the exact anatomical site determined		
Differential diagnosis: having regard to possible organ or tissue in which the lump has arisen		

Patient referrals

Human disease allows learners to develop skills in receiving and making referrals (see Chapter 1.13). Exposure in outpatient medical and dental departments and ward based referrals allow them to gain insight into a process and build on their knowledge until they become fully competent to make their own referrals.

References and further reading

Fortune F. (2004) *Human Disease for Dentistry*. Oxford, Oxford University Press.

GDC (2002) *The First Five Years: a framework for undergraduate dental education*, 2nd edn. London, The General Dental Council. Also availabe at: http://www.gdc-uk.org/NR/rdonlyres/4B6221BD-6224-415A-AOC3-8AD241DE249D/15158/first_five_years_2002.pdf

Kurtz S. M. and Silverman J. D. (1996) The Calgary–Cambridge Referenced Observation Guides: An aid to defining the curriculum and organising the teaching in communication training programmes. *Med Education* 30, 83–9.

Mofidi M, Strauss R., Pinter L. L. and Sandler E. S. (2003) Dental students' reflections on their community-based experiences: the use of critical incidents. *Journal of Dental Education* 67(5) 515–23.

QAA (2002) *Dentistry: academic standards*. Subject benchmark statements. Gloucester, Quality Assurance Agency for Higher Education.

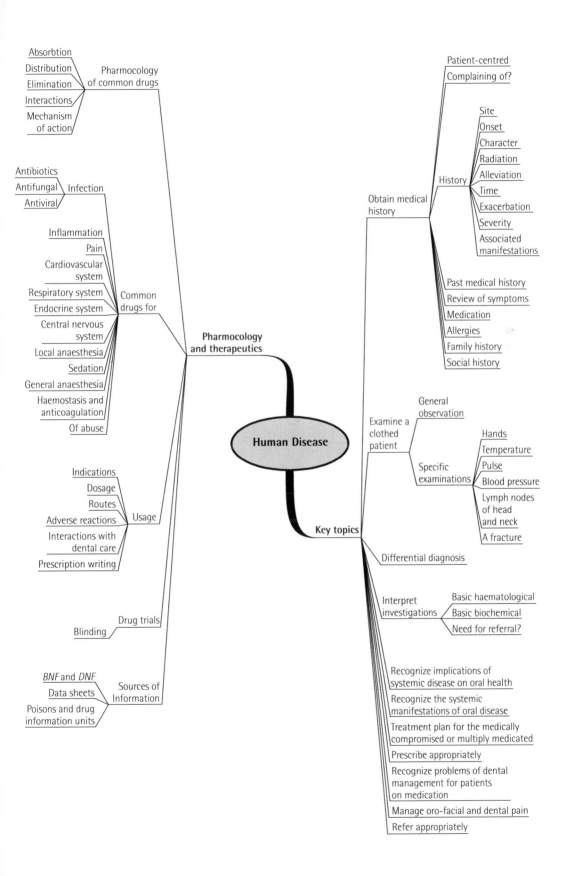

Pharmocology and therapeutics

Human Disease

Pharmacology of common drugs
- Absorbtion
- Distribution
- Elimination
- Interactions
- Mechanism of action

Infection
- Antibiotics
- Antifungal
- Antiviral

Common drugs for
- Inflammation
- Pain
- Cardiovascular system
- Respiratory system
- Endocrine system
- Central nervous system
- Local anaesthesia
- Sedation
- General anaesthesia
- Haemostasis and anticoagulation
- Of abuse

Usage
- Indications
- Dosage
- Routes
- Adverse reactions
- Interactions with dental care
- Prescription writing

Drug trials
- Blinding

Sources of Information
- BNF and DNF
- Data sheets
- Poisons and drug information units

Key topics

Obtain medical history
- Patient-centred
- Complaining of?
- History
  - Site
  - Onset
  - Character
  - Radiation
  - Alleviation
  - Time
  - Exacerbation
  - Severity
  - Associated manifestations
- Past medical history
- Review of symptoms
- Medication
- Allergies
- Family history
- Social history

Examine a clothed patient
- General observation
- Specific examinations
  - Hands
  - Temperature
  - Pulse
  - Blood pressure
  - Lymph nodes of head and neck
  - A fracture

Differential diagnosis

Interpret investigations
- Basic haematological
- Basic biochemical
- Need for referral?

- Recognize implications of systemic disease on oral health
- Recognize the systemic manifestations of oral disease
- Treatment plan for the medically compromised or multiply medicated
- Prescribe appropriately
- Recognize problems of dental management for patients on medication
- Manage oro-facial and dental pain
- Refer appropriately

1.9 Pharmacological management of pain and anxiety

Andrew Mason

Key points

- Management of pain and anxiety can be considered to be a cornerstone of good patient management and dental practice.

- The mainstay of pain management in dental practice is local anaesthesia.

- Dental training should include practical experience in the administration of inhalational and intravenous conscious sedation including assessment and preparation, care under treatment, and recovery/discharge.

- Management of pain and anxiety requires full awareness of the social and psychological needs of the individual patient.

- An understanding of the applied science of local anaesthesia is essential for the safe administration of a local anaesthetic today but also will allow the graduate to evaluate new drugs and techniques that may be developed during their practising career objectively.

- This chapter will attempt to define the competencies (a) for local anaesthesia and (b) for the pharmacological management of dental anxiety via conscious sedation and general anaesthesia.

Introduction

Safe and effective management of pain and anxiety can be considered to be a cornerstone of good patient management and dental practice. Delivering this requires a level of background, theoretical knowledge that underpins a sound clinical technique. The requirements for undergraduate training are explicitly laid out in *The First Five Years*:

> The control of anxiety and pain is fundamental to the practice of dentistry and requires full awareness of the social and psychological needs of the individual patient. Building on a sound knowledge of the prevalence and nature of dental phobias and anxieties in respect of dental treatment and the relevant basic sciences, students should be able to assess the suitability of the various methods of managing and controlling anxiety. They should recognise those patients requiring

referral for specialist care. In addition students should be able to advise patients on the advantages, limitations and advisability of different forms of pain and anxiety control appropriate to treatment to be undertaken.

GDC (2002, paragraph 101)

In addition, professional standards for pain and anxiety management are defined in the GDC (2001) document *Maintaining Standards*.

Dentists have a duty to provide and patients have a right to expect adequate and appropriate pain and anxiety control. Pharmacological methods of pain and anxiety control include local anaesthesia and conscious sedation techniques.

GDC (2001, paragraph 4.8)

Obviously, the mainstay of pain management is local anaesthesia. However, students must be able to assess individual patient needs in terms of dental anxiety and/or their ability to co-operate during treatment to be able to make decisions with respect to employing non-pharmacological (behavioural) management techniques (see Chapter 1.10) or pharmacological adjuncts (conscious sedation or even general anaesthesia). This chapter will attempt to define the competencies, first for local anaesthesia and then for pharmacological management of dental anxiety.

Local anaesthesia

By the end of the undergraduate programme students should be competent to administer all forms of local and regional analgesia for dental operations and procedures and have been trained in the management of the complications which may arise in the application of such methods of pain control.

GDC (2002, paragraph 103)

Table 1.9.1 Intended learning outcomes for pharmacological management of pain and anxiety

Be competent at	Have knowledge of	Be familiar with
Infiltration and regional block analgesia in the oral cavity	Inhalational and intravenous conscious sedation techniques	
Recognizing and managing potential complications relating to use of local anaesthetic	Conscious sedation techniques in clinical practice	
When, how and where to refer a patient for general anaethesia	The indications, contraindications, limitations, risks and benefits of conscious sedation and general anaesthesia	

Among the specific learning outcomes is the following: 'Be competent in infiltration and block local anaesthesia in the oral cavity' (GDC 2002, paragraph 111).

To achieve these outcomes, the student must have a level of foundation knowledge on to which the clinical skills can be acquired.

Foundation knowledge and understanding

An understanding of the applied science of local anaesthesia is essential for the safe administration of a local anaesthetic today but also will allow the graduate to objectively evaluate new drugs and techniques that may be developed during their practising career.

For basic *anatomy and physiology*, the student should:

◆ Have a detailed knowledge of the anatomy of orofacial structures

◆ Have a detailed working knowledge of the innervation of the orofacial tissues – in particular the distribution of the trigeminal nerve and possible accessory nerves supplying dental structures

◆ Have an understanding of the ionic basis of the action potential

◆ Have an understanding of the peripheral and central mechanisms involved in the process of nociception.

For the *pharmacology* of local anaesthetic (LA), the student should:

◆ Have an understanding of the potential modes of action for LA drugs, and the mechanisms of metabolism and excretion

◆ Be aware of the physicochemical properties of LA drugs (e.g. dissociation and partition coefficients) and how they affect the performance of the drug. In particular, this is important in evaluating the properties of new drugs

◆ Have an understanding of the reason for the use of vasoconstrictors as part of the LA preparation

◆ Have an understanding of the mode of action of vasoconstrictor agents

◆ For the commonly available LA preparations (e.g. those containing lidocaine, priolocaine, articaine, mepivacaine, and bupivacaine), the student should know the maximum safe dose that can be administered in both adults and children

◆ Have a knowledge of the potential systemic side effects and/or drug interactions that may relate to local anaesthetic preparations

◆ Have knowledge of systemic conditions that may affect the local administration of a local anaesthetic preparation

◆ Have a working knowledge of systemic conditions that may be an absolute or relative contraindication to a particular local anaesthetic preparation.

Anaesthetic techniques

General skills

- The student should be able to take a medical/dental history so as to elicit possible systemic disorders of medication that may affect the choice of pain control method and/or drug

- The student should understand the importance of patient's previous anaesthetic history when deciding on an appropriate drug or technique to use

- The student should be able to identify specific local or systemic conditions when it would not be appropriate to administer an local anaesthetic

- The student should be able to employ the appropriate patient management skills to provide psychological support before, during and after, in particular, the administration of a local anaesthetic injection.

Topical/surface anaesthesia

The student should:

- Know the indications for the use of topical anaesthetics

- Know what drugs and which modes of delivery are available

- Demonstrate the safe, appropriate usage of topical anaesthetics.

Injection techniques, general considerations

The student:

- Must have knowledge of the equipment required for safe administration of a local anaesthetics injection

- Must be able to demonstrate the safe assembly and disassembly of a syringe and needle with particular reference to the handling and disposal of sharps

- Must demonstrate how to prevent needle stick injuries by:

  - The use of needle guards/sheath holders

  - The use of safety syringes

  - Where appropriate using for example a mirror, or similar instrument, to retract the soft tissues rather than a finger prior to an injection

- Must demonstrate how to minimize the risk of intravascular injection by:

  - Understanding how aspiration works

  - Identifying and correctly using only syringes with the ability to aspirate

  - Describing how to manage a positive blood aspiration

- Should be able to identify a healthy and safe injection site

- Should be able to demonstrate techniques that will minimize any discomfort from the administration of a local anaesthetic injection

- Should be able to demonstrate how to determine whether the local anaesthetic injection has been successful prior to commencing the proposed treatment.

Injection techniques: infiltration

The student must:

- Have knowledge of the mode of action of infiltration injections
- Have knowledge of the regions of the maxilla and mandible in which infiltration local anaesthesia is appropriate to achieve dental anaesthesia
- Have knowledge of the local anatomy of the mouth and jaws that may affect the outcome of an infiltration local anaesthetic
- Demonstrate the clinical technique for safe infiltration local anaesthesia with particular regard to:
  - Safe retraction of the soft tissues
  - The orientation of the needle, including the bevel of the needle
  - The site of needle penetration
  - The depth of needle penetration
  - Aspiration
  - Speed of injection
  - Safe withdrawal of the needle
  - Re-sheathing of the needle
  - Support of the patient
- Have knowledge as to appropriate dosage of drug to use for infiltration anaesthetic injections
- Demonstrate infiltration techniques for dento-alveolar procedures (i.e. labial/buccal and palatal infiltrations) and soft tissue procedures (e.g. for soft tissue biopsy).

Injection techniques: regional anaesthesia

The student must be proficient at achieving anaesthesia of the following nerves:

- Inferior alveolar
- Lingual
- Long buccal
- Mental and incisive.

For each of the above nerve blocks, the student should:

- Be able to describe, in detail, the anatomy of the regions involved, in particular the location of the nerve trunks in relation to other important structures, e.g. blood vessel, motor nerves, muscle, and salivary glands

- ◆ Have knowledge of the indications and contraindications for each of the block techniques

- ◆ Demonstrate the clinical technique for each of the nerve blocks with particular regard to:
  - Safe retraction of the soft tissues
  - Identification of the anatomical landmarks
  - The orientation of the needle, including the bevel of the needle
  - The site of needle penetration
  - The depth of needle penetration
  - Aspiration
  - Speed of injection
  - Dosage of drug usually required
  - Safe withdrawal of the needle
  - Re-sheathing of the needle
  - Support of the patient

- ◆ Be able to interpret the outcome of a particular injection in terms of the nerves blocked relative the soft tissue anaesthesia reported by the patient.

For the inferior alveolar nerve block, the student should, in addition:

- ◆ Be aware of the alternative methods of approach to the nerve – the direct technique vs.:
  - The indirect technique
  - The Akinosi–Vazirani technique
  - Gow–Gates technique

- ◆ Be able to describe how to safely manage a possible motor nerve paralysis (in particular that of the facial (VII) nerve) that may result from the local anaesthetic injection.

The student should, in addition, have an understanding of the use and techniques for the following nerve blocks:

- ◆ Superior alveolar nerves (posterior, middle and superior)
- ◆ Nasopalatine
- ◆ Mylohyoid.

Supplemental local anaesthetic techniques

The student should have an understanding of the indications, contraindications and limitations of local anaesthetic techniques that may supplement the above conventional techniques. In particular:

- Intra-osseous anaesthesia via the periodontal approach – intraligamentary technique
- Intra-osseous anaesthesia via the direct approach – e.g. using a perforator
- Intrapulpal anaesthesia
- Intrapapillary anaesthesia.

  For each technique, the student should:
- Be able to describe any special equipment required
- Demonstrate the clinical technique.

Local anaesthetic problems

The student should be proficient at identification/diagnosis and management of the common local or systemic problems that may arise as result of the administration of a local anaesthetic injection. In particular:

- Failure to achieve local anaesthesia. The student should:
  - Understand why a local anaesthetic may fail
  - Be able to systematically assess the potential causes of an individual failure
  - With strict adherence to safe local anaesthetic drug dosages, be able to develop a safe strategy for the management of a failed local anaesthetic that may utilize modifications to injection technique, a different technique and/or different drug.
- Management/prevention of local post-anaesthetic problems e.g. trauma, trismus
- Diagnosis and management of common systemic problems that may occur before, during or after local anaesthetic, e.g. faint
- Management of allergy or suspected allergy. The student should:
  - Understand the importance of a history of true allergy to an administered local anaesthetic (including the anaesthetic drug and any other constituent of an anaesthetic solution or cartridge component)
  - Be able to recognize either clinically or from a history, the signs of allergy and ensure appropriate investigation by a specialist prior to administering further anaesthetics

Conscious sedation

The General Dental Council defines conscious sedation as:

A technique in which the use of a drug or drugs produces a state of depression of the central nervous system enabling treatment to be carried out, but during which verbal contact with the patient is maintained throughout the period of sedation. The drugs and techniques used to provide conscious sedation for dental treatment should carry a margin of safety wide enough to render loss of consciousness unlikely.

GDC (2001, paragraph 4.11)

Implicit in both *The First Five Years* and *Maintaining Standards* is the need for further 'relevant postgraduate education and training' for dentists willing to provide sedation as either operator/sedationist or as a sedationist working along side another operating dentist. However, the undergraduate dental course must deliver sufficient experience of sedation techniques to allow graduates to be able to consider sedation as an adjunct to their treatment plans.

All dental students must have a range of practical experience in the administration of inhalational and intravenous conscious sedation including assessment and preparation, care under treatment, and recovery and discharge of patients receiving conscious sedation. All dental students should also have practical experience of providing different forms of treatment for sedated patients and be familiar with the drugs, techniques and equipment for the safe sedation of adults and children. Dental students should graduate with a full recognition of their limited experience in the use of conscious sedation techniques and of the necessity for postgraduate study and instruction in such forms of pain and anxiety control.

GDC (2002, paragraph 104)

The GDC therefore defines the specific learning outcome as: 'The dental graduate should: have knowledge of inhalational and intravenous sedation techniques' (GDC 2002, paragraph 111).

General considerations

◆ Students should have a knowledge of the problem of dental anxiety, in particular they should:

  ▪ Understand the potential aetiological factors for dental anxiety

  ▪ From their history of dental experience, be able to identify patients who are anxious

  ▪ Be able to identify, from a history, aspects of dental treatment that may trigger a patient's anxiety

◆ Students must have a clear understanding of all potential methods of anxiety management, both pharmacological and behavioural

◆ Students must be aware of the advantages and limitations of different methods of anxiety management and identify those patients who may benefit from conscious sedation

◆ On graduation, students must be and remain familiar with the current guidelines regarding the provision of sedation in dentistry.

To satisfy the current GDC regulations, the student must have a level of foundation knowledge on which to build their postgraduate clinical development.

Foundation knowledge of basic anatomy, physiology and pharmacology. The student must:

◆ Have an understanding of respiratory physiology – with particular reference to gaseous exchange in the lungs and the control of respiration

- Have an understanding of cardiovascular physiology
- Understand the principles of monitoring of vital signs
- Have a detailed knowledge of the anatomy of potential venepuncture sites: the dorsum of the hand and the antecubital fossa
- Have knowledge of the principle drugs available for intravenous sedation – midazolam and diazepam:
  - their potential for anxiolysis and amnesia and lack of analgesia
  - their mode of action, metabolism and excretion
  - their effects on the respiratory and cardiovascular systems
  - the mode of delivery – intravenous incremental titration
  - safe maximum dosages
- Be aware of the existence advanced sedation techniques (e.g. Propofol) that may be administered by appropriately trained specialists working in specialist centres.
- Have knowledge of drugs that may be used to reverse the effects of intravenous sedatives (e.g. flumazenil)
- Have a knowledge of the pharmacokinetics of inhalational sedation – nitrous oxide
- Be aware of the risks of chronic exposure to nitrous oxide and therefore the importance of scavenging
- Have a detailed knowledge of medical conditions that may affect the safe provision of intravenous or inhalational sedation
- Have knowledge of the potential drug interactions with sedative agents.

For patient assessment, the student should:
- Be able to elicit a comprehensive medical history and identify factors (medical problems or current medication) that may impact on the provision of intravenous sedation
- Be familiar with the American Society of Anaesthesiologists (ASA) classification of systemic illness and its relevance to the decision whether to, and where to administer sedation
- Be able to elicit a comprehensive past dental treatment history to evaluate a patient's potential dental anxiety, its scope and precipitating factors
- Be able to carry out an appropriate dental examination of a dentally anxious patient and prioritize treatment need
- Be able to appropriately incorporate pharmacological methods of anxiety management in to a treatment plan
- Be able to present the treatment plan and options to the dental patient
- Be able to realistically explain to a patient how a sedative agent may affect them and facilitate treatment

- Be able to identify patients who fall out with their experience and capabilities that require referral to specialist centres as a result of dental treatment needed, medical problems or potential psychological problems
- Know the importance and legal obligation for informed consent and written pre- and post-operative instructions for both the patient and escort.

For the clinical administration of conscious sedation, the student should:

- Be able to obtain written consent from a patient, parent or guardian
- Be able to record a patient's pulse and blood pressure pre-operatively
- Understand that the dentist must be 'assisted by a second appropriately trained person who is present throughout and is capable of monitoring the clinical condition of the patient and assisting the dentist in the event of any complication' GDC (2001, paragraph 4.14.vi)
- Understand the importance of monitoring cardio-respiratory parameters
- Appreciate the importance of behavioural management and support as part of treatment with intravenous or inhalation sedation
- Be able to identify the signs of an appropriately sedated patient and indeed an over-sedated patient
- Be aware of the potential for impaired protective reflexes as a result of the sedative and therefore the importance of airway management in the prevention of the inhalation or ingestion of foreign bodies
- At the end of a procedure, be able to objectively determine when a patient has recovered sufficiently to be able to leave the surgery with an escort
- Be aware of the obligation to give written an verbal instructions to both patient and escort at the end of the appointment.

In addition, for intravenous sedation, the student should:

- Know what equipment is required to administer intravenous sedation and to manage any problem that may arise as a result of the treatment
- Have experience of venepuncture
- Understand the importance of maintaining venous access throughout the procedure until the patient has sufficiently recovered
- Understand the importance of titration of the sedative agent
- Understand the importance of monitoring cardio-respiratory parameters of using, at minimum, a pulse oximeter, including:
  - Experience of monitoring a sedated patient
  - Ability to identify and manage changes in blood oxygenation or pulse rate
- Be aware of the indications for the use of a reversal agent.

In addition, for inhalational sedation, the student should:

◆ Have knowledge of the equipment required and set up for the administration of inhalational sedation

◆ Have experience of administration of nitrous oxide/oxygen inhalational sedation, in particular:

- Introduction of the equipment to the patient

- Appropriate gaseous flow rates

- Administration of pure oxygen followed by titration of nitrous oxide

- Importance of the use of pure oxygen at the end of treatment

- Monitoring of vital signs – an awareness of patients who may require pulse oximetry

General anaesthesia

The use of general anaesthesia for dental procedures is reducing. Since the revised guidance published in the GDC's *Maintaining Standards* document in November 2001:

> The theoretical principles of general anaesthesia should be taught to students and they should have this knowledge reinforced by attachment to an anaesthetist who is administering general anaesthesia to dental patients. Practical experience should be gained in operating on patients under general anaesthesia and in their care, including management of the airway. Practical experience should also be gained in the pre- and post-operative care of patients requiring treatment under general anaesthesia. All dental students should receive instruction in the referral of patients for treatment under general anaesthesia in a hospital setting.
>
> **GDC (2002, paragraph 105)**

The GDC therefore defines the specific learning outcome as: 'The dental graduate should: be competent at when, how and where to refer a patient for general anaesthesia' (GDC 2002, paragraph 111).

The principal role of the dental graduate with respect to general anaesthesia is to be able to identify patients who require general anaesthesia and importantly be able to where possible suggest alternative management strategies to keep the need for general anaesthesia to an absolute minimum. To be able to achieve this, students possess a level of knowledge and understanding and experience of general anaesthesia.

Foundation knowledge of anatomy, physiology and pharmacology. The student must:

◆ Have a knowledge and understanding of the anatomy and physiology of the cardio-vascular and respiratory systems.

◆ Have knowledge of the drugs used both by inhalation and intravenous routes to induce and maintain general anaesthesia.

◆ Have a knowledge of the different stages/planes of anaesthesia.

For patient assessment, the student must:

◆ Have a clear knowledge of the obligations and responsibilities placed upon the referring dentist and defined in the GDC document *Maintaining Standards*:

The decision to refer a patient for treatment under general anaesthesia should not be taken lightly. As part of this decision, a full medical history of the patient must be taken and agreement to refer obtained following a thorough and clear explanation of the risks involved and the alternative methods of pain control available. Clear justification for the use of general anaesthesia, together with details of the relevant medical and dental histories of the patient, must be contained in the referral letter.

GDC (2001, paragraph 4.18)

◆ Be able to elicit a comprehensive medical history and identify factors (medical problems or current medication) that may impact on the provision of a general anaesthetic.

◆ Be familiar with the American Society of Anaesthesiologists (ASA) classification of systemic illness and its relevance to the decision whether to refer for a general anaesthetic.

◆ Be able to elicit a comprehensive past dental treatment history to evaluate a patient's potential dental anxiety or ability to cope/co-operate with dental treatment.

◆ Be able to explain to the patient (and, if appropriate, the parent/escort) in light of the risks of general anaesthetia, the alternativemanagement strategies available.

◆ Be able to realistically explain to a patient what can be achieved under a general anaesthetic.

◆ Know the importance and legal obligation for informed consent and written pre- and post-operative instructions for both the patient and escort.

◆ Be able to appropriately refer a patient to a hospital centre for treatment under general anaesthetic and be aware of the legal/ethical obligations of the referring dentist.

For management of patients under general anaesthesia

Students should have experience of operating on patients who are under general anaesthesia. In particular, they should:

◆ Have observed the stages of patient preparation prior to administration of the general anaesthetic

◆ Be aware of the roles of the anaesthetist, dentist, nurses and other support staff before, during and after the treatment of a patient under a general anaesthetic

◆ Have experience of operating on a patient who is under a general anaesthetic – in particular the management/protection of the airway

◆ Have observed the immediate after care of a patient who has received a general anaesthetic.

Checklist 18 **Administration of a local anaesthetic injection**

	YES	NO
Review of relevant medical history		
Identification of the most appropriate technique		
Selection of the safest, most efficacious local anaesthetic drug*		
Know the safe maximum dosage of the chosen drug*		
Explanation of procedure to patient		
Operator in correct position		
Patient in appropriate position		
Patient with bib and glasses		
Topical anaesthesia applied – if appropriate		
Operator correctly accepts syringe from assistant		
Operator checks patency of needle		
Safe retraction of tissues		
Identification of landmarks and injection site*		
Administers the injection with correct injection site and needle orientation*		
Correctly aspirates prior to, and intermittently during, the injection of the drug*		
Correct dose and rate of drug administration*		
Operator removes needle from injection site without risk of needle touching patient or of stick injury		
Needle re-sheathed safely following correct procedure*		
Post-injection instructions given to patient		
Syringe disposed of appropriately		
Appropriate assessment of efficacy of injection		
Operator maintained correct position throughout		
Operator maintained communication with patient throughout		

* Indicates a veto assessment.

References and further reading

General Dental Council (2001) *Maintaining Standards: guidance to dentists, dental hygenists and dental therapists on professional and personal conduct*. London, General Dental Council. Also available at www.gdc-uk.org, accessed 8 December 2004.

General Dental Council (2002) *The First Five Years: a framework for undergraduate dental education*, 2nd edn. London, The General Dental Council.

Hill C. M. and Girdler N. M. (1998) *Sedation in Dentistry*. Oxford, Wright.

Malamed S. F. (2004) *Handbook of Local Anaesthesia*, 5th edn. St Louis, Mosby/Elsevier.

Meechan J. G. and Seymour R. A. (1998) *Pain and Anxiety Control for the Conscious Dental Patient*. Oxford, Oxford University Press.

Meechan J. G. and Nairn H. F. (2002) *Practical Dental Local Anaesthesia*. Quintessentials: Oral Surgery and Oral Medicine. London, Wilson Quintessence Publishing Co. Ltd

QAA (2002) *Dentistry: academic standards*. Subject benchmark statements. Gloucester, Quality Assurance Agency for Higher Education.

Robinson P. D., Pitt-Ford T. R. and McDonald F. (2000) *Local Anaesthesia in Dentistry*. Oxford, Wright.

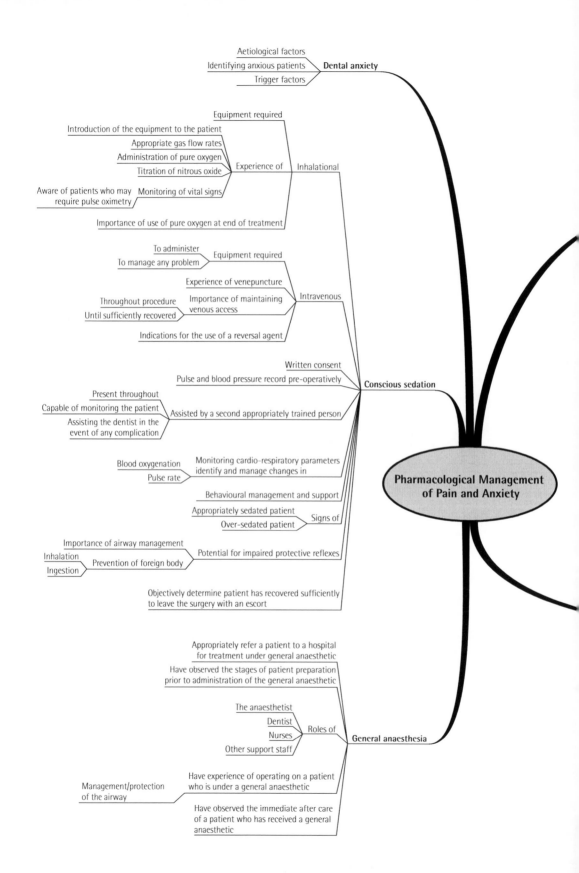

Dental anxiety
- Aetiological factors
- Identifying anxious patients
- Trigger factors

Conscious sedation

Inhalational
- Equipment required
- Experience of
  - Introduction of the equipment to the patient
  - Appropriate gas flow rates
  - Administration of pure oxygen
  - Titration of nitrous oxide
  - Monitoring of vital signs — Aware of patients who may require pulse oximetry
  - Importance of use of pure oxygen at end of treatment

Intravenous
- Equipment required
  - To administer
  - To manage any problem
- Experience of venepuncture
- Importance of maintaining venous access
  - Throughout procedure
  - Until sufficiently recovered
- Indications for the use of a reversal agent

- Written consent
- Pulse and blood pressure record pre-operatively
- Assisted by a second appropriately trained person
  - Present throughout
  - Capable of monitoring the patient
  - Assisting the dentist in the event of any complication
- Monitoring cardio-respiratory parameters identify and manage changes in
  - Blood oxygenation
  - Pulse rate
- Behavioural management and support
- Signs of
  - Appropriately sedated patient
  - Over-sedated patient
- Potential for impaired protective reflexes
  - Importance of airway management
  - Prevention of foreign body
    - Inhalation
    - Ingestion
- Objectively determine patient has recovered sufficiently to leave the surgery with an escort

General anaesthesia
- Appropriately refer a patient to a hospital for treatment under general anaesthetic
- Have observed the stages of patient preparation prior to administration of the general anaesthetic
- Roles of
  - The anaesthetist
  - Dentist
  - Nurses
  - Other support staff
- Have experience of operating on a patient who is under a general anaesthetic
  - Management/protection of the airway
- Have observed the immediate after care of a patient who has received a general anaesthetic

Pharmacological Management of Pain and Anxiety

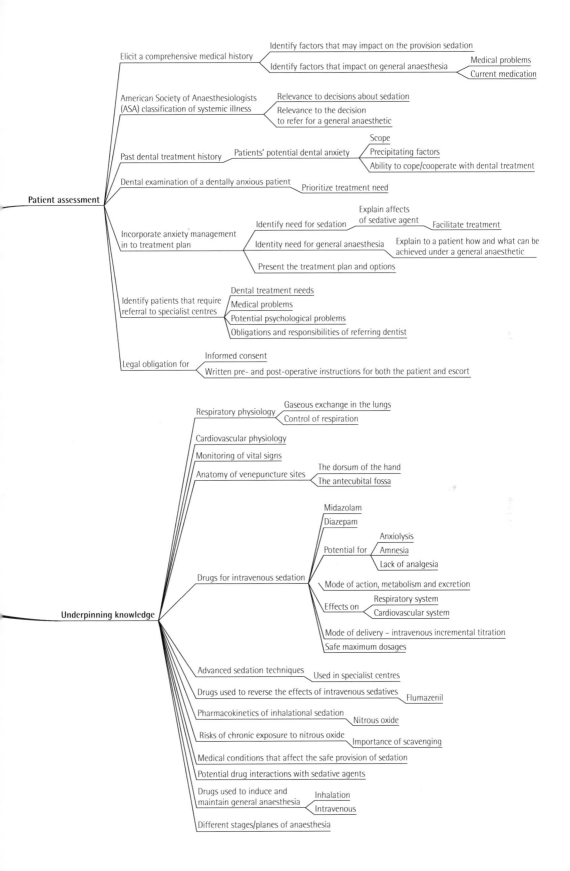

Patient assessment

- Elicit a comprehensive medical history
  - Identify factors that may impact on the provision sedation
  - Identify factors that impact on general anaesthesia
    - Medical problems
    - Current medication
- American Society of Anaesthesiologists (ASA) classification of systemic illness
  - Relevance to decisions about sedation
  - Relevance to the decision to refer for a general anaesthetic
- Past dental treatment history
  - Patients' potential dental anxiety
    - Scope
    - Precipitating factors
    - Ability to cope/cooperate with dental treatment
- Dental examination of a dentally anxious patient
  - Prioritize treatment need
- Incorporate anxiety management in to treatment plan
  - Identify need for sedation
    - Explain affects of sedative agent
      - Facilitate treatment
  - Identity need for general anaesthesia
    - Explain to a patient how and what can be achieved under a general anaesthetic
  - Present the treatment plan and options
- Identify patients that require referral to specialist centres
  - Dental treatment needs
  - Medical problems
  - Potential psychological problems
  - Obligations and responsibilities of referring dentist
- Legal obligation for
  - Informed consent
  - Written pre- and post-operative instructions for both the patient and escort

Underpinning knowledge

- Respiratory physiology
  - Gaseous exchange in the lungs
  - Control of respiration
- Cardiovascular physiology
- Monitoring of vital signs
- Anatomy of venepuncture sites
  - The dorsum of the hand
  - The antecubital fossa
- Drugs for intravenous sedation
  - Midazolam
  - Diazepam
  - Potential for
    - Anxiolysis
    - Amnesia
    - Lack of analgesia
  - Mode of action, metabolism and excretion
  - Effects on
    - Respiratory system
    - Cardiovascular system
  - Mode of delivery – intravenous incremental titration
  - Safe maximum dosages
- Advanced sedation techniques
  - Used in specialist centres
- Drugs used to reverse the effects of intravenous sedatives
  - Flumazenil
- Pharmacokinetics of inhalational sedation
  - Nitrous oxide
- Risks of chronic exposure to nitrous oxide
  - Importance of scavenging
- Medical conditions that affect the safe provision of sedation
- Potential drug interactions with sedative agents
- Drugs used to induce and maintain general anaesthesia
  - Inhalation
  - Intravenous
- Different stages/planes of anaesthesia

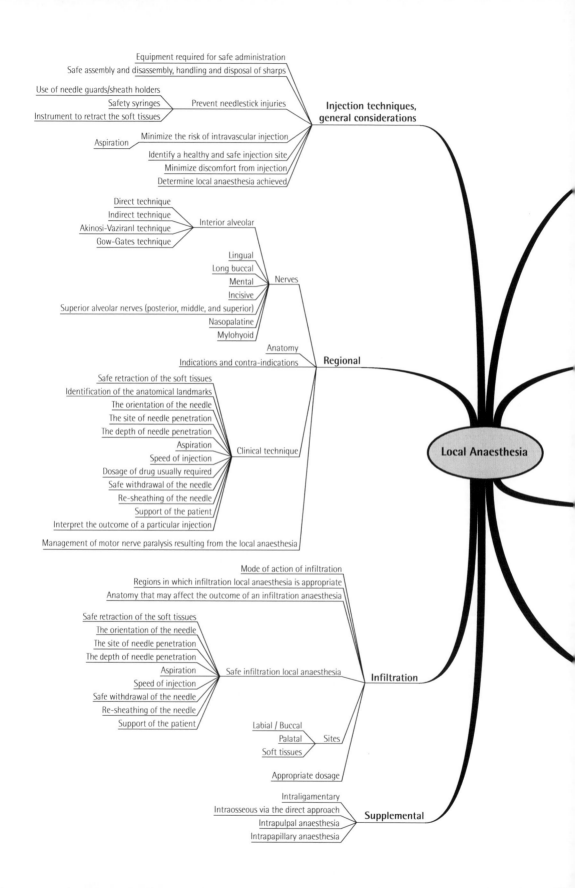

Equipment required for safe administration
Safe assembly and disassembly, handling and disposal of sharps
Use of needle guards/sheath holders
Safety syringes — Prevent needlestick injuries
Instrument to retract the soft tissues
Aspiration — Minimize the risk of intravascular injection
Identify a healthy and safe injection site
Minimize discomfort from injection
Determine local anaesthesia achieved

Injection techniques, general considerations

Direct technique
Indirect technique
Akinosi-Vaziranl technique — Interior alveolar
Gow-Gates technique

Lingual
Long buccal
Mental — Nerves
Incisive
Superior alveolar nerves (posterior, middle, and superior)
Nasopalatine
Mylohyoid

Anatomy
Indications and contra-indications — **Regional**

Safe retraction of the soft tissues
Identification of the anatomical landmarks
The orientation of the needle
The site of needle penetration
The depth of needle penetration
Aspiration — Clinical technique
Speed of injection
Dosage of drug usually required
Safe withdrawal of the needle
Re-sheathing of the needle
Support of the patient
Interpret the outcome of a particular injection
Management of motor nerve paralysis resulting from the local anaesthesia

Mode of action of infiltration
Regions in which infiltration local anaesthesia is appropriate
Anatomy that may affect the outcome of an infiltration anaesthesia

Safe retraction of the soft tissues
The orientation of the needle
The site of needle penetration
The depth of needle penetration
Aspiration — Safe infiltration local anaesthesia
Speed of injection
Safe withdrawal of the needle
Re-sheathing of the needle
Support of the patient

Infiltration

Labial / Buccal
Palatal — Sites
Soft tissues

Appropriate dosage

Intraligamentary
Intraosseous via the direct approach
Intrapulpal anaesthesia — **Supplemental**
Intrapapillary anaesthesia

Local Anaesthesia

Pharmacology
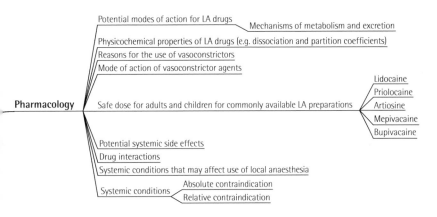
- Potential modes of action for LA drugs — Mechanisms of metabolism and excretion
- Physicochemical properties of LA drugs (e.g. dissociation and partition coefficients)
- Reasons for the use of vasoconstrictors
- Mode of action of vasoconstrictor agents
- Safe dose for adults and children for commonly available LA preparations
  - Lidocaine
  - Priolocaine
  - Artiosine
  - Mepivacaine
  - Bupivacaine
- Potential systemic side effects
- Drug interactions
- Systemic conditions that may affect use of local anaesthesia
- Systemic conditions
  - Absolute contraindication
  - Relative contraindication

Anatomy and physiology of oro-facial structures
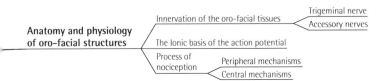
- Innervation of the oro-facial tissues
  - Trigeminal nerve
  - Accessory nerves
- The Ionic basis of the action potential
- Process of nociception
  - Peripheral mechanisms
  - Central mechanisms

Topical
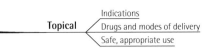
- Indications
- Drugs and modes of delivery
- Safe, appropriate use

Problems
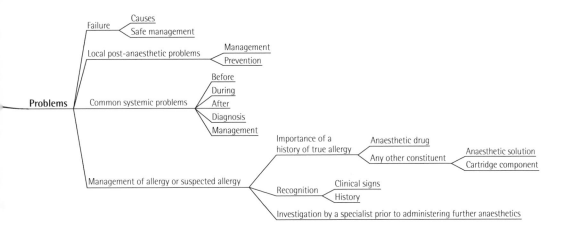
- Failure
  - Causes
  - Safe management
- Local post-anaesthetic problems
  - Management
  - Prevention
- Common systemic problems
  - Before
  - During
  - After
  - Diagnosis
  - Management
- Management of allergy or suspected allergy
  - Importance of a history of true allergy
    - Anaesthetic drug
    - Any other constituent
      - Anaesthetic solution
      - Cartridge component
  - Recognition
    - Clinical signs
    - History
  - Investigation by a specialist prior to administering further anaesthetics

1.10 The identification and behavioural management of the dentally anxious adult and child patient

Ruth Freeman

Key points

- Competence in dental practice implies the ability to establish and maintain a healthy oral environment for the dentally anxious patient.
- Communication and behavioural management are essential elements in the competent management of dental anxiety.
- Dental students need to be familiar with the ethnic, social and psychological issues relevant to the care of such patients.
- The ability to communicate effectively with patients, their families and other professionals is the key to management of oral health promotion.
- Dental students should be competent in behavioural management techniques in the treatment of the dentally anxious adult or child patient.
- Familiarity with alternative methods of behavioural management is also important as is competence at making appropriate referrals based on assessment.

Introduction

The General Dental Council's document *The First Five Years* (GDC 2002) describes the management of dental anxiety within an interlinking rubric of behavioural sciences, pain and anxiety control. The document stresses the importance of patient-centred care, implying that it is the behavioural management of the patient which is the cornerstone of pain and anxiety control.

The requirements for behavioural management of the dentally anxious adult and child patient are outlined in *The First Five Years*:

Paragraph 65 (Law, ethics and professionalism) Students should understand the importance of communication between practitioner and patient. This helps to develop attitudes of empathy and insight in the student and provides the opportunity for discussion of contemporary ethical issues. Students should also be encouraged to understand their own responses to work pressures and their management. There may be opportunities for integrated or complementary teaching with other basic sciences on topics such as pain, stress and anxiety and with clinical specialties on topics such as social class, poverty and the needs of children and the elderly.

Paragraph 101 (Pain and anxiety control) The control of anxiety and pain is fundamental to the practice of dentistry and requires full awareness of the social and psychological needs of the individual patient. Building on a sound knowledge of the prevalence and nature of dental phobias and anxieties in respect of dental treatment and the relevant basic sciences, students should be able to assess the suitability of the various methods of managing and controlling anxiety. They should recognize those patients requiring referral for specialist care. In addition students should be able to advise patients on the advantages, limitations and advisability of different forms of pain and anxiety control appropriate to treatment to be undertaken.

Paragraph 102 (Pain and anxiety control) The value and range of behavioural non-pharmacological methods of anxiety management must be emphasized. In order to assess and manage an anxious patient, dental students should have learnt a range of methodologies that can be reasonably matched to individual circumstances.

The intended learning outcomes for behavioural management of the dentally anxious adult and child patient from paragraph 111 of *The First Five Years* are summarized in Table 1.10.1.

Behavioural management is perceived as the fundamental element and cornerstone in controlling pain and anxiety. The need for dental students to be competent in identifying and distinguishing patients who can be treated within the practice setting and those who require referral is also emphasized.

The requirement for dental students on qualification to have a familiarity and competency of the key skills in order to maintain the oral health of patients has been recognized. Being familiar with psychological issues and competent in communication allows the qualifying dentist to have an understanding appropriate to the patient's needs as well as the skills to identify, manage and treat the dentally anxious patient.

The dentistry Benchmarking Statements (QAA 2002) stated that qualifying dentists must have:

Table 1.10.1 Intended learning outcomes for the for behavioural management of the dentally anxious adult and child patient

Be competent at	Have knowledge of	Be familiar with
Recognizing the common signs and symptoms of anxiety and apprehension	Applying the principles of pharmacological dental anxiety management to the treatment of the anxious dental patient	The social and psychological issues relevant to the care of dentally anxious patients
Communication with patients	Using recognized psychological inventories	Alternative methods of behavioural management
Empathizing with patients in stressful situations		
Assessing the level of anxiety in adult and child patients		
Making appropriate referrals based on assessment		
Managing fear and anxiety with behavioural techniques		

The knowledge and understanding of:

◆ communication between dentists and patients [and] their families

◆ patients' responses to dental care and an understanding of how these may be affected by experience, psychological, social and cultural influences.

The skills and attributes to:

◆ appreciate the importance of psychological and social factors in the delivery and acceptance of dental care by patients

◆ apply the principles of dental anxiety management (behavioural and pharmacological) to the treatment of the anxious dental patient.

and establish and maintain a healthy oral environment by being able to:

◆ recognise the common signs and symptoms of ... anxiety and apprehension

◆ assess the level of anxiety in adult and child patients and have experience of using recognised psychological inventories

◆ manage fear and anxiety with behavioural techniques.

The First Five Years (GDC 2002) closes the loop by reflecting the dentistry benchmarking statements (QAA 2002) as dental students on qualification must have the competency to manage 'fear and anxiety with behavioural techniques'. Behavioural management has come of age and is the key competency required for the holistic dental health care of anxious dental patients (see Table 1.10.1).

The aim of this chapter is to provide a checklist of key competencies necessary for the graduating dentist to care for the dentally anxious patient. The competencies will be described within the framework of knowledge and understanding and skills and attributes and how they connect with the key competencies necessary to establish and maintain a health oral environment for the dentally anxious patient.

Be competent at communication

Communication is the basis of a patient-centred approach in health care. A knowledge of the basic communication skills is therefore essential in order to recognize and identify dentally anxious patients and differentiate them from those who are dentally phobic and require referral for specialist care. There are two aspects of communication: non-verbal and verbal.

♦ **Non-verbal communication**: an understanding of the patient's appearance and non-verbal cues will provide the dentist with clues as to their dental anxiety status. Non-verbal cues include: body language; eye contact; pitch, tone, speed of speech; filled pauses (ahs, errs and uhms).

♦ **Verbal communication**: the awareness of the need to discover all about the patient's previous dental and medical experiences will enable the dentist to understand the patient's responses to dental care. A knowledge of communication will allow the dentist to ask open questions (to glean information) to move to focus questions (to focus the interview) and finally to use closed questions (to clarify) aspects of the patient's story which will allow the dentist to make a diagnosis with regard to the patient's dental anxiety status and treatment requirements (see Figure 1.10.1). Leading questions must be avoided as they can result in the patient providing inaccurate information in an attempt to agree or please the clinician.

At the centre of the communication process is the requirement for the dentist to have an understanding of active listening. Active listening (Figure 1.10.2) is listening to what is being said and what remains unsaid (listening with the 'third ear').

The importance of reflecting back the patients' statements provides a means of clarification – that the dentist has understood what the patient has said and the patient

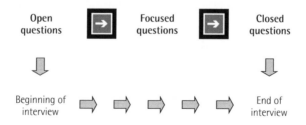

Figure 1.10.1 The questioning continuum

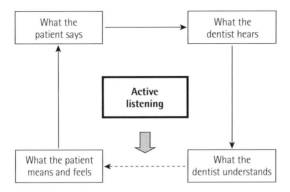

Figure 1.10.2 Active listening

- Clarifying and summarizing
    - Checking you understand what the patient has said
    - Checking that the patient understands what you have said
- Reflective listening
    - These statements reflect and confirm the patient's statement
    - Reduce the gap between patient and dentist

Figure 1.10.3 Clarifying, summarizing and reflective listening

has understood the dentist. This allows the dentist to close the gap between what the patient's words mean and what the dentist understands the patient is saying. This is known as reflective listening (Figure 1.10.3).

- The dentist must also have an understanding or awareness of the effects of the environment where the communication occurs. For non-anxious patients they may be able to talk in the surgery but for those with dental anxiety the surgery equipment, the smells and noises may inhibit their ability to communicate freely. In such instances it is necessary to consider interviewing the anxious patient away from the dental chair in 'non-threatening' surroundings in order to elicit the details of the patient's history and negotiate a treatment plan.

- Thus a knowledge and understanding of communication within the dental surgery will assist the dentist in deciphering the patient's story – from the perspective of the patient's previous dental experiences; life experiences (e.g. hospitalization); psychological (e.g. personality) and social (e.g. cultural background) view points. This information will enable the dentist to formulate a treatment plan (e.g. behavioural management) specifically on the needs of the individual patient.

- Communicating with children may often be through their parents. In this sense the parent acts as an advocate for the child and so much of what has been stated here in relation to the anxious adult is applicable to the parent who accompanies the child.

In this situation the dentist needs to have an understanding of the parent's own difficulties and anxieties not only in relation to dentistry but also with regard to how their child will respond to dental treatment. The dentist must allow the parent to ventilate these fears in order to obtain a clear and concise history of the child's dental and life experiences. In this way the dentist will be in a position to formulate a diagnosis and patient management treatment plan.

Be familiar with psychological issues relevant to the care of patients

Psychological issues and dental anxiety

+ A continuum of dental anxiety: it has been proposed that dentally anxious patients are not a homogeneous group of patients – since there are some who despite of their considerable fears attend for care whereas other avoid dental treatment, suggesting that this latter group represent those with a dental phobia. The commonality between them is their presenting symptomatology of dental anxiety (emotional) with its accompanying cognitive and physiological manifestations (see Table 1.10.2).

An awareness and understanding of the differences between patients with dental anxiety in contrast with dental phobia would allow the dentist to provide appropriate patient management and referrals for secondary level care (Burke and Freeman 2004).

+ **Dental anxiety:** The term dental anxiety was first mentioned Coriat (1946). He stated that dental anxiety was a fear of the unknown: an anticipatory anxiety in which previous frightening dental experiences were relived and experienced as if they were happening in the present. Dental anxiety may also be thought of in terms of trait (personality) and state anxiety (situation-specific). Dentally anxious patients are often able to link their present day dental fears to painful and/or distressing dental treatments experiences in childhood (see Figure 1.10.4).

+ **Dental phobia:** A phobia is an irrational fear of a place or an object with avoidance of the place or object. The intensity of anxiety is such that the individual avoids that place or object rather than experiencing the emotional and physiological manifestations of

Table 1.10.2 The presenting symptomatology of a patient with dental anxiety

Emotional manifestations	Cognitive manifestations	Physiological manifestations
	Treatment experiences	
Anxiety	Difficulty in accessing care	High heart rate
	Difficulty in speaking	Feeling nauseated
	Easily moved to tears	Dry mouth
		Sweating
		High respiratory rate

➤ Diagnosis dental anxiety

> [1] **Qualitative information**
> From patient's history
> Experiences of painful/unpleasant dental treatment
> [2] **Quantitative information**
> From dental anxiety questionnaires
> DAS score: >8<17
> MDAS score: >10 but <19

Figure 1.10.4

➤ Diagnosis dental phobia 1

> [1] **Qualitative information**
> From patient's history
> Assessment: history of false connections with past dental treatment experiences
> [2] **Quantitative information**
> From dental anxiety questionnaires
> DAS score: >17
> MDAS score: >19

Figure 1.10.5

their fear. Dental phobia differentiated from to dental anxiety by the patient's history. Often a hospitalization experience with a memory of painful injections is displaced (shifted) and falsely connected (mistakenly associated with dental treatment as the two situations have an element [the injection] in common) with the local anaesthetic injection which the patient remembers as being painful. The dentist's awareness of the possibility of shifting life experiences from outside to inside the surgery can assist in helping phobic patients accept dental treatment (see Figure 1.10.5).

A second group of phobic adult and child patients exist for whom there appears to be no obvious false connection. These patients do not remember a frightening or distressing experience only that something unpleasant happened. Listening carefully uncovers that this dental phobia, rather than being a 'disease entity in its own right' is in fact a symptom of an underlying emotional problem (see Figure 1.10.6).

A third group of dentally phobic individuals exist. These are children and adults with profound learning difficulties. Their responses to dental care may or may not be a consequence of previous frightening experiences but may be due to not being able to understand what is happening – a failure in communication (see Figure 1.10.7).

Psychological issues: assessing anxiety in adults and child patients using recognized psychological inventories

Dental anxiety may be quantified using psychological questionnaires or inventories which have been designed for the purpose. There are a number inventories which are

➤ Diagnosis dental phobia 2

> [1] **Qualitative information**
> From patient's history
> Assessment: no apparent history of painful/unpleasant experience: other emotional problems
> [2] **Quantitative information**
> From dental anxiety questionnaires
> DAS score: >17
> MDAS score: >19

Figure 1.10.6

➤ Diagnosis dental phobia 3

> **Qualitative information**
> From patient's history
> Assessment: dental phobic patient with learning difficulties

Figure 1.10.7

available for both adults and children. They are simple, easy to administer and complete as well as providing the dentist with the means of confirming the anxiety or phobia diagnosis.

- The Dental Anxiety Scale (DAS) (Corah 1969): This was the first questionnaire to assess adult dental anxiety status. It is a four-item inventory. The questions ask about the intensity of anxiety when waiting for, first the day of the appointment, second in the waiting room, third for drilling and finally for scaling. Each question has 5 possible responses from feeling relaxed (scoring 1) to feeling anxious (scoring 5). This gives a possible range of scores from 4 to 20 with the score of 8.89 representing the population average score. Scores between 17 and 20 correspond to dental phobia.

- The Modified Dental Anxiety Scale (MDAS) (Humphris *et al.* 1995): The MDAS is a modification of the DAS and includes a question about local anaesthesia. The questions assess the intensity of dental anxiety when waiting for, first the day of the appointment, second in the waiting room, third for drilling, growth for scaling and finally for local anaesthesia. The scoring system is the same as the DAS. Total scores range from 5 to 25. A score of 10.97 is the population average. Scores over 19 indicate dental phobia.

- The Child Fear Survey Schedule (Alvesalo *et al.* 1993): Children are asked to rate their level of dental fear on a five-point scale covering 15 situations such as drilling, injections etc. The possible responses range from 'not at all afraid' to 'very much afraid'. Scores range from 15 to 75.

Be competent at making appropriate referrals based on assessment

With the completion of the dental history and examination the dentist will be in the position to formulate a diagnosis of dental anxiety or dental phobia. The treatment decision and whether to refer the patient for secondary care will be dependent upon:

1. Previous treatment experiences (from the dental history)
2. The intensity of anxiety experienced by the patient (from the dental anxiety inventories)
3. The dentist's ability to provide a behavioural management regime appropriate to the patient's needs
4. The patient's ability to understand what is being said and what is happening.

The dentists' communication skills will provide the basis of a successful interaction by allowing the patient or relative the time to speak freely of previous frightening treatment experiences. The dentist is now cognisant of the information necessary and armed with this knowledge and understanding can decide to refer the patient for secondary level care or decide to negotiate the options with the patient as a prelude to treatment.

The Dental Anxiety Scale (Corah 1969)

If you had to go to the dentist tomorrow, how would you feel?
Would look forward to it as a:

Reasonably enjoyable experience	❑ [1]
Wouldn't care one way or the other	❑ [2]
Would be uneasy about it	❑ [3]
Would be afraid	❑ [4]
Would be very frightened	❑ [5]

While you are waiting in the waiting room for your turn in the dentist's chair, how do you feel?

Relaxed	❑ [1]
Uneasy	❑ [2]
Tense	❑ [3]
Anxious	❑ [4]
So anxious, I feel sick and break out in a sweat	❑ [5]

While you are sitting in the dentist's chair and he is getting his instruments out to drill your teeth, how do you feel?

Relaxed	❑ [1]
Uneasy	❑ [2]
Tense	❑ [3]
Anxious	❑ [4]
So anxious, I feel sick and break out in a sweat	❑ [5]

While you are sitting in the dentist's chair and he is getting his instruments out to scale your teeth, how do you feel?

Relaxed	❑ [1]
Uneasy	❑ [2]
Tense	❑ [3]
Anxious	❑ [4]
So anxious, I feel sick and break out in a sweat	❑ [5]

Modified Dental Anxiety Scale (Humphris *et al.* 1995)

If you went to your dentist for **TREATMENT TOMORROW**, how would you feel: (please check ☑)

Not anxious	❏
Slightly anxious	❏
Fairly anxious	❏
Very anxious	❏
Extremely anxious	❏

If you were sitting in the **WAITING ROOM** (waiting for treatment), how would you feel: (please check ☑)

Not anxious	❏
Slightly anxious	❏
Fairly anxious	❏
Very anxious	❏
Extremely anxious	❏

If you were about to have your **TEETH DRILLED**, how would you feel: (please check ☑)

Not anxious	❏
Slightly anxious	❏
Fairly anxious	❏
Very anxious	❏
Extremely anxious	❏

If you were about to have your **TEETH SCALED AND POLISHED**, how would you feel? (please check ☑)

Not anxious	❏
Slightly anxious	❏
Fairly anxious	❏
Very anxious	❏
Extremely anxious	❏

Modified Dental Anxiety Scale (Humphris *et al.* 1995)   continued

If you were about to have a **LOCAL ANAESTHETIC INJECTION** in your gum, above an upper back tooth, how would you feel? (please check ☑)

Not anxious	❏
Slightly anxious	❏
Fairly anxious	❏
Very anxious	❏
Extremely anxious	❏

Patients who fall into dental phobia categories 2 and 3 may be best served with referral for secondary level and specialist dental and medical care (Burke and Freeman 2004). For the dentally anxious patient and those who may be described as dentally phobic where a clear 'false connection' has been discovered then the dentist must use his communication skills within a framework of motivational interviewing to negotiate treatment and referral options (Figure 1.10.8, Figure 1.10.9).

Be competent at managing fear and anxiety with behavioural techniques

This section describes an applied model of motivational interviewing and the various behavioural management techniques used in dental practice (Figure 1.10.9).

Communication skills

Motivational interviewing (Rollnick *et al.* 2000) is an assessment of the patients' ambivalence, the associated resistance and their readiness to change or accept dental treatment. The basis of motivational interviewing is that the dentist must make few assumptions about the patient and adhere to the principles of good practice. The communication techniques used in motivational interviewing are appropriate when managing and negotiating treatment for patients in general (Figure 1.10.9).

Ambivalence and resistance

Many people feel ambivalent or in conflict about the idea of accepting dental treatment. This is due to the intensity of their anxiety (acting as a resistance to the forward movement to the acceptance of treatment) and the dentist needs to use his communication skills to appreciate that it is the patient's fears that are prohibitive and to accept that the patient is not yet ready for treatment. The underlying anxieties can be explored in an attempt to reduce the patient's worries and anxieties and enable them to accept the treatment which is being offered.

Child Fear Survey Schedule (Alvesalo *et al.* 1993)

How afraid are you of:	Not afraid at all	A little amount afraid	A fair amount afraid	Pretty much afraid	Very much afraid
	1	2	3	4	5
1. Dentists	O	O	O	O	O
2. Doctors	O	O	O	O	O
3. Injection	O	O	O	O	O
4. Having somebody examine your mouth	O	O	O	O	O
5. Having to open your mouth	O	O	O	O	O
6. Having a stranger touch you	O	O	O	O	O
7. Having somebody look at you	O	O	O	O	O
8. The dentist drilling	O	O	O	O	O
9. The sight of the dentist's drill	O	O	O	O	O
10. The noise of the dentist drilling	O	O	O	O	O
11. Having somebody put instruments in your mouth	O	O	O	O	O
12. Choking	O	O	O	O	O
13. Having to go to the hospital	O	O	O	O	O
14. People in white uniforms	O	O	O	O	O
15. Having the nurse clean your teeth	O	O	O	O	O

Readiness to change

The patient's state of readiness is a critical factor in the patient's acceptance of treatment. Associated with this process are the various behavioural management techniques. For some patients simply using 'tell-show-do' will suffice to reduce their dentally anxiety: at

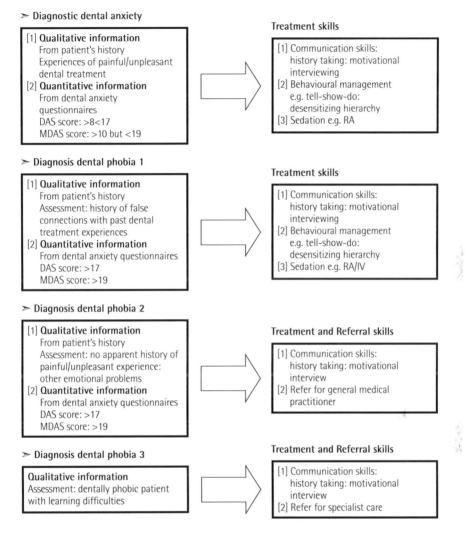

➤ Diagnostic dental anxiety

[1] **Qualitative information**
From patient's history
Experiences of painful/unpleasant
dental treatment
[2] **Quantitative information**
From dental anxiety
questionnaires
DAS score: >8<17
MDAS score: >10 but <19

Treatment skills

[1] Communication skills:
history taking: motivational
interviewing
[2] Behavioural management
e.g. tell-show-do:
desensitizing hierarchy
[3] Sedation e.g. RA

➤ Diagnosis dental phobia 1

[1] **Qualitative information**
From patient's history
Assessment: history of false
connections with past dental
treatment experiences
[2] **Quantitative information**
From dental anxiety questionnaires
DAS score: >17
MDAS score: >19

Treatment skills

[1] Communication skills:
history taking: motivational
interviewing
[2] Behavioural management
e.g. tell-show-do:
desensitizing hierarchy
[3] Sedation e.g. RA/IV

➤ Diagnosis dental phobia 2

[1] **Qualitative information**
From patient's history
Assessment: no apparent history of
painful/unpleasant experience:
other emotional problems
[2] **Quantitative information**
From dental anxiety questionnaires
DAS score: >17
MDAS score: >19

Treatment and Referral skills

[1] Communication skills:
history taking: motivational
interview
[2] Refer for general medical
practitioner

➤ Diagnosis dental phobia 3

Qualitative information
Assessment: dentally phobic patient
with learning difficulties

Treatment and Referral skills

[1] Communication skills:
history taking: motivational
interview
[2] Refer for specialist care

Figure 1.10.8 Scheme for assessment, management and referral for the dentally anxious patient

the other end of the continuum are those who will need assistance in the form of relative analgesia or IV sedation.

Two agendas and dangerous assumptions

Difficulties arise in the clinical management of the dentally anxious patient because dentists can misjudge the patient's attitudes and behaviours because the dentist and patient have two differing treatment agendas. When the dentist ignores the agenda of the patient it is unlikely that the patient will be able to accept the treatment which is being offered, however, when the patient is directly involved in identifying treatment options and has a feeling of control then they are more likely to accept the treatment which is provided.

Dangerous assumptions to avoid include:

1. This patient ought to accept treatment
2. This patient is ready for treatment
3. This patient's dental health must be a prime motivating factor
4. If the patient does not decides not to have treatment then consultation has failed
5. Patients are either motivated or not
6. Now is the right time for treatment
7. A frightening approach is always best
8. The patient must follow the dentist's advice.

Principles of good practice when negotiating treatment options include:

1. Respect for the autonomy of the patients and that their choices are important
2. Readiness to change must be taken into account
3. Ambivalence is common and reasons for conflict need to be explored and understood
4. Target/goals should be identified by the patient
5. The dentist must provide information and support
6. The patient makes the final decision.

Behavioural management

Iatrosedation

Iatrosedation, along with effective communication and history taking, forms the first part of the behavioural management of the dentally anxious patient. In a non-clinical setting the dentist establishes rapport with the patient using effective communication. This allows the patient to ventilate their anxieties, tell of their previous experiences and to be reassured. Effective communication is the cornerstone of non-pharmacological techniques, such as iatrosedation, 'tell-show-do', desensitizing hierarchy, relaxation, hypnosis, and so forth.

Tell-show-do

This is a simple means of preparing children and anxious adults for dental care. The dentist tells the patient what is to be done, shows the patient what will be done and then does it. The ability of the dentist to use language that the patient can understand assists in reducing anticipatory fears. It has been shown that a simple tell-show-do scenario prior to general anaesthesia can reduce dental anxiety and heart rate prior to the extraction of teeth in children (Carson and Freeman 1998).

Desensitizing hierarchy

This procedure is based upon effective communication and motivational interviewing techniques to negotiate dental treatment. The patient and dentist negotiate a treatment plan based upon the patient's least feared dental treatment item through to their most feared. In this way treatment starts with the least feared treatment (for example prophylaxsis) working through those items of treatment which are less feared (for example infiltration anaesthetic and filling) to the most feared (for example an extraction of a lower molar). As the treatment continues the patient gains confidence not only in the dentist but also in their ability to cope with their anxiety.

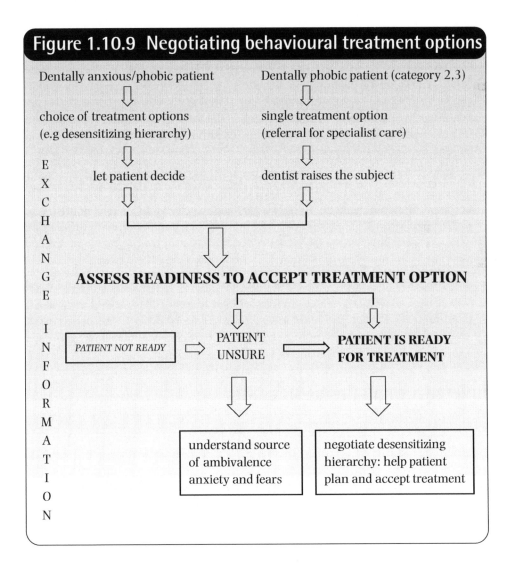

Figure 1.10.9 Negotiating behavioural treatment options

Dentally anxious/phobic patient

⇩

choice of treatment options
(e.g desensitizing hierarchy)

⇩

let patient decide

⇩

Dentally phobic patient (category 2,3)

⇩

single treatment option
(referral for specialist care)

⇩

dentist raises the subject

⇩

E X C H A N G E

ASSESS READINESS TO ACCEPT TREATMENT OPTION

I N F O R M A T I O N

| *PATIENT NOT READY* | ⇨ | PATIENT UNSURE | ⇨ | **PATIENT IS READY FOR TREATMENT** |

⇩

⇩

understand source
of ambivalence
anxiety and fears

negotiate desensitizing
hierarchy: help patient
plan and accept treatment

Familiarity with alternative methods of behavioural management

Another set of behavioural techniques exists which are used to reduce anxiety by inducing muscle relaxation. These include:

♦ Relaxation: relaxation is associated with biofeedback and hypnosis and provides a common link between these various techniques. The principle behind it is that relaxation will inhibit anxiety. McGoldrick and Pine (2000) provide an excellent description of applied relaxation techniques in the dental chair. They (McGoldrick and Pine 2000) state that there are two aims – which are assisting the patient to recognize anxiety and secondly to help the patient cope and contain their dental fear. This is achieved by teaching the patients to progressively relax all groups of muscles by either tense-release or imagery-based techniques. The patient gradually attains a relaxed state as they are asked to tense and release each group of muscles resulting in complete relaxation on demand (cue-controlled relaxation). The patient can be taught to relax on cue and this means that it is easily incorporated into the dental treatment scenario. For instance, when the patient sees the injection they can be instructed to relax on cue, leading to relaxation of the body as a whole and containment of anxiety.

♦ Hypnosis: This is an altered state of consciousness that characterized by muscle relaxation and suggestibility. Patients in the hypnotic state can recovery memories and emotions (abreaction). Hypnosis has been used extensively in dentistry to reduce anxiety and induce states of relaxation. Disadvantages of hypnosis are that with increased anxiety it is harder for patient to relax and enter the hypnotic state and that the technique is time-intensive with new patients.

• Biofeedback: This involves the training of patients to control their physiological responses to anxiety provoking situations. The technique is based upon the premise that that through monitoring an individual can gain voluntary control over what are thought as being involuntary physiological processes. Biofeedback has been used successfully in the treatment of stress-related disorders.

References and further reading

Alvesalo H., Murtomaa H., Milgrom P., Honkanen A., Karjalainen M. and Tay K. M. (1993) The dental fear survey schedule: a study with Finnish children. *Int J Paed Dent* 3, 193–8.

Burke F. J. T. and Freeman R. (2004) *Preparing for Dental Practice*. Oxford, Oxford University Press.

Carson P. and Freeman R. (1998) Tell-show-do: reducing anticipatory anxiety in emergency paediatric dental patients. *International Journal of Health Promotion and Education* 36, 87–90.

Corah N. L. (1969) Development of a dental anxiety scale. *Journal of Dental Research* 48, 596.

Coriat I. H. (1946) Dental anxiety: fear of going to the dentist. *Psychoanalytical Review*, 33, 365–7.

Freeman R. (2000) *The Psychology of Dental Patient Care*. London, BDJ Books.

GDC (2002) *The First Five Years: a framework for undergraduate dental education*, 2nd edn. London, The General Dental Council.

Humphris G. M., Morrison T. and Lindsay S. J. (1995) The modified dental anxiety scale: validation and United Kingdom norms. *Community Dental Health* 12, 143–50.

McGoldrick P. M. and Pine C. M. (2000) Teaching and assessing behavioural techniques of applied relaxation for reduction of dental fear using a controlled chairside simulation model. *European Journal of Dental Education* 4, 176–82.

QAA (2002) *Dentistry: academic standards*. Subject benchmark statements. Gloucester, Quality Assurance Agency for Higher Education.

Rollnick S., Mason P. and Butler C. (2000) *Health Behaviors Change: a guide for practitioners*. London, Churchill Livingstone.

Swallow J. N. (1970) Fear and the dentist. *New Society* 5, 819–21.

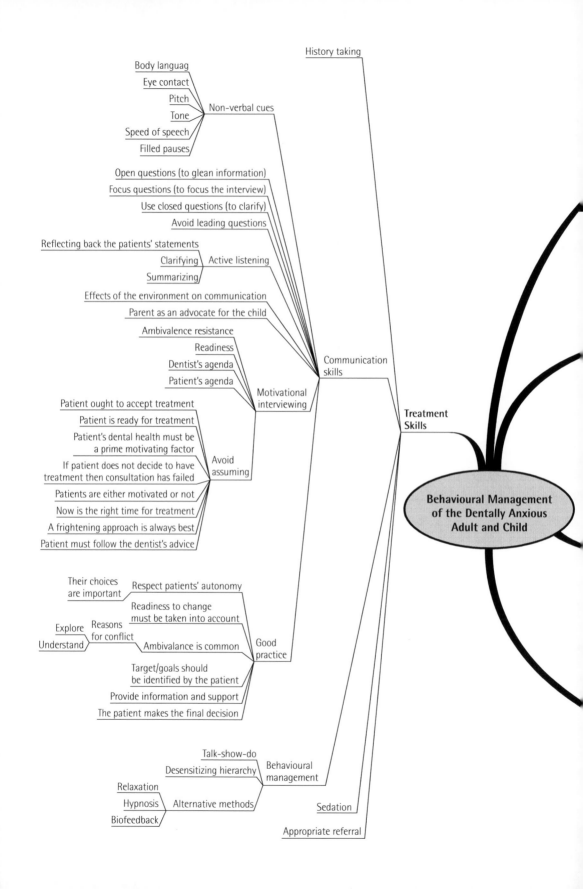

History taking

Body languag
Eye contact
Pitch
Tone
Speed of speech
Filled pauses

Non-verbal cues

Open questions (to glean information)
Focus questions (to focus the interview)
Use closed questions (to clarify)
Avoid leading questions

Reflecting back the patients' statements
Clarifying
Summarizing

Active listening

Effects of the environment on communication
Parent as an advocate for the child

Ambivalence resistance
Readiness
Dentist's agenda
Patient's agenda

Motivational
interviewing

Communication
skills

Treatment
Skills

Patient ought to accept treatment
Patient is ready for treatment
Patient's dental health must be
a prime motivating factor
If patient does not decide to have
treatment then consultation has failed
Patients are either motivated or not
Now is the right time for treatment
A frightening approach is always best
Patient must follow the dentist's advice

Avoid
assuming

**Behavioural Management
of the Dentally Anxious
Adult and Child**

Their choices
are important

Respect patients' autonomy

Readiness to change
must be taken into account

Explore
Understand

Reasons
for conflict

Ambivalance is common

Good
practice

Target/goals should
be identified by the patient
Provide information and support
The patient makes the final decision

Talk-show-do
Desensitizing hierarchy

Behavioural
management

Relaxation
Hypnosis
Biofeedback

Alternative methods

Sedation

Appropriate referral

Dental anxiety

- Is
  - Trait (personality)
  - State anxiety (situation-specific)
  - Often linked to experiences in childhood
- Diagnosis
  - Qualitative information — From patient's history
  - Quantitative information — Dental anxiety questionnaires:
    DAS score: >8<17
    MDAS score: >10 but <19

Dental phobia

- Is — Irrational fear with avoidance
- Diagnosis
  - From patient's history
    - False connections with past dental treatment experiences
    - No obvious false connection — Emotional problems
    - Or dental trauma
    - Learning difficulties — Communication problems
  - Quantitative information — From dental anxiety questionnaires
    DAS score: >17
    MDAS score: >19

Presenting symptomatology of dental anxiety

- Emotional — Anxiety
- Cognitive
  - Treatment experiences
  - Difficulty in accessing care
  - Difficulty in speaking
  - Easily moved to tears
- Physiological
  - High heart rate
  - Feeling nauseated
  - Dry mouth
  - Sweating
  - High respiratory rate

Quantification

- " The Dental Anxiety Scale (DAS)
- " The Modified Dental Anxiety Scale (MDAS)
- " The Child Fear Survey Schedule – Dental Scale (CFSS – DS)

1.11 Dental radiology
Laetitia Brocklebank

Introduction

Radiography and radiology are in all the dental clinical disciplines, to aid in diagnosis, treatment planning and management of patients. Dentists usually undertake their own radiography and therefore require to be competent at producing images, and interpreting the findings. They have a duty under the regulations currently in force to comply with legal requirements, and to be aware of those requirements, and any changes made to them.

The specific requirements to be fulfilled at graduation are specified in *The First Five Years* (GDC 2002), and the QAA Benchmark document (QAA 2002). Relevant sections in *The First Five Years* are:

Paragraph 96 Students should receive instruction and practical experience in the referral criteria, taking, processing and interpretation of intra- and extra-oral radiographs and the writing of radiology reports. They should be aware of alternative imaging techniques. It is highly desirable that instruction in this part of the programme is under the direction of a registered specialist in dental radiology.

Paragraph 97 Students should understand the principles which underlie dental radiographic techniques, the equipment employed and the methods of processing films and the practice of digital radiography. They should be fully instructed in the hazards of ionising radiation and understand the current UK/European regulations pertaining to those hazards so they can undertake proper radiation protection measures for their patients, staff and themselves.

Paragraph 98 The programme must provide 'adequate training' as specified in the Ionising Radiation (Medical Exposure) Regulations, 2000 or in any subsequent regulations. This includes the nature of ionising radiation and its interaction with tissues, principles of quality control and quality assurance applied to equipment and technique, justification and optimisation of all radiation exposures (including the importance of utilising previous radiographic information and that available from other diagnostic techniques) and the current safety regulations affecting general dental practice.

Paragraph 99 Students must undergo practical instruction in radiographic technique using equipment normally available to dental practitioners, and in taking the various film views used in general dental practice. They should also be aware of digital imaging techniques. Opportunities should be readily available for students to take radiographs under close supervision for the patients they are treating. Trusts with dental teaching hospitals should be aware of this requirement and ensure that sufficient equipment and staff are available for the purpose and that this may be in addition to service needs.

Paragraph 100 Students should understand the appearance of normal structures on a radiograph, and be able to assess image quality, apply differential diagnosis to abnormal appearances, write informative reports of findings, and apply clinical audit procedures to the process. This part of the course should be well integrated with the teaching of other clinical dental disciplines so that students appreciate the relevance of radiology to treatment.

The QAA (2002) Benchmark statement says:

Paragraph 3.9 Oral radiology prescribe, take and process appropriate intra-oral and dental panoramic radiographs; derive diagnoses by interpreting and relating findings from the history, clinical and radiographic examinations and other diagnostic tests.

Intended learning outcomes in dental radiology

The dental graduate should:

♦ be competent at taking and processing the various film views used in general dental practice;

♦ be competent at radiographic interpretation and be able to write an accurate radiographic report;

♦ have knowledge of the hazards of ionizing radiation and regulations relating to them, including radiation protection and dose reduction;

♦ be familiar with the principles which underlie dental radiographic techniques.

Outline description and generic points

Radiographic views taken in general dental practice may be intra-oral, where the image receptor is positioned inside the mouth, or extra-oral, where the imaging receptor is positioned outside.

- Intra-oral:
  - Bitewings
  - Periapicals, including endodontic views
  - Occlusals
- Extra-oral:
  - Panoramic or Dental Panoramic Radiograph (DPR)
  - Lateral cephalometric radiograph – usually only in specialist orthodontic practices
  - Lateral oblique views of the jaws – not common

The graduating dentist should be competent at taking all of the intra-oral views and panoramic radiographs, and should have knowledge of the theory for producing the other views. *The Guidance Notes for Dental Practitioners on the Safe Use of X-ray Equipment* (Health Protection Agency 2001) include a number of references to legal requirements, or good practice in relation to production and utilization of dental radiographic views: these will be reproduced in this chapter in text boxes.

> Whenever practicable, techniques using film holders incorporating beam-aim devices should be adopted for bitewing and periapical radiography.

> If rectangular collimation is being used, a beam-aiming device is essential for accurate alignment with the intra-oral film.

Image receptors

Film and digital detectors are available for production of radiographic images.

> Intra-oral film should be undertaken with the fastest film consistent with satisfactory diagnostic results. Intra-oral films of ISO speed group E, or faster, are preferred. Speed F is now available which offers a further dose reduction over E, provided automatic processing systems are used.

> For extra-oral radiography the fastest film and intensifying screen combination consistent with satisfactory results should be used. The speed of the system should be at least 400.

Direct digital radiographic procedures are available for all intra-oral views and panoramic and cephalometric views. Patient preparation and position is not affected by the use of digital detectors, but modified film holders may be required.

Two systems are available:

1. Direct – use of CCD (charge-coupled device) or CMOS (complementary metal-oxide semiconductor) technology where the digital sensor is linked to the computer by a cable. The image appears virtually instantaneously.

2. Indirect – use of PSP (photo stimulable phosphor, also called SPP storage phosphor plates) imaging plates. These plates store the pattern of X-ray energy and release it when scanned by an appropriate laser beam.

Intra-oral digital systems require less radiation than film, as do extra-oral CCD systems. Extra-oral PSP systems have a speed equivalent to rare earth screen systems. It is recommended to use DC intra-oral X-ray machines. Users should also be aware that the PSP systems have a wide latitude – this means that they will produce acceptable images over a very wide exposure range and care must be taken to ensure that a dose reduction for the patient is achieved.

Processing

With the exception of direct digital images which are available on a computer screen virtually instantly all radiographic images require a processing stage to make the latent image visible, and archiveable. Film images are processed using chemicals, and advice is given in the Guidance Notes, which stress the importance of appropriate quality assurance protocols to ensure optimum image quality.

> Strict attention should be paid to correct and consistent film processing so as to produce good quality radiographs and avoid the necessity for examinations to be repeated.

> The developer should be changed at regular intervals in accordance with the manufacturer's instructions.
>
> The overall performance of the processing also needs to be monitored. One of the simplest ways of achieving this is with the use of a test object such as a step-wedge.

> Routine checks should be made to ensure that darkrooms remain light tight and that safelights do not produce fogging of films.

Testing for white light leakage can be carried out by standing in the room with all lights off, and looking at edges of doors and windows, and any equipment passing through the wall, for signs of white light. Safelight testing is carried out using a sheet of extra-oral film and a series of coins placed on top in complete darkness; uncovering one at a time in safelight conditions at timed intervals, and then processing the film will enable information to be obtained about the time period before fogging starts to occur (Brocklebank 1998).

Indirect digital systems utilize a special laser scanner to read the information contained in the phosphor plate. These sensors are sensitive to white light, exposure to which will result in a degradation of image quality, and care needs to be taken about the location of the scanner, to ensure that the image will not be degraded during the period of unwrapping the sensor and positioning it in the scanner.

Indications and contraindications

Before any radiographic exposure can take place it must be justified by an IRMER Practitioner and authorized as a means of demonstrating that it has been justified. In deciding whether an individual exposure is justified appropriate weight must be given to:

- the availability and findings of previous radiographs;
- the specific objectives of the exposure in relation to the history and examination of the patient;
- the total potential diagnostic benefit to the individual;
- the radiation risk associated with the radiographic examination;
- the efficacy, benefits and risk of available alternative techniques having the same objective but involving no, or less, exposure to ionizing radiation.

A number of documents are available to assist with the decision making, giving guidance on the suitability of selection criteria in various clinical situations:

1. *Selection Criteria in Dental Radiography* (Faculty of General Dental Practitioners 2004)

2. *Orthodontic Radiographs Guidelines* (British Orthodontic Society 2001)

3. *European Guidelines on Radiation Protection in Dental Radiography* (European Commission (2004).

In addition to published guidelines, the legal person in a practice or institutional situation, must establish guidelines for referral criteria for radiographic examinations and ensure that these are available to all referrers.

When considering selection criteria for dental radiography it is appropriate to consider whether the possibility of a female patient being pregnant is relevant to the proposed examination. Based on the guidance notes the following advice is relevant:

- The possibility of a female of child-bearing age and the impact on a radiographic examination is relevant only if the pelvic region is to be irradiated – in such a case the patient should be asked. The only dental radiographic view in which this would be relevant is the no longer used vertex occlusal view.

♦ The risk to the foetus is negligible for all other dental views.

♦ The importance of emotions is acknowledged and it is recommended to delay if considered prudent – this is a decision to be made together with the patient, and taking into account the need for a radiograph in relation to certain treatments, e.g. the surgical removal of an impacted third molar.

Common indications for the standard views can be summarized:

Bitewing

1. Detection of proximal carious lesions
2. Determination of depth of carious lesions
3. Detection of secondary caries
4. Demonstration of alveolar bone level in cases of mild to moderate chronic inflammatory periodontal disease (vertical orientation suitable for middle-range bone loss)
5. Demonstration of restorative excesses and defects.

Periapical

1. Detection of periapical or pararadicular bone change, related to pulpal disorders
2. Endodontic treatment and pre-extraction evaluation – number and morphology; proximity to anatomical structures
3. Determination of alveolar bone support in periodontal disease
4. Localization of unerupted teeth, pathological lesions or foreign objects
5. Post-trauma
6. Review of clinical/surgical procedures.

Occlusal – oblique

1. Determination of presence of developing teeth, or supernumerary or absent teeth
2. Situations where periapicals are desired but cannot be obtained
3. Situations where periapical pathology is present, and of such a size that it is not demonstrated on a single periapical view, e.g. cystic lesions.

Occlusal – true or cross-sectional – mandible only

1. Bucco-lingual localization of unerupted teeth, pathology, horizontal displacement of alveolar fractures, and foreign objects
2. Demonstration of buccal/lingual expansion caused by pathological change
3. Demonstration of radiopaque calculi in submandibular gland salivary ducts.

Panoramic

Dental panoramic radiograph (DPR)

Demonstration of the complete dentition and supporting structures for:

1. Determination of dentition presence or absence

2. Determination of pathology within the bone and the extent of such pathology

3. Demonstration of height of supporting alveolar bone

4. Demonstration of fractures, their presence and displacement

5. Review following surgery or treatment of fracture cases.

Lateral cephalometric radiograph

1. Orthodontic treatment, planning and evaluating in cases with marked vertical or antero-posterior discrepancy

2. Orthognathic surgery, planning and follow-up

3. Cleft palate patients.

Oblique lateral

Also called the lateral oblique. Demonstration of one part of the jaws:

1. When panoramic radiography is not possible

2. To provide a full thickness image of extensive pathology (e.g. impacted third molars when intra-oral views are not possible).

Further information

Information concerning current procedures relating to the use of film holders and beam-aiming devices, rectangular collimators, and the speed of the selected imaging receptor in dental radiography can be found in Faculty of General Dental Practitioners (2004). A summary of key points concerning the production of each radiographic view can be found in Brocklebank (1997). Reminder points are available in the *Oxford Handbook of Clinical Dentistry* (Mitchell and Mitchell 1995).

Assessment

For each of the views listed an appropriate form of assessment involves observation of the student carrying out the procedure on a patient. It should include assessment of the quality of the final image. The checklist and assessment sheet can be modified for each of the different views, amending any highlighted points noted in the checklist.

A separate checklist is provided for panoramic radiography as this involves quite different equipment, although many of the generic points are common.

This checklist approach can also be applied to assessing a student's ability to adequately assess a radiographic image, in order to determine the presence of abnormalities, and make an initial judgment about any such finding.

Intra-oral radiographic examination

The checklist should include:

♦ Introduction of student by themselves to patient, and other persons present

♦ Identification of the patient:

   1. name

   2. date of birth

   3. address

♦ Confirmation with patient of region to be X-rayed: e.g. site of pain, reason for X-rays being taken

♦ Appropriate cross-infection control procedures, prior to, during and after carrying out the procedure according to standard procedures in use in the clinic:

   1. Prior to: own hands, preparation of equipment, selection of appropriate film-holder and image receptor, selection of exposure factors

   2. During: avoidance of contamination, selection of any additional requirements, placement of exposed films

   3. After: procedures specific to imaging receptors, surfaces, equipment control panel, own hands

♦ Preparation of X-ray facility, preferably prior to patient entry: selection of required accessories, setting of exposure factors

♦ Patient preparation: outdoor clothing; seated or prone position with appropriate head support; removal of relevant jewellery and hair ornaments, and dentures

♦ Explanation of procedure to patient

♦ Procedure:

   1. placement of imaging receptor including correct relationship to teeth, stability – receptor to always be parallel to line of teeth being examined

   2. alignment of X-ray tube-head including rectangular collimator, correct distance, *and for occlusals vertical angulation*

   3. exposure including continued observation of patient

   4. relocation of X-ray tube-head and removal of all accessories from patient's mouth

   5. explanation to patient of what will happen next

♦ Recording of examination details including, as a minimum, type and number of films, exposure settings

♦ Appropriate assessment of film quality using the standard ratings as detailed in the Dental Guidance Notes.

Checklist 19 **For intra-oral radiographic examination**

	Superior	Adequate	Inadequate
Introduction of student by themselves to patient, and other persons present			
Identification of the patient			
• name			
• date of birth			
• address			
Confirmation with patient of region to be X-rayed: e.g. site of pain, reason for X-rays being taken			
Cross-infection control prior to:			
own hands, preparation of equipment, selection of appropriate film-holder and image receptor, selection of exposure factors			
Cross-infection control during:			
avoidance of contamination, selection of any additional requirements, placement of exposed films			
Cross-infection control after:			
procedures specific to imaging receptors, surfaces, equipment control panel, own hands			
Preparation of X-ray facility, preferably prior to patient entry: selection of required accessories, setting of exposure factors			
Patient preparation: outdoor clothing; seated or prone position with appropriate head support, removal of relevant jewellery etc., and dentures			
Explanation of procedure to patient			
Procedure:			
• placement of imaging receptor including correct relationship to teeth (parallel), stability			
• alignment of X-ray tube-head including rectangular collimator, correct distance			
• exposure including continued observation of patient			

Checklist 19 **For intra-oral radiographic examination** – *continued*

	Superior	Adequate	Inadequate
• relocation of X-ray tube-head and removal of all accessories from patient's mouth			
• explanation to patient of what will happen next			
Recording of examination details including as a minimum, type and number of films, exposure settings			
Appropriate film quality rating using the standard ratings as detailed in the Dental Guidance Notes			

Signing off will be declined for an 'Inadequate' score; it will be necessary to complete this procedure in its entirety to the satisfaction of the examiner in order to be signed off as competent in the performance of this task.

Student name:

Staff signature:

Date: ....

Panoramic radiographic examination

The checklist should include:

◆ Introduction of student by themselves to patient, and other persons present

◆ Identification of the patient:

1. name

2. date of birth

3. address

◆ Confirmation with patient of reason for X-ray examination

◆ Appropriate cross-infection control procedures, prior to, during and after carrying out the procedure according to standard procedures in use in the clinic:

1. Prior to: own hands, preparation of equipment, selection of appropriate positioning device/s, selection of exposure factors

2. During: avoidance of contamination, selection of any additional requirements

3. After: procedures specific to equipment and accessories: cassette, surfaces, equipment control panel, own hands

♦ Preparation of X-ray facility, preferably prior to patient entry: selection of required accessories, initial selection of programme and exposure factors

♦ Patient preparation: outdoor clothing, and/or bulky top; removal of jewellery, hair ornaments, dentures

♦ Explanation of procedure to patient

♦ Procedure:

1. height adjustment of machine

2. placement of cassette

3. initial positioning of patient, with straight neck, hands on supports

4. correct use of bite-peg and/or chin support

5. correct positioning with the aid of lights or other guides

6. Frankfort plane horizontal (porion-orbitale – top of external auditory meatus to lower border of visible orbit)

7. final explanation to patient and request to stay still

8. request to place tongue against the roof of the mouth

9. check of correct programme and exposure settings

10. observation of patient throughout exposure

♦ Post-procedure:

1. Assisting patient out of machine; returning all possessions; explanation of what will happen next

2. returning machine to start position

3. removal of cassette and transfer to darkroom/daylight processor with appropriate identification

♦ Recording of examination details including as a minimum: programme selected and exposure settings

♦ Appropriate assessment of film quality using the standard ratings as detailed in the Dental Guidance Notes.

Processing

The checklist for intra-oral film should include:

♦ Demonstration of awareness to carry out procedures in a safe-light environment (at least until the film is fixed)

- Correct removal of film from an intra-oral film packet and identification of component parts, with an explanation of their function:

  (a) outer plastic cover – waterproof, light protection

  (b) inner paper with flap – additional light protection; flap to aid in removal of film

  (c) lead foil – prevent secondary X-rays reaching film; removes some of the primary beam

  (d) film – for image formation

- Handling of film without touching the flat surfaces
- Correct use of automatic film processor
- Appropriate assessment of film quality using the standard ratings as detailed in the Dental Guidance Notes
- Correct orientation on the viewing box
- Labelling requirements to include at least name, and other identifier (hospital number or date of birth) and date of film/s.

The student should be able to explain or demonstrate the use of a daily test object for checking the efficacy of the developer. Details of the use of a test object can be found in Brocklebank (1998).

Daily test film for quality assurance of chemical processing

The checklist should include adequate explanation of the following:

- Suitable test objects, and how to make a simple step-wedge from discarded lead foil
- Relationship of test object, film and X-ray tube-head
- Selection of appropriate exposure setting
- Exposing and processing a film in fresh chemicals on each change (control film)
- Exposing and processing a film regularly (ideally daily) as a test
- Comparison of test film with control film, and assessment of status of chemicals.

Safelight testing

The checklist should include:

- Selection of a sheet of extra-oral film in darkness
- Placing of a number of coins along the length of the film
- Covering the film and coins with card
- Switching on the safelights
- Uncovering a coin at 30 second intervals, until one coin remains covered
- Switching off the safelights and transferring the film to the processor on complete darkness

◆ Assessment of the resultant image, where any coin visible indicates that the safelights are not safe for that period of time. The test can be carried out with shorter time intervals as appropriate.

Be competent at radiographic interpretation and be able to write an accurate radiographic report

Outline description

The ability to recognize that a radiographic image includes features which may be due to developmental or acquired abnormalities is founded on a sound anatomical knowledge, and knowledge of those features which should be demonstrated in any particular radiographic view.

The graduating dentist should be competent at examining a radiograph, recognizing normal features, recognizing the presence of abnormalities, and describing any such findings in an appropriate way in order to demonstrate a degree of knowledge about the processes which may be involved in causing the image.

The Guidance Notes make it explicit that a clinical evaluation of the outcome of each exposure is carried out and recorded.

Clinical evaluation does not necessarily have to be a full radiology report, but should show that each radiograph has been evaluated and should provide enough information so that it can be subject to a later audit. For example, this information may include:

◆ the charting of caries;

◆ the patient's management or prognosis;

◆ in the case of a pre-extraction radiograph, it may be sufficient to record either 'root form simple' or 'nothing abnormal diagnosed'.

Step by step description

Radiographic examination should be carried out with the aid of a proper viewing box in a room where the ambient light can be dimmed. Masking facilities should be available, and a magnifying glass is sometimes useful.

An examination checklist is useful, in order to ensure that no part of the image is overlooked – this is particularly important when using panoramic and other extra-oral views.

The following checklist is reproduced from Brocklebank (1998), and a detailed explanation of how to use this is available in Chapter 3 of that book.

Examination of radiographs – checklist and order

Background to examination:

1. Patient profile – sex, age, racial/ethnic origin, home environment, diet, dental health care, etc.

2. Reason for taking radiograph: patient's complaint

3. Radiographic view(s) – expectation of anatomical features that should be demonstrated

4. Technical acceptability – quality 1, 2 or 3, with reasons for allocation of 2 or 3

5. Correct viewing conditions:
   - quiet and concentration
   - bright white backlight
   - dim room
   - blackout availability
   - (magnifying glass)

Detailed examination:

6. Symmetry

7. Margins:
   - intact
   - thickness

8. Bone consistency

9. Teeth:
   - number
   - eruption status
   - morphology
   - condition

10. Supporting bone:
    - alveolar margins
    - periapical

11. Any other features:
    - radiolucent/radiopaque
    - site
    - shape
    - size

- ◆ margins
- ◆ relation to other structures
- ◆ aetiological factors
- ◆ effect on other structures
- ◆ provisional/differential diagnosis

12. Summary

13. Proposals to meet patient's requirements, including other investigations.

Assessment

Assessment of this component may be separated into:

1. Recognition of normal features

2. Recognition and interpretation of abnormal features.

Recognition of normal features is best carried out by a tracing of a full panoramic radiograph, in order that the full extent of the jaws is included in the field of view, and peripheral structures such as the vertebrae.

The student should be able to accurately identify and label the following features, provided they are included in the field of view:

- ◆ hard palate
- ◆ maxillary sinus
- ◆ nasal cavity
- ◆ nasal septum
- ◆ nasal conchae
- ◆ ID canal
- ◆ tongue
- ◆ lips
- ◆ soft palate
- ◆ ear lobe
- ◆ mental foramen
- ◆ zygomatic buttress
- ◆ pharynx:
  - ■ naso
  - ■ oro
  - ■ laryngo

- epiglottis
- vertebrae – named
- hyoid
- styloid process
- external auditory meatus
- zygomatic arch
- pterygo-maxillary fissure.

The checklist approach can also be applied to assessing a student's ability to adequately assess a radiographic image, in order to determine the presence of abnormalities, and make an initial judgment about any such finding.

Radiological assessment

The checklist should include:

- Orientation of the radiograph on the viewing box
- Identification of the patient:

   1. name
   2. date of birth
   3. address

- Reason for radiograph/s being taken – justification, demonstrating appropriate knowledge of selection criteria
- Assessment of quality of the radiograph/s
- An overview of the status of the dentition
- Accurate recording of teeth present and absent
- Recognition of caries and other coronal abnormalities
- The status of the supporting bone, both in relation to the periodontium and the periradicular bone
- Recognition of the presence of other abnormalities, with a logical description of each abnormality, and evidence of an understanding of the significance of the features described
- Evidence of the ability to apply the principles of parallax
- Correct proposals for appropriate further investigations
- Differential diagnosis of the described abnormalities.

Suitable images for use in radiological assessment would include:

1. A developing dentition with unerupted canines
2. A classical presentation of a radicular cyst

3. A dentigerous cyst

4. An aggressive, destructive lesion.

Have knowledge of the hazards of ionizing radiation and regulations relating to them, including radiation protection and dose reduction

The Health Protection Agency web-site has a number of useful references concerning the nature of ionizing radiations, the relevant hazards and associated risks, including publications appropriate for the general public, at http://www.hpa.org.uk/radiation.

The regulations relating to the use of ionizing radiation in dental practice are all incorporated in the Dental Guidance Notes (Health Protection Agency 2001). This is available both online and as a paper document direct from the HPA, and should be studied in order to obtain the information relating to radiation protection and dose reduction.

The regulations refer to personnel in specific terms and the student should be able to explain the legal responsibilities of each of them:

- the Employer (Legal Person)

- the Referrer

- the (IRMER) Practitioner

- the Operator

- the Radiation Protection Supervisor

- the Radiation Protection Advisor

- the Medical Physics Expert.

Details of all these persons and their responsibilities can be found in the Dental Guidance Notes, together with the current requirements for achieving doses as low as reasonably practicable.

The student should be able to detail the various methods of reducing the dose to the patient, whilst producing an image of adequate diagnostic value, in relation to the following physical parameters related to image production:

- Tube operating voltage

- Film speed: intra-oral and extra-oral

- Use of film holders and beam-aiming devices

- Collimation: intra-oral, and extra-oral (panoramic and lateral cephalometric), and the importance of programme selection in panoramic radiography.

Justification is an important component of dose reduction, and cross-reference may be made to the issue of application of appropriate, and preferably evidence-based, selection criteria in this respect.

References and further reading

Isaacson K. G. and Thom A. R. (eds) (2001) *Guidelines for the use of Radiographs in Orthodontics*, 2nd edn. London, British Orthodontic Society.

Brocklebank, L. (1997) *Dental Radiology – understanding the x-ray image*. Oxford, Oxford University Press.

Brocklebank L. M. (1998) Dental radiology: capture your image. *Dental Update* 25, 94–102.

European Commission (2004) *European Guidelines on Radiation Protection in Dental Radiography*. Brussels, The European Commission. Also available at
http://europa.eu.int/comm/energy/nuclear/radioprotection/publication/136_en.htm

Pendlebury M. E., Horner K. and Eaton K. A. (2004) *Selection Criteria in Dental Radiography*, 2nd edn. London, Faculty of General Dental Practice (UK).

GDC (2002) *The First Five Years: a framework for undergraduate dental education*, 2nd edn. London, The General Dental Council.

Mitchell and Mitchell (1995) *Oxford Handbook of Clinical Dentistry*, 2nd edn. Oxford, Oxford University Press.

Health Protection Agency (2001) *Guidance Notes for Dental Practitioners on the Safe Use of X-ray Equipment*. Didcot, Health Protection Agency. Also available at
http://www.hpa.org.uk/radiation/publications/misc_publications/dental_guidance_notes.htm

Health Protection Agency (2001) *X-rays: how safe are they?* Didcot, Health Protection Agency. Also available at http://www.hpa.org.uk/radiation/publications/misc_publications/x-ray_safety_leaflet.htm

QAA (2002) *Dentistry: academic standards*. Subject benchmark statements. Gloucester, Quality Assurance Agency for Higher Education.

Dental Radiology and Imaging

Selection criteria

- Decision to be made jointly with a pregnant patient, and taking into account the need for a radiograph and urgency of treatment
- The risk to the foetus is negligible for all normal dental views

Bilewing
- Detection of proximal carious lesions
- Determination of depth of carious lesions
- Detection of secondary caries
- Demonstration of alveolar bone level in periodontal disease
- Demonstration of restorative excesses and defects

Periapical
- Detection of periapical or para radicular bone change, related to pulpal disorders
- Endodontic treatment and pre extraction evaluation
  - Root number
  - Root morphology
  - Proximity to anatomical structures
- Determination of alveolar bone support in periodontal disease
- Localization of
  - Unerupted teeth
  - Pathological lesions
  - Foreign objects
  - Post trauma
- Review of clinical/surgical procedures

Occlusal-oblique
- Presence and localization of
  - Developing and supernumerary teeth
  - Absence of teeth
- Situations where periapicals are desired but cannot be obtained
- Where periapical pathology is present, and of such a size that it is not demonstrated on a single periapical view

Occlusal true or cross-sectional-mandible only
- Bucco-lingual localization of unerupted teeth
- Pathology
  - Demonstration of buccal/lingual expansion
- Horizontal displacement of alveolar fractures
- Foreign objects
- Demonstration of radiopaque calculi in submandibular gland salivary ducts.

Panoramic
- Demonstration of the complete dentition and supporting structures
- Teeth
  - Presence
  - Absence
- Pathology within the bone
  - Presence
  - Extent
- Height of supporting alveolar bone
- Fractures
  - Presence
  - Displacement
  - Review

Lateral cephalometric radiograph
- Orthodontics
  - Marked vertical discrepancy or antero-posterior discrepancy
- Orthognathic surgery
  - Planning
  - Follow-up
- Cleft palate patients

Oblique lateral (lateral oblique)
- Demonstration of one part of the jaws
  - When panoramic radiography is not possible
  - To provide a full thickness image of extensive pathology

Good practice
- Film holders with beam-aiming devices
  - Bitewing
  - Periapical radiography
- Fastest film consistent with satisfactory diagnostic results
  - Intra-oral ISO speed group E, or faster
  - Extra-oral, fastest available film/intensifying screen combination, at least system speed 400

Skills
- Taking and processing views used in general dental practice
- Radiographic interpretation
- Radiographic reporting
- Knowledge of
  - The hazards of ionizing radiation
  - Regulations
    - Radiation protection
    - Dose reduction
  - Principles underlying dental radiographic techniques

Radiographic views used in dental practice
- Intra-oral
  - Bitewings
  - Periapicals, including endodontic views
  - Occlusals
- Extra-oral
  - Panoramic or dental panoramic radiograph (DPR)
  - Lateral cephalometric radiograph – usualy only in specialist orthodontic practices
  - Lateral oblique views of the jaws – not common
- Before any radiographic exposure can take place it must be justified by an IRMER practitioner and authorized

Processing
- To make the latent image visible and archiveable
- Digital images on a computer screen
- Quality assurance protocols to ensure optimum image quality

Digital radiography
- Direct
  - CCD (charge-coupled device)
  - CMOS (complementary metal-oxide semiconductor)
- Indirect
  - PSP (photo stimulable phosphor) imaging plates also called SPP (storage phosphor plates)
    - Acceptable images over a very wide exposure range
- Intra-oral digital systems require less radiation than film

1.12 Prevention and interception

Anne Maguire

Key points

- Knowledge and understanding of the principles of health promotion and disease prevention is essential for preventive and interceptive dental care.

- Competence in preventive techniques forms a cornerstone for the practice of dentistry based on an ethos of evidence-based prevention and health promotion.

- The key elements for prevention are dietary control, oral hygiene, appropriate use of fluoride, fissure sealing, and regular review.

- Interception in relation to orthodontics aims to minimize the total amount of treatment needed, primarily through the maintenance of space and early treatment of local irregularities.

- Every patient contact provides an opportunity for preventive care.

- The rationale for all preventive treatments and an awareness of their success and limitations should be evidence-based.

- The ability to evaluate the efficacy of preventive measures is an important part of continuing care provision for patients.

- Collaboration with other health care professionals and with patients themselves is fundamental in the prevention, diagnosis, treatment and management of disease.

Introduction

There are a number of generic skills required of the graduate in the area of prevention and interception. Prevention of disease should form an integral part of any comprehensive treatment plan in clinical practice. A dentist has a fundamental role to play in the prevention of dental diseases and conditions including dental caries, periodontal disease and tooth surface loss as well as a contributory role in the prevention of oral cancer and other smoking- and alcohol-related diseases. In addition, a dentist's interceptive role is particularly important in the management of the developing dentition, especially with regard to space maintenance, and timely management of local irregularities, such as single tooth crossbites. The graduate should also recognize how an increased overjet increases risk of dental trauma and be proactive in its timely and appropriate management, through specialist referral where necessary. The dental graduate also has a contributory role in reducing the dental effects of trauma by being able to provide well-fitting mouthguards and instructing patients in their use for contact sports.

The First Five Years (GDC 2002) requires the attainment of a number of generic learning outcomes by dental graduates in relation to prevention and interception:

PREVENTIVE DENTISTRY

Paragraph 83 Dental students should be made aware of the successes and limitations of preventive dentistry, and the potential for further progress. The ethos of preventive dentistry should prevail in every clinical dental department, so that new preventive dentistry techniques are taught to students as they become available. Students should be conversant with the practice of preventive care including oral health education and oral health promotion. Students should recognise the increasing evidence-based approach to treatment and should be able to make appropriate judgements. The student should appreciate the need for the dentist to collaborate in prevention, diagnosis, treatment and management of disease with other healthcare professionals and with patients themselves. The student should be aware of the economic and practical constraints affecting the provision of healthcare.

CHILD DENTAL HEALTH

Paragraph 80 The study of child dental health should encompass the interrelationships between orthodontics and paediatric dentistry together with the general growth and development of the individual. It should be related to social and psychological factors and to the recognition, preventive treatment and operative management of the common disease processes.

Paragraph 82 Students should be able to ... recognise and manage those problems of the mixed dentition where interceptive treatment is indicated, including space maintenance.

DENTAL PUBLIC HEALTH

Paragraph 85 Dental students should learn that health promotion involves helping individuals and communities to benefit from increased control over their own health with the intention of improving it. Although many groups and organisations in addition to those composed of healthcare professionals are involved, doctors and dentists can play an important role. Dental students should understand the principles of health promotion and apply them when in contact with patients and at other times, particularly in matters of tooth brushing with fluoridated dentifrices, diet and nutrition, tobacco avoidance and public health measures such as fluoridation.

RESTORATIVE DENTISTRY

Paragraph 74 Restorative dentistry is concerned with the management of the plaque-related diseases (dental caries and periodontal diseases), tooth wear and tooth loss. Management includes preventive, non-operative care as well as the restoration of teeth using the well-established techniques of conservative dentistry, including crowns and endodontics, the replacement of teeth by means of prostheses, and the treatment and maintenance of the supporting structures of the teeth by the procedures of periodontology. In restorative dentistry students should have continuous responsibility for the care of a number of adults in order to assess their overall needs, the efficacy of preventive measures, their behaviour, management and long term success or failure of restorative treatment.

ORAL PATHOLOGY AND ORAL MICROBIOLOGY

Paragraph 95 The course in oral pathology and oral microbiology should integrate with pathology and medical microbiology. Initially the processes underlying the common oral diseases and methods of their diagnosis, prevention and management should be described.

Prevention and interception are also key elements in the Subject Benchmark for Dentistry:

Paragraph 3.6 Oral health promotion

Recognise predisposing and aetiological factors that require intervention to promote oral health.

Understand the pattern of oral disease in society and be able to contribute to health promotion.

Assess the need for, and provide, preventive procedures and instruction in oral health methods that incorporate sound biological principles in order to preserve oral hard and soft tissues, and to prevent disease.

Use and provide appropriate therapeutic agents and treatment modalities.

Paragraph 3.13 Dental caries and tooth surface loss – the restoration of teeth

Assess patient risk for dental caries and non-bacterial tooth surface loss and be able to provide dietary counselling and nutritional education for the patient relevant to oral health and disease, based upon knowledge of disease patterns and aetiology.

Paragraph 3.18 Orthodontics

Recognise abnormalities of facial growth and development in dental patients and arrange appropriate management of such disorders either within the dental practice or by referral to the relevant specialist.

> **Paragraph 2.6** Knowledge and understanding of:
>
> Diseases and disorders of the oral cavity and associated structures, their causes and sequelae together with the principles of their prevention, diagnosis and management.
>
> **Paragraph 2.13** Knowledge and understanding of:
>
> The principles and importance of health promotion, health education and prevention in relation to dental disease, and how these principles are applied.

In addition, the European Academy of Paediatric Dentistry (2002) in their first draft of a 'Golden Standard' for a European Undergraduate teaching programme, emphasize the need for graduates to be competent to:

◆ Initiate and co-operate in organisation and performance of preventive dental care.

◆ Evaluate the effect and cost/value of preventive programmes and methods within dental care for children and adolescents.

and to have knowledge of:

◆ Interpretation of data on caries prevention, interaction of factors in disease.

◆ Estimation of single and combined measures, prediction of future caries development and cost/value of preventive measures.

Intended learning outcomes for prevention and interception

These generic learning outcomes are supported by current undergraduate teaching and directed by specific learning outcomes in a number of subject areas.

The general principles of health promotion and disease prevention are described in Dental public health (Chapter 1.6), which also focuses on health care beliefs and how these vary both between individuals and between communities, based on social, ethnic and environmental factors.

The role of the dental graduate in the prevention of oral cancer, on an individual patient basis as well as from a practice and community perspective, is covered in Oral pathology (Chapter 2.10) and Oral medicine (Chapter 2.9), while the skills and underpinning knowledge required to provide a positive contribution in the health promotion and disease prevention aspects of smoking cessation is covered in Periodontology (Chapter 2.4).

The skills and knowledge required for interception in orthodontics are described in Chapter 2.3, while the diagnostic and planning aspects of preventive non-operative care for the individual patient who presents with dental caries, periodontal diseases and tooth surface loss are covered in Chapters 2.1a, 2.4, and 2.5 respectively.

A graduate dentist should be able to do the following:

Table 1.12.1 Intended learning outcomes for prevention

Be competent at	Have knowledge of	Be familiar with
Diagnosing and planning preventive non-operative care for the individual patient who presents with dental caries, periodontal diseases and tooth wear	The principles of health promotion and disease prevention	The prevalence of certain dental conditions
Diagnosing active caries and planning appropriate non-operative care	The causes and effects of oral disease, needed for their prevention, diagnosis and management	The importance and cost-effectiveness of community-based preventive measures
Oral hygiene instruction, dietary analysis, and fluoride therapy	The design, insertion and adjustment of space maintainers and	The social, cultural and environmental factors which contribute to health or illness
Fissure sealing, preventive resin restorations and pit and fissure restoration	The design, insertion and adjustment of active removable appliances to move a single tooth or correct a crossbite	The complex interactions between oral health, nutrition, general health, drugs and diseases that can have an impact on dental care and disease
A range of clinical procedures which are within a dentist's area of competence, including techniques for preventing and treating oral and dental diseases and disorders	Of the prevention and management of trauma in both dentitions	Principles of recording oral conditions, and the evaluation and interpretation of data
Providing dental health education for patients, parents and carers		
Using laboratory and imaging facilities appropriately and efficiently		
Sharing with patients, or parents and carers, a provisional assessment of their problems and formulating plans for their further investigation and management		

Table 1.12.1 Intended learning outcomes for prevention – *continued*

Be competent at	Have knowledge of	Be familiar with
Applying an evidence-based approach to prevention and treatment		
Initiating and co-operating in the organization and performance of preventive dental care		

Clinical skills

♦ Be competent at diagnosing and planning preventive non-operative care for the individual patient who presents with:

 ▪ dental caries

 ▪ periodontal disease

 ▪ tooth wear.

 Be competent at diagnosing active caries and planning appropriate non-operative care.

Practical procedures

♦ Be competent at oral hygiene instruction, dietary analysis, and topical fluoride therapy.

♦ Be competent at fissure sealing, preventive resin restorations and pit and fissure restoration.

♦ Undertake a range of clinical procedures which are within a dentist's area of competence, including techniques for preventing and treating oral and dental diseases and disorders.

♦ Be competent at providing dental health education for patients, parents and carers.

Patient investigation

♦ Be competent at using laboratory and imaging facilities appropriately and efficiently.

Patient management

♦ Share with patients, provisional assessment of their problems and formulate plans for their further investigation and management.

♦ Have knowledge to manage patients from different social and ethnic backgrounds.

Health promotion and disease prevention

♦ Understand the principles of health promotion and disease prevention.

♦ Be competent in evaluating and applying evidence-based prevention and treatment.

♦ Have knowledge of the organization and provision of health care in the community and in hospital.

- Be familiar with the complex interactions between oral health, nutrition, general health, drugs, and diseases that can have an impact on dental care and disease.
- Be familiar with the prevalence of certain dental conditions.
- Be familiar with the importance and cost-effectiveness of community-based preventive measures.
- Be familiar with the social, cultural and environmental factors which contribute to health or illness.

How the dentist approaches practice

Communication

- Have knowledge to be able to explain and discuss treatments with patients and their parents/carers.

Data and information handling skills

- Be familiar with the principles of recording oral conditions, and the evaluation and interpretation of data.

Understanding of basic and clinical sciences and underlying principles

- Understand the scientific basis of dentistry, including the relevant biomedical sciences, the mechanisms of knowledge acquisition, scientific method and evaluation of evidence.
- Have knowledge of anatomy, physiology and biomedical sciences relevant to dentistry.
- Have knowledge of the aetiology and processes of oral diseases.
- Have knowledge of the causes and effects of oral disease needed for their prevention, diagnosis and management.
- Be familiar with those aspects of biomaterial safety that relate to dentistry.

Appropriate attitudes, ethical understanding and legal responsibilities

- Be competent in initiating and co-operating in the organization and performance of preventive dental care.

Appropriate decision-making, clinical reasoning and judgement

- Be competent in applying an evidence-based approach to prevention and treatment.
- Be familiar with an evidence-based approach to prevention and treatment.

The dentist as a professional

Professional development

- Have knowledge of the permitted activities of DCPs.

Personal development

- Have knowledge of working as part of the dental team.
- Be familiar with the obligation to practise in the best interest of the patient at all times.
- Therefore, with regard to prevention and interception, the graduate is required to have competence in:

1. Diagnosing and planning preventive non-operative care for the individual patient who presents with:
   - ◆ Dental caries (see Chapters 2.1a, 2.5)
   - ◆ Periodontal disease (see Chapter 2.4)
   - ◆ Tooth wear (see Chapter 2.5)

2. Diagnosing active caries and planning appropriate non-operative care (see Chapters 2.1a and 2.5).

3. Oral hygiene instruction, dietary analysis and advice and fluoride therapy.

4. Fissure sealing, preventive resin restorations and pit and fissure restoration (see Chapter 2.1a).

5. A range of clinical procedures which are within a dentist's area of competence, including techniques for preventing and treating oral and dental diseases and disorders (see Chapters 2.1a, 2.3–2.5, 2.7, 2.9, 2.10).

6. Providing dental health education for patients, parents and carers (see Chapters 1.6, 2.1a).

7. Using laboratory and imaging facilities appropriately and efficiently (see Chapter 1.11).

8. Sharing with patients, parents/carers, provisional assessment of their problems and formulating plans for their further investigation and management (see Chapters 1.1, 1.13, 2.1a, 2.2 and 2.3).

9. Applying an evidence-based approach to prevention and treatment (using and having knowledge of) (see Chapter 1.6).

10. Initiating and co-operating in the organization and performance of preventive dental care (see Chapters 1.6 and 2.1a).

The 'pillars of prevention' include dental plaque control, dietary control, appropriate use of fluorides, fissure sealing and regular review. The evidence base for determining appropriate review intervals according to disease risk is outlined in Chapters 1.6 and 2.4 while fissure sealing is considered in Chapter 2.1a.

The core competencies required in oral hygiene instruction, dietary history analysis and advice, and fluoride therapy are each considered below, together with their associated underpinning skills and knowledge.

Oral hygiene instruction
- ◆ The student should be competent in assessing the need for and providing oral hygiene instruction in a child, adolescent and adult.

Dietary history, analysis and advice
There is overwhelming evidence that sugars, in particular, non-milk extrinsic sugars, are the main dietary cause of dental caries. In addition, extrinsic sources of acid in the diet may increase a patient's risk of dental erosion. The student should be competent in assessing a patient's need for dietary advice, obtaining an accurate diet history,

analysing the diet in terms of risk of dental caries and dental erosion as well as its general nutritional features, and providing the patient/parent/carer with dietary advice based on its analysis that is personal, positive and practical.

Fluoride therapy

A sound knowledge of an individual's total exposure to fluoride as well as thorough assessment of their caries risk is key to appropriate fluoride therapy, maximizing the dental health benefits, while minimizing risk.

All sources of systemic (drinks, food, toothpaste, dietary fluoride supplements) and topical fluorides (self-applied and professionally applied) should be included in baseline assessment of need for fluoride therapy.

Underpinning skills for oral hygiene instruction, dietary history, analysis and advice, and fluoride therapy

The student should:

- Be competent in history taking, including medical, dental, family, social and fluoride histories.

- Be competent in dental examination including the use of appropriate indices for recording dental caries, tooth surface loss, gingival and periodontal disease.

- Demonstrate knowledge of behavioural sciences and communication to be able to explain, discuss and manage prevention and treatment with patients, parents/carers from different social and ethnic backgrounds, encouraging them to assume responsibility for their oral health (see Chapters 1.2 and 1.3).

- Have knowledge of team working and the permitted activities of DCPs (see Chapters 2.6 and 3.3). The dentist has a pivotal role in team-leading as well as being an integral team member and need to be able to direct and utilize the skills of DCPs appropriately in the provision of preventive and operative dental care.

- Initiate and co-operate in the organisation and performance of preventive dental care, both in the community and on an individual patient basis.

Underpinning knowledge for oral hygiene instruction, dietary history, analysis and advice, and fluoride therapy

- Familiarity with the prevalence of certain dental conditions in all age groups (see Chapter 1.6), as well as the demography of the community in which they practise in terms of age, socio-economic status and ethnicity.

Targeting for primary prevention and developing individual and community-based preventive strategies based on accurate assessment of disease risk is key to oral health promotion. The contributory factors for increased risk of dental caries, periodontal disease and tooth surface loss should be known and used routinely for determining level of risk of disease as part of treatment planning.

- Knowledge of the scientific basis of dentistry includes the aetiology, processes and effects of dental caries, gingival and periodontal diseases needed for their prevention, diagnosis and management. This should include an understanding of:

- the development, structure and functional biology of the dental tissues,
- the principles of microbial ecology and its relationship to dental plaque formation,
- the contribution of dental plaque to caries and periodontal disease and,
- the importance of saliva and the role it plays in maintaining oral health.

It is important that health education messages given to patients and the public are consistent and scientifically correct.

- The complex interactions between oral health, nutrition, general health, drugs and diseases that can have an impact on dental care and disease (see Chapter 1.8). This should include an understanding of:
- the influence of diet and nutritional status on general health,
- the influence of specific nutrients and nutritional status on the dentition's development.
- The principles of health promotion and disease prevention and the social, cultural and environmental factors which contribute to health or illness (see Chapter 1.6). Disease prevention is as pivotal to the graduate's role as treatment and an understanding of the factors which influence a patient's choice and actions is essential if a dentist is going to be effective in helping to reduce inequalities in oral health.
- Organization and provision of health care in the community and in hospital (see Chapter 1.6) including knowledge of current health issues in the community, as well as local and national preventive strategies for dental and general health.
- Appropriate special investigations, including the role of laboratory tests in diagnosis, and the interpretation of their results (see Chapters 1.1, 1.11, 3.3). This should include familiarity with clinical aids to diagnosis of caries and caries risk assessment as well as the knowledge to be able to estimate total fluoride exposure when planning fluoride therapy.
- Using an evidence-based approach to prevention and treatment (see Chapter 1.2).

It is important that clinical decisions are based on a critical appraisal of the scientific evidence. Selection of a preventive technique requires knowledge of its clinical effectiveness, its accessibility and acceptability to those individuals or populations who need it (see Chapters 1.2, 1.6).

- Familiarity with the obligation to practise in the best interest of the patient at all times (see Chapter 1.2). Prevention should be a key contribution to every patient contact.
- The importance and cost-effectiveness of community-based preventive measures (see Chapter 1.6) and the advantages and disadvantages of different modes of delivery; for example, water fluoridation in comparison with individual fluoride therapies.
- Those aspects of biomaterial safety that relate to dentistry (see Chapters 1.4, 1.5, 1.16), including the safe and effective use of materials for the prevention of dental caries (e.g. fissure sealants, toothpastes, professionally applied topical fluorides, self-applied topical fluorides, dietary fluoride supplements) and the prevention of periodontal disease (toothpastes and mouthwashes).

Checklists for skills in prevention and interception
Key clinical skills
Competence in these particular skills would need to be formally assessed. For three of these assessments, sample checklists are provided.

◆ Diagnosing, planning and evaluating preventive, evidence-based non-operative care for an individual patient who presents with active dental caries.

◆ Diagnosing, planning and evaluating preventive, evidence-based non-operative care for an individual patient who presents with periodontal disease.

Checklist 20 **Oral hygiene instruction in a child/adolescent/adult**

Task	Yes	No	N/A
Take histories			
• Medical			
• Dental			
• Family			
• Social			
• Fluoride			
Dental examination			
• Teeth present			
– Caries			
– Toothwear			
• Periodontal condition (BPE)*			
• Malocclusion			
• Soft tissues			
Provide OHI			
• Assess			
• Toothbrush			
• Toothpaste			
• Frequency			
• Technique			
• Additional aids			
Review and monitor			
• Baseline indices			
• Subsequent visits			

BPE: basic periodontal examination

- Diagnosing, planning and evaluating preventive, evidence-based non-operative care for an individual patient who presents with tooth wear.

- Assessing the need for and providing oral hygiene instruction.

- Assessing the need for dietary advice, collecting an accurate dietary history, analysing it and providing appropriate dietary advice based on its analysis (See **Checklist 21**)

- Assessing the need for fluoride therapy based on an evidence-based assessment of risk/benefit, prescribing and providing fluoride therapy (See **Checklist 22**)

- Assessing the need for, (based on an evidence-based assessment of risk/benefit) and providing fissure sealant.

- Using laboratory and imaging facilities appropriately and efficiently.

Checklist 21 **Collection and analysis of diet history and provision of dietary advice for child or adult**

Task	Yes	No	N/A
Take histories			
• Medical			
• Dental			
• Family			
• Social			
• Fluoride			
Dental examination			
• Caries			
• Toothwear			
Collect diet history			
• Issue 3 day diary			
• Confirm 3 day diary			
Analyse diary and derive appropriate dietary recommendations with regard to:			
• Sugars control			
• Acid control			
• General diet			
Communicate dietary recommendations to patient			
Arrange appropriate review/monitoring			

Checklist 22 Assessment of the need for, and provision of, fluoride therapy

Task	Yes	No	N/A
Take histories			
• Medical			
• Dental			
• Family			
• Social			
• Fluoride			
Dental examination			
• Caries			
– DMFT*			
– +/– radiographic			
• Toothwear			
Justify, prescribe and undertake special investigations and interpret results			
Consideration of caries 'risk' status and current exposure to fluoride			
Discussion and explanation of fluoride use with patient /carer			
Discuss use of toothpaste as a topical fluoride therapy			
Prescribe systemic fluoride supplements (if appropriate – mainly for 'at risk' children)			
Provide topical fluoride therapy (if appropriate – mainly for 'at risk' patients)			
Arrange appropriate review and monitoring			

*DMFT: decayed, missing and filled permanent teeth.

References and further reading

Daly B., Watt R. G., Batchelor P. and Treasure E. T. (2002) *Essential Dental Public Health*. Oxford, Oxford University Press. Part 1: Principles of dental public health, and Part 3: Prevention and oral health promotion.

Holt R. D., Nunn J. H., Rock P. and Page J. (1996) British Society of Paediatric Dentistry. A policy document on fluoride dietary supplements and fluoride toothpastes for children. *Int J Paed Dent* 6, 139–42.

Kelly M., Steele J. G., Nuttall N., Bradnock G., Morris J., Nunn J. H., Pine C., Pitts N. Treasure E. T. and White D. (2000) *Adult Dental Health Survey: Oral health in the UK 1998*. Government Statistical Service. London, The Stationery Office.

Kidd E. A. M. and Joyston-Bechal S. (2002) *Essentials of dental caries*, 2nd edn. Oxford, Oxford University Press. Chapter 8, Prevention of caries by plaque control, Chapter 6, Dietary history taking, analysis and advice, and Chapter 9, Patient motivation.

Marthaler T. M. *et al.* (2004) Changes in dental caries 1953–2003. *Caries Research* **38**(3), 173–81.

Murray J. J., Nunn J. H. and Steele J. G. (2003) *Prevention of Oral Disease*, 4th edn. Oxford, Oxford University Press. See Chapter 8, Prevention of periodontal disease, Chapter 7, Toothwear: aetiology, prevention, clinical implications, and Chapter 3, Fluoride and dental caries.

Nunn J., Crawford P. J., Page J. and Winter G. (1997) Dental needs of children. *Int J Paed Dent 7*, 203–7.

Office of National Statistics (2003) *UK Children's Dental Health Survey 2003*. Available at http://www.statistics.gov.uk/downloads/theme_health/Executive_Summary-CDH.PDF Accessed 6 June 2005.

Rugg-Gunn A. J. (1992) Sugars and dental health in children. *Int J Paed Dent 2*, 177–80.

Rugg-Gunn A. J. and Nunn J. H. (2003) *Nutrition, Diet and Oral Health*. Oxford, Oxford University Press. See Chapter 4, Diet and dental erosion, and Chapter 10, Dietary advice in the dental surgery.

Scottish Intercollegiate Guidelines Network (SIGN) (2000) *Preventing Dental Caries in Children at High Caries Risk*, Number 47, December. Edinburgh, Royal College of Physicians.

Shaw L. British Society of Paediatric Dentistry (1997) UK National Clinical Guidelines in Paediatric Dentistry. Prevention of dental caries in children. *Int J Paed Dent 7*, 267–72.

Shaw L. and O'Sullivan E. (2000) British Society of Paediatric Dentistry. UK National Clinical Guidelines in Paediatric Dentistry. Diagnosis and prevention of dental erosion in children. *Int J Paed Dent 10*, 356–65.

Welbury R. R., Duggal M. S. and Hosey M. T. (2005) *Paediatric Dentistry*, 3rd edn. Oxford, Oxford University Press. See Chapter 3, History, examination, risk assessment and treatment planning, and Chapter 6, Diagnosis and prevention of dental caries.

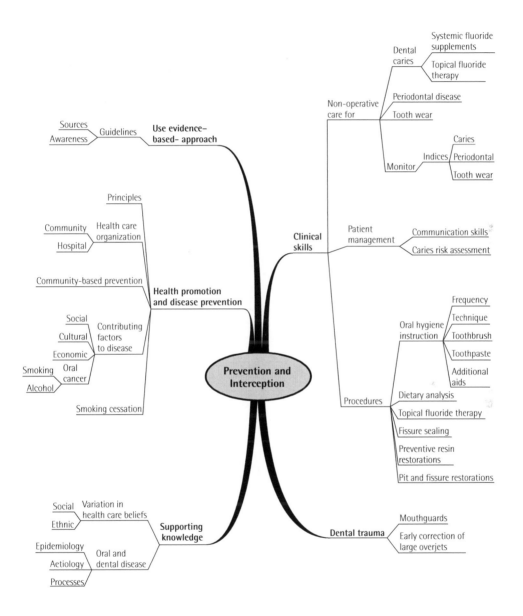

Use evidence-based-approach
- Guidelines
  - Sources
  - Awareness

Health promotion and disease prevention
- Principles
- Health care organization
  - Community
  - Hospital
- Community-based prevention
- Contributing factors to disease
  - Social
  - Cultural
  - Economic
  - Oral cancer
    - Smoking
    - Alcohol
- Smoking cessation

Supporting knowledge
- Variation in health care beliefs
  - Social
  - Ethnic
- Oral and dental disease
  - Epidemiology
  - Aetiology
  - Processes

Prevention and Interception

Clinical skills
- Non-operative care for
  - Dental caries
    - Systemic fluoride supplements
    - Topical fluoride therapy
  - Periodontal disease
  - Tooth wear
  - Monitor
    - Indices
      - Caries
      - Periodontal
      - Tooth wear
- Patient management
  - Communication skills
  - Caries risk assessment
- Procedures
  - Oral hygiene instruction
    - Frequency
    - Technique
    - Toothbrush
    - Toothpaste
    - Additional aids
  - Dietary analysis
  - Topical fluoride therapy
  - Fissure sealing
  - Preventive resin restorations
  - Pit and fissure restorations

Dental trauma
- Mouthguards
- Early correction of large overjets

1.13 Patient Referral
Peter Mossey

Key points

+ Referral of patients from primary care to secondary care is an indispensable part of clinical practice.
+ Examination/diagnostic skills, underpinning knowledge, clinical judgement, self-awareness and recognition of own limitations are implied underpinning skills.
+ A competent letter of referral requires an ability to communicate effectively and appropriately by the written word.

Introduction

Among the aims of undergraduate dental education both the General Dental Council and the Quality Assurance Agency recognize that referral of patients to colleagues in the dental profession is an integral part of clinical practice.

This is likely to become more commonplace with increasing emphasis on specialism, increased public awareness of what services and alternatives are available and increasingly specialized equipment and expertise are required. Referral is also a quality of care issue, and appropriate referral requires a range of professional, knowledge and attitudinal skills.

Under 'The aim of undergraduate dental education' the *First Five Years* (GDC 2002) states that:

> The undergraduate dental curriculum must allow students to acquire the clinical understanding in competence to practise without supervision, on graduation and at the same time to allow them to be aware of their limitations and need to refer for specialist advice.
>
> **GDC (2002, paragraph 17)**

> The dental graduate must be able to communicate effectively with patients, their families and associates and with other health professionals involved in their care.
>
> **GDC (2002, paragraph 19)**

It is essential that graduating dentists understand the limitations of their current knowledge and clinical abilities. They should be aware of the range of treatments available, and of the current evidence to support their choices, but not be expected to be able to provide them all. In such circumstances they must be able to refer for an opinion on treatment and management by a suitably experienced/qualified individual.

QAA (2002, paragraph 1.6)

Furthermore among the transferable skills outlined, the same document states that the graduating dentist should have the ability to communicate effectively at all levels in both scientific and professional contexts using verbal, non-verbal and written means.

QAA (2002, paragraph 3.1)

Intended learning outcomes

Exposure to integrated oral care units, outreach, outpatient medical and dental departments and ward-based referrals allows undergraduates to gain insight into a process and build on their knowledge until they become fully competent to make their own referrals.

The essential components of a competent referral

Letter from a general dental practitioner in primary care to a colleague in secondary care or in specialist practice should include the following:

1. Referrer's details – the information should include name of referring dentist:

   ◆ Address (essential)

   ◆ Telephone number (desirable)

   ◆ Email address (optional)

2. Name of the person to whom you are referring the patient. This may be a specific person, or a department in secondary care without specifying the individual.

3. Patient's details must include name, address, telephone number and date of birth.

4. Presenting complaint: it is important to record the patient's own perception of the problem for which they are being referred. On occasion, views of a parent, guardian, older sibling or partner may be sought to obtain an accurate assessment of how the patient perceives the problem for which they are being referred.

5. Medical history: comment on whether there is any relevant medical history and whether or not the patient is on any drugs or medication. If so, this should be elaborated upon. Those aspects that are important for the general welfare of the patient or that may have an impact on the dental treatment should be specifically mentioned. Women of reproductive age should be asked if they might be pregnant,

Table 1.13.1 Intended learning outcomes for referral

Be competent at	Have knowledge of	Be familiar with
Making and accepting referrals to and from colleagues	Systemic conditions that require appropriate referral for dental treatment	Complex cases that require referral with recognition of personal limitations)
Responding to a referral letter, fax, e-mail, telephone call, and grade the degree of urgency	Reasons for referral to specialist, hospital dental practitioner	
Writing a referral letter to a colleague with demographic data, reason for referral, relevant background information including dental, medical and social information		

and if not whether they are using contraceptive measures. Other relatively common instances include allergies, diabetes, congenital heart problems or infective endocarditis (requiring antibiotic cover for invasive dental treatment), and whether consultation with the patient's medical practitioner would be advisable.

6. Dental history: in all disciplines, oral hygiene status, caries experience, teeth of doubtful prognosis and any areas of hypoplasia or decalcification will be relevant. In the dental history it may also be relevant to record previous exposure to anaesthesia and radiography. The frequency of attendance and any concerns you may have about patient attitude, motivation or compliance based on your own experience of the patient in the past.

7. Social history: should record patient's social habits that may impact on dental health such as smoking, alcohol consumption (particularly if it is felt that this may be excessive), other siblings and ability to attend. For example, orthodontic treatment requires regular attendance over a prolonged time period and the level of parental support and ability to attend should be recorded. It may also be useful to advise if the patient can attend at short notice.

8. Family history may also be included, particularly if the condition for whom the patient is being referred may have a familial or genetic contribution. Examples of common conditions that may have some genetic contribution are malocclusion, periodontal disease, hypodontia, rarer conditions with a genetic contribution such as cleft lip and/or palate or hereditary gingival fibromatosis and even more rare

single gene disorders such as dentinogenesis imperfecta, amelogenesis imperfecta, and cleidocranial dysostosis.

9. Reason for referral: provide appropriate detail on your examination, diagnosis, severity and differential diagnosis (if appropriate). Also describe the condition, perceived problem or aspect of treatment for which the patient is being referred. The oral soft tissues should also be examined and anything unusual reported and well known indices such as DMF, plaque and gingival indices might be noted.

10. Specify whether advice only is being sought or if the reason for referral is to have treatment carried out in secondary care. It is helpful to indicate what aspects of the treatment you might be willing to do, e.g. extractions or restorative treatment that is within the scope of your own skills. There may be positive advantages to doing so such as avoiding a treatment waiting list.

11. Enclosures: any previous records may be extremely helpful in the diagnosis and treatment planning related to the presenting complaint. It is also regarded as unethical clinical practice to repeat invasive procedures or records. The type of record will depend on the nature of the referral but radiographs, study models, photographs or, on occasion, previous appliances, dentures or components of treatment. The referral letter should be signed and if the signature is illegible or difficult to interpret, a stamp can be used or the name may be printed in bold underneath.

Checklist 23 **Letter of referral**

Marking scheme	Yes	No	Not relevant
Date of referral			
GDP details (name, address and phone number)			
Name, address and DOB of patient			
Reason for referral (advice and/or treatment requested)			
Key details of clinical problem			
Medical history and drugs			
Dental history			
Relevant social and family history			
Indication of urgency of referral			
Radiograph or other supporting documentation enclosed			
Signature and printed name of referring practitioner			
Letter reasonably clear and legible			

12. Abbreviations and jargon: while jargon and abbreviations should generally be avoided or explained, it is acceptable to use jargon or abbreviations that would reasonably be expected in the repertoire of the specialist to whom the referral is addressed.

Hospital practitioners, specialist practitioners or those who limit their practise to particular aspects of dental care such as oral surgery, endodontics, orthodontics or implantology may receive referrals from colleagues in primary care. Upon receipt of such referrals they should respond to acknowledge receipt, and also to provide feedback on how their patient is to be managed, or to provide the advice or assistance requested. This reply will vary according to the nature of the referral received. For further information on specialty specific referrals, references such as White *et al.* (2004) concerning referral for oral cancer and Djemal *et al.* (2004) for restorative dentistry are useful. Details of these is beyond the scope of this chapter.

References and further reading

Djemal S., Chia M. and Ubaya-Narayange T. (2004) Quality improvement of referrals to a department of restorative dentistry following the use of a referral proforma by referring dental practitioners. *Br Dent J* 197(2), 85–8.

GDC (2002) *The First Five Years: a framework for undergraduate dental education,* 2nd edn. London, The General Dental Council.

QAA (2002) *Dentistry: academic standards.* Subject benchmark statements. Gloucester, Quality Assurance Agency for Higher Education.

White D. A., Morris A. J., Burgess L., Hamburger J. and Hamburger R. (2004) Facilitators and barriers to improving the quality of referrals for potential oral cancer. *Br Dent J* 197(9), 537–40.

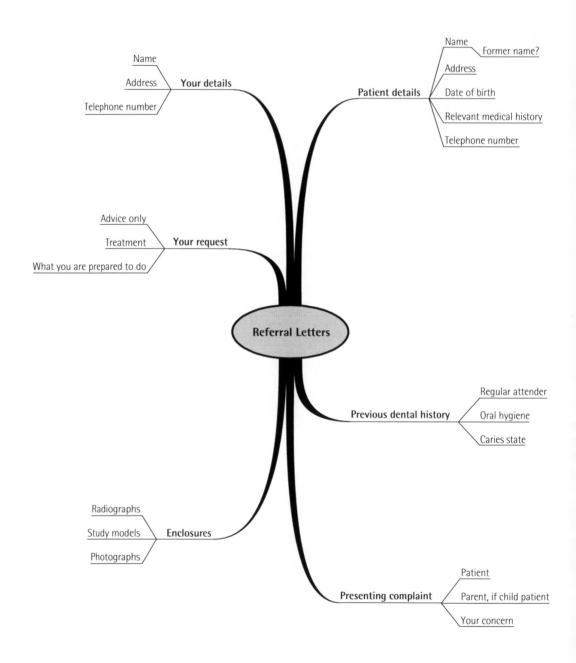

Name

Address   **Your details**

Telephone number

Name

Former name?

Address

Patient details   Date of birth

Relevant medical history

Telephone number

Advice only

Treatment   **Your request**

What you are prepared to do

Referral Letters

Regular attender

Previous dental history   Oral hygiene

Caries state

Radiographs

Study models   **Enclosures**

Photographs

Patient

Presenting complaint   Parent, if child patient

Your concern

1.14 Isolation and moisture control

Francis Burke

Key points

- Isolation and moisture control are desirable for many restorative procedures.
- Isolation and moisture control can enhance patient comfort and protection.
- For most restorative procedures the use of a rubber dam is the most appropriate means of isolation.
- Effective isolation and moisture control is best achieved using four-handed dentistry.

Introduction

During operative care copious amounts of fluid can accumulate in the patient's mouth. These fluids can come from handpieces and the three-in-one syringe. Furthermore there can be increased levels of saliva as well as gingival exudate and even blood. Such accumulation of fluids can be uncomfortable for the patient and obscure the operating site. Moisture contamination can have an effect on the quality of adhesive restorations (Summitt 2001). A lack of appropriate isolation can not only lead to potential contamination of the root canal system in endodontic therapy but can also heighten the medico-legal exposure of the operator.

In 2003 the Dental Practice Board for England and Wales reported that 6.3 million adhesive restorations were placed, as well as one million courses of endodontic treatment. Therefore the ability to carry out appropriate isolation and moisture control is likely to play an essential role in the undergraduate curriculum. Provision of such care will also need to encompass an understanding of behaviour management (Chapter 1.10), infection control (Chapter 1.5), law and ethics (Chapter 1.2), dental materials (Chapter 1.16), endodontics (Chapter 2.6), paediatric dentistry (Chapter 2.1) and restorative dentistry (Chapter 2.5).

Provision of adequate isolation involves working as part of a dental team and such activity is outlined in the General Dental Council's *The First Five Years: a framework for dental undergraduate education* (GDC 2002):

> **Paragraph 37** Dental students must learn the principles and practice of assisted-operating dentistry, which is the normal method used in clinical practice to ensure safety and provision of high quality care for patients.
>
> **Paragraph 88** For the provision of comprehensive oral care dental students should have the opportunity to work with all members of the dental team. They should appreciate the benefit of working with a dental nurse and learn the principles and practice of assisted operating practice.

Appropriate moisture control and isolation have been considered by the Subject Benchmark for Dentistry (QAA 2002) which says that the undergraduate should:

> **Paragraph 2.11** Demonstrate interpersonal skills appropriate for working within a multi-skilled team.
>
> **Paragraph 2.14** Demonstrate the safe and effective management of patients.
>
> **Paragraph 3.23** Implement and perform satisfactory infection control and prevent physical, chemical or microbiological contamination in the practice of dentistry.

Intended learning outcomes

Table 1.14.1 summarizes the intended learning outcomes for isolation and moisture control, incorporating those outlined in *The First Five Years* (GDC 2002) and recommendations from the European Society of Endodontology (2001).

Reasons to undertake isolation and moisture control procedures

Isolation and moisture control

While carrying out an operative or endodontic procedure the undergraduate should obtain the optimum isolation and moisture control. This will facilitate patient comfort, protection and delivery of treatment.

The undergraduate should demonstrate knowledge of the rationale for isolation and moisture control. This should include:

+ enhance patient comfort, relaxation and acceptance;
+ reduce the risk of cross-infection between the patient and the dental team;
+ retraction of the soft tissues during operative procedures;
+ protection of the soft tissues during operative procedures;
+ minimize moisture contamination from saliva, gingival crevicular fluid water or blood of the operative site;

Table 1.14.1 Intended learning outcomes for isolation and moisture control

Be competent at	Have knowledge of	Be familiar with
Choosing the most appropriate isolation technique for a specific clinical situation	Reasons for isolation and moisture control	Recognition and management of latex allergy
Explaining to a patient the rationale of rubber dam isolation and communicate with them during the procedure	Consequences of inadequate isolation	
Working as a dental team in carrying out isolation	Different isolation techniques	
Using a rubber dam for the isolation of teeth	Circumstances when different isolation techniques could be used	
Modifying rubber dam isolation for specific circumstances		
Using isolation techniques other than a rubber dam for moisture control		

+ facilitate visualization of the operative site;

+ increase operator efficiency;

+ reduce the potential for the inhalation/ingestion of debris, restorations or instruments during operative procedures;

+ minimize salivary contamination during direct and indirect pulp capping.

Adhesive restorations

In the provision of adhesive dentistry, especially in the surface treatment of enamel, the critical phase is the preservation of the etched surface of enamel from contamination, in particular from moisture. This applies to a variety of adhesive procedures including the placement of fissure sealants, composites, veneers, or resin-bonded bridges.

The undergraduate should demonstrate an understanding of the rationale for isolation and moisture control for adhesive restorations, including:

+ minimize moisture contamination of the operative site;

+ preservation of the etch pattern;

◆ increase bond strength of adhesive materials to enamel (Summitt 2001);

◆ minimize microleakage of adhesive materials to enamel.

Endodontics

Endodontic therapy for the deciduous and permanent dentitions places a particular onus on the operator to provide isolation to ensure patient safety and facilitate the optimum delivery of treatment.

The undergraduate should have a detailed knowledge of the principles and practice of the use of the rubber dam in endodontic therapy (European Society of Endodontology 2001). This should include knowledge of the rationale for the use of the rubber dam in endodontic therapy including;

◆ the acceptability of its use by patients (Stewardson and McHugh 2002);

◆ isolation of the endodontic site;

◆ retraction of the soft tissues;

◆ protection of the soft tissues;

◆ enhance vision of endodontic site;

◆ minimize microbial contamination of the pulp chamber and canal;

◆ minimize moisture contamination of the pulp chamber and canal;

◆ reduce the potential for inhalation/ingestion of endodontic instruments;

◆ reduce the potential for inhalation/ingestion of endodontic irrigants.

Consequences of inadequate isolation and moisture control

A lack of isolation or moisture control may have deleterious consequences for both the patient and operator. While some of the consequences may appear immediately some may manifest themselves in the long term.

The undergraduate should demonstrate knowledge of the consequences of inadequate isolation and moisture control. Such consequences would include:

◆ trauma to the soft tissues;

◆ moisture contamination of the operative site;

◆ reduced adhesion and increased microleakage of adhesive materials;

◆ inhalation/ingestion of oral debris;

◆ contamination of the root canal system;

◆ inhalation/ingestion of endodontic instruments/irrigants;

◆ increased operator fatigue and difficulty in executing operative and endodontic procedures.

Isolation techniques

There are a range of materials and techniques available for isolation and moisture control.

The undergraduate should demonstrate knowledge of the range of isolation materials and techniques available, including their properties and the clinical circumstances under which they are used, and they should also demonstrate an ability to carry out the following isolation techniques:

◆ rubber dam

◆ cotton wool

◆ gauze

◆ cellulose pads

◆ suction.

Rubber dam

The rubber dam for isolation and moisture control was developed by Dr Barnum in 1864. It is essentially a sheet of rubber used to isolate the teeth. The efficient placement, use and removal of rubber dam are greatly enhanced by the application of four-handed dentistry working as a team with a dental nurse.

The undergraduate should demonstrate knowledge of the following:

◆ rationale for the application of rubber dam;

◆ factors in a medical history indicative of latex allergy;

◆ in cases of latex allergy alternatives to latex for rubber dam isolation;

◆ rationale for colour contrast between rubber dam and oral tissues;

◆ differences in thickness of rubber dam and their use;

◆ ideal features of a rubber dam clamp;

◆ relative merits of winged and wingless rubber dam clamps;

◆ disadvantages of rubber dam application including:

   ■ potential latex allergy (European Society of Endodontology 2001);

   ■ reduced patient to dentist communication;

   ■ some patients may dislike rubber dam;

   ■ may be time-consuming to place and remove;

   ■ clamped tooth may be uncomfortable subsequently;

   ■ loss of orientation for endodontic access cavity preparation when a single tooth is isolated with rubber dam;

   ■ modification of radiographic technique during endodontic therapy when the rubber dam is *in situ;*

- alteration in tooth colour when dried under rubber dam.

The undergraduate should demonstrate ability to:

◆ utilize alternatives to latex for rubber dam isolation in cases of latex allergy;

◆ select the shade for an adhesive restoration prior to rubber dam application;

◆ explain to a patient the rationale of rubber dam isolation;

◆ apply appropriate anaesthesia prior to rubber dam application;

◆ identify and explain the functions of the different components of a rubber dam kit including sheets of rubber dam, rubber dam stamp, rubber dam punch, rubber dam lubricant (water-based), rubber dam clamp forceps, the different types of clamp and the teeth to which they are applied, dental floss, gauze napkin and the rubber dam frame;

◆ distinguish between winged and wingless rubber dam clamps;

◆ select an appropriate rubber dam clamp for a specific clinical situation;

◆ apply appropriate safety procedures during rubber dam isolation;

◆ apply a rubber clamp to a tooth;

◆ assess the fit of a rubber dam clamp;

◆ apply a rubber dam to isolate an appropriate number of teeth to ensure adequate isolation and access;

◆ communicate with a patient the during the isolation procedure;

◆ work with other members of the dental team during rubber dam isolation;

◆ evaluate the fit of a rubber dam in the patient's mouth;

◆ place a matrix band on a tooth which has been clamped;

◆ remove a rubber dam safely.

The undergraduate should demonstrate a familiarity with:

◆ recognition and management of latex allergy.

Rubber dam modification

Conventional rubber dam application is a straightforward procedure. This occurs when the patient has what could be described as a regular dentition. However there are situations when modification of rubber dam technique is required. The undergraduate should demonstrate an understanding of the circumstances of when it is appropriate to modify the rubber dam application technique. Such circumstances would include application of rubber dam for:

◆ missing teeth;

◆ children, especially in the mixed dentition;

◆ insufficient tooth structure for a clamp;

- inadequate tooth structure for clamping;
- gross proximal overhangs;
- gross calculus deposits;
- tooth build-up prior to isolation;
- abutment teeth for rubber dam with ceramic crowns or veneers;
- fixed prostheses;
- roots;
- tilted teeth;
- loss of orientation for endodontic access cavity preparation when a single tooth is isolated with rubber dam;
- modification in radiographic technique during endodontic treatment of a clamped tooth.

The undergraduate should demonstrate an ability to apply rubber dam under the following clinical circumstances when it is appropriate for technique modification including:

- missing teeth;
- children, especially in the mixed dentition;
- tooth build-up prior to isolation where possible;
- removal of calculus deposits;
- removal of overhangs;
- abutment teeth for rubber dam with ceramic crowns or veneers;
- fixed prostheses;
- roots;
- tilted teeth;
- possible access cavity preparation prior to rubber dam application;
- modification of radiographic technique during endodontic treatment of a clamped tooth.

Other isolation techniques

There are circumstances when it is not reasonable or possible to apply rubber dam. The undergraduate should demonstrate knowledge of when it is appropriate to use other isolation techniques or carry out treatment prior to rubber dam application. Such circumstances would include:

- latex allergy;
- gag reflex;

- insufficient tooth structure for clamp;
- inadequate tooth structure for clamping;
- fitting an indirect restoration such as a post and core or crown.

Demonstrate an ability to use other isolation techniques including:
- latex-free rubber dam;
- cotton wool rolls;
- cellulose pads;
- gauze;
- suction;
- work with other members of the dental team during isolation and moisture control.

Checklist 24 **Placement of rubber dam**

Task	Yes	No
Appropriate choice of clamp		
Floss applied to clamp		
Contacts flossed		
Appropriate lubricant applied to dam		
Clamp application		
Appropriate number of teeth isolated		
Gauze placed		
Rubber dam frame placed		
Everted dam around teeth		
Removed dam completely and safely		

References and further reading

Dental Practice Board (2003) http://www.dpb.nhs.uk/download/digest/digest_2003.pdf

European Society of Endodontology (2001) Undergraduate Curriculum Guidelines for Endodontology. *International Endodontic Journal* 34, 574–80.

GDC (2002) *The First Five Years: a framework for undergraduate dental education*, 2nd edn. London, The General Dental Council.

QAA (2002) *Dentistry: academic standards*. Subject benchmark statements. Gloucester; Quality Assurance Agency for Higher Education.

Stewardson D. A. and McHugh E. S. (2002) Patients' attitude to rubber dam. *International Endodontic Journal* 35, 812–19.

Summitt J. B. (2001) Field isolation. In J. B. Summitt, J. W. Robbins and R. S. Schwartz (eds) *Fundamentals of Operative Dentistry: a contemporary approach*, 2nd edn, pp. 149–77. Chicago, Quintessence Books.

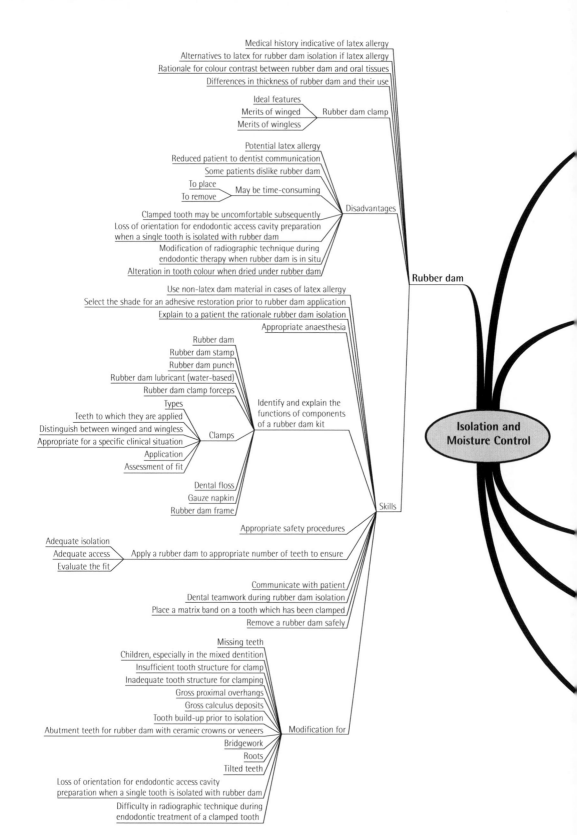

Isolation and Moisture Control

Rubber dam

Medical history indicative of latex allergy
Alternatives to latex for rubber dam isolation if latex allergy
Rationale for colour contrast between rubber dam and oral tissues
Differences in thickness of rubber dam and their use

Rubber dam clamp
Ideal features
Merits of winged
Merits of wingless

Disadvantages
Potential latex allergy
Reduced patient to dentist communication
Some patients dislike rubber dam
May be time-consuming
To place
To remove
Clamped tooth may be uncomfortable subsequently
Loss of orientation for endodontic access cavity preparation when a single tooth is isolated with rubber dam
Modification of radiographic technique during endodontic therapy when rubber dam is in situ
Alteration in tooth colour when dried under rubber dam

Skills
Use non-latex dam material in cases of latex allergy
Select the shade for an adhesive restoration prior to rubber dam application
Explain to a patient the rationale rubber dam isolation
Appropriate anaesthesia

Identify and explain the functions of components of a rubber dam kit
Rubber dam
Rubber dam stamp
Rubber dam punch
Rubber dam lubricant (water-based)
Rubber dam clamp forceps
Clamps
Types
Teeth to which they are applied
Distinguish between winged and wingless
Appropriate for a specific clinical situation
Application
Assessment of fit
Dental floss
Gauze napkin
Rubber dam frame

Appropriate safety procedures
Apply a rubber dam to appropriate number of teeth to ensure
Adequate isolation
Adequate access
Evaluate the fit

Communicate with patient
Dental teamwork during rubber dam isolation
Place a matrix band on a tooth which has been clamped
Remove a rubber dam safely

Modification for
Missing teeth
Children, especially in the mixed dentition
Insufficient tooth structure for clamp
Inadequate tooth structure for clamping
Gross proximal overhangs
Gross calculus deposits
Tooth build-up prior to isolation
Abutment teeth for rubber dam with ceramic crowns or veneers
Bridgework
Roots
Tilted teeth
Loss of orientation for endodontic access cavity preparation when a single tooth is isolated with rubber dam
Difficulty in radiographic technique during endodontic treatment of a clamped tooth

Consequences of inadequate isolation and moisture control
- Trauma to the soft tissue
- Moisture contamination of the operative site
- Reduced adhesion and increased microleakage of adhesive materials
- Inhalation/ingestion of oral debris
- Contamination of the root canal system
- Inhalation/ingestion of endodntic instruments/irrigants
- Increased operator fatigue and difficulty

General indications
- Enhance patient comfort, relaxation and acceptance
- Reduce the risk of cross infection from patient to the dental team
- Retraction of the soft tissues during operative procedures
- Protection of the soft tissues during operative procedures
- Minimize moisture contamination from saliva, gingival crevicular fluid, water or blood of the operative site
- Facilitate visualization of the operative site
- Increase operator efficiency
- Reduce the potential for the inhalation/ingestion of
  - Debris
  - Restorations
  - Instruments
  - Endodontic irrigants
- Minimize salivary contamination during direct and indirect pulp capping

Additional indications for adhesive restorations
- Preservation of the etch pattern
- Increase bond strength of adhesive materials to enamel
- Minimize microleakage of adhesive materials to enamel

Additional indications for endodontics
- Isolation of the endodontic site
- Enhance vision of endodontic site
- Minimize contamination of the pulp chamber and canal
  - Moisture
  - Microbial

Other isolation techniques
- Cotton wool
- Suction
- Cellulose pads
- Gauze
- Indications for other techniques
  - Latex allergy
  - Gag reflex
  - Insufficient/or inadequate tooth structure for clamp
  - Fitting an indirect restoration
    - Post and core
    - Crown

1.15 Impression-making
General and special circumstances
Francis Burke

Key points

+ Appropriate and precise impression-making is essential for accurate diagnosis and provision of treatment.
+ The selection and handling of impression materials is based on sound knowledge of their composition and physical properties.
+ Precise communication with dental technicians is necessary for optimal results in the provision of care.

Introduction

An impression is a 'negative likeness or copy in reverse of the surface of an object; an imprint of the teeth and adjacent structures for use in dentistry' (Journal of Prosthetic Dentistry 1999). From this negative likeness a cast is made which can be used in the planning and/or provision of care.

In 2003 the Dental Practice Board for England and Wales reported that 1.7 million units of crown and bridge work were placed as well as one million dentures and 470,000 courses of orthodontic treatment. For all of these procedures as well as for diagnostic reasons impressions were necessary (DPB 2003).

The ability to carry out appropriate impression-making is likely to continue to play an essential role in the undergraduate curriculum. Provision of such care will also need to encompass an understanding of behaviour management (Chapter 1.10), infection control (Chapter 1.5), law and ethics (Chapter 1.2), dental materials (Chapter 1.16), removable prostheses (Chapter 2.7), and restorative dentistry (Chapter 2.5).

An understanding of the properties of impression materials prior to and during their use are outlined in the General Dental Council's *The First Five Years: a framework for dental undergraduate education* (GDC 2002):

Paragraph 79 Instruction in the properties, correct manipulation and the science underpinning the correct use of dental materials is needed to equip the student with the knowledge to select and handle those materials safely and effectively. Dental students need to understand how such materials, and the biological response to them, are evaluated.

Intended learning outcomes

Table 1.15.1 summarizes the intended learning outcomes for impression-making, incorporating those outlined in *The First Five Years* (GDC 2002) and recommendations from the British Society for Restorative Dentistry (1999).

Table 1.15.1 Intended learning outcomes for impression-making

Be competent at	Have knowledge of	Be familiar with
Choosing the most appropriate impression material for a specific clinical situation	Reasons for making impressions	Developments in impression techniques
	Properties of impression materials	
Choosing and modifying appropriately an impression tray	Appropriate characteristics of an impression tray	
Explaining to a patient the rationale for an impression-making and communicating with them during the procedure		
Carrying the process of making an impression		
Critically evaluating the quality of an impression		
Disinfecting impressions appropriately		
Prescribing laboratory work		

Specific skills in impression-making

Reasons to make impressions

The undergraduate should demonstrate knowledge of the rationale for making impressions. This should include:

1. Study models that can be used to:
   - Educate the patient
   - Monitor tooth wear
   - Monitor tooth position
   - Prepare pre-orthodontic records
   - Construct post-orthodontic records
   - Plan provision of fixed or removable prostheses including influence of opposing arch
   - Trial wax-up
   - Trial tooth preparation
   - Evaluate tooth preparation.

2. Primary or secondary models fabricated for:
   - Splint
   - Special tray
   - Pull down for temporization
   - Stent fabrication prior to implant placement.

3. Prostheses including:
   - Partial coverage restorations such as inlays or onlays
   - Crowns
   - Bridges
   - Primary partial denture impression
   - Master partial denture impression
   - Primary full denture impression
   - Master full denture impression
   - Additions to dentures
   - Denture repair.

4. Temporary prostheses:
   - Temporary crown
   - Temporary bridge.

Properties of impression materials

The undergraduate should demonstrate knowledge of the characteristics of the ideal impression material.

Such properties would include:

- Biocompatibility;
- Working time – the period of time that it is possible to manipulate the impression material without an adverse effect on its properties;
- Setting time – the period of time measured from the start of mixing the impression material until it has set;
- Record detail;
- Mucocompressive, mucostatic, dimensionable stability;
- Permanent deformation;
- Stress relaxation;
- Tear strength;
- Elasticity;
- Sterilizable/disinfectable;
- Pouring time;
- Wettability;
- Compatibility with gypsum model materials;
- Hydrophilic;
- Ease of manipulation;
- Compatible taste;
- Unaffected by latex.

Impression materials

The undergraduate should demonstrate knowledge of the range of impression materials available including their properties, the difference between elastic and non-elastic materials, the functions of the different viscosities of materials including light, medium, heavy and putty consistencies and the clinical circumstances under which they are used.

The materials under consideration should include:

- Alginate
- Agar
- Zinc oxide and eugenol
- Impression compound
- Polysulphide

- Polysilicone, condensation and addition
- Polyether
- Plaster of Paris
- Wax
- Acrylic
- Gutta percha.

The undergraduate should demonstrate an ability to prepare, dispense and use the following impression materials:

- Alginate
- Zinc oxide and eugenol
- Impression compound
- Polysulphide
- Polysilicone, condensation and addition
- Polyether
- Plaster of Paris
- Wax.

Impression trays

The undergraduate should demonstrate knowledge of the British Society for Restorative Dentistry (1999) guidelines concerning the:

- Rationale for the selection of a specific tray type;
- Relative merits of stock trays and special trays;
- Design features for a special tray;
- Ideal features of a stock impression tray;
- Rationale for the application of an adhesive to the impression tray.
  The undergraduate should also demonstrate the ability to:
- Fabricate a special tray for a dentate patient incorporating spacing, occlusal stops and an appropriate handle;
- Fabricate a special tray for an edentulous patient incorporating an appropriate handle;
- Evaluate the fit of a tray in the patient's mouth;
- Modify an edentulous special tray with greenstick;
- Apply adhesive to the tray at the appropriate time.

Soft tissue management and moisture control

The undergraduate should demonstrate knowledge of the:

+ Relevance of gingival health prior to impression-making in the dentate patient;
+ Relevance of soft tissue health prior to impression-making in an edentulous patient;
+ Influence of moisture on impression accuracy;
+ Techniques available for moisture control;
+ Techniques available for gingival retraction;
+ Properties of gingival retraction cord and associated chemicals;
+ Effect of gingival retraction techniques on gingival health.

The undergraduate should demonstrate ability to:

+ Obtain optimal gingival health prior to impression-making in a dentate patient;
+ Obtain optimum soft tissue health prior to impression-making in an edentulous patient;
+ Control moisture during impression-making;
+ Retract the gingiva appropriately during impression-making.

The undergraduate should demonstrate a familiarity with:

+ The principles of electrosurgery including aspects of health and safety.

Impression techniques

The undergraduate should demonstrate knowledge of the:

+ Circumstances of when it is appropriate to make a mucostatic impression;
+ Circumstances of when it is appropriate to make a mucocompressive impression;
+ Technique and limitations of the putty and wash impression technique.

The undergraduate should demonstrate ability to:

+ Make a mucostatic impression;
+ Make a mucocompressive impression;
+ Communicate to a patient the rationale for impression-making and use appropriate communication techniques during the impression procedure.

The undergraduate should demonstrate a familiarity with:

+ The principles of copper ring impressions;
+ Impression techniques for the direct provision of restorations such as a direct wax impression for an inlay or an acrylic impression for a post and core.

Occlusal registration

The undergraduate should demonstrate knowledge of the:

- Rationale for occlusal registration;
- Different positions of the mandible which can be used during occlusal registration;
- Materials used to make an occlusal record;
- Rationale for a facebow record;
- Principles of articulator use;
- Differing types of articulator.

    The undergraduate should demonstrate ability to:

- Make an occlusal registration;
- Make a facebow record;
- Mount casts on an articulator using a facebow and occlusal registration.

Evaluation of impressions

The undergraduate should demonstrate ability to:

- Carry out appropriate care for the patient on removal of the impression from their mouth;
- Clean the impression appropriately of oral fluids;
- Critically evaluate the impression for the presence of the relevant intra-oral structures and tooth preparation features where appropriate;
- Identify defects in the impression, be aware of their cause and rectify them appropriately prior to remaking the impression (Wassell *et al.* 2002).

Shade selection

The undergraduate should demonstrate knowledge of the:

- Influence of hue, chroma and value on shade selection;
- Influence of factors including patient age, make-up, ambient lighting, tooth hydration, tooth staining and operator fatigue on shade selection;
- Rationale for determining different shades for different portions of the tooth including incisal, body and cervical shades;
- Relationship between the degree of tooth reduction and the resultant shade for ceramic restorations;
- Relationship between face shape and size and the selection of denture teeth.

    The undergraduate should demonstrate ability to:

- Select the most appropriate shade for a crown, veneer, bridge abutment or denture;

- Select the most appropriate mould and size for denture teeth;
- Provide a prescription for tooth and shade selection for a dental technician.

Disinfection

The undergraduate should demonstrate knowledge of the:

- Rationale for disinfection of impressions;
- Effects of disinfection techniques on different impression materials;
- Effects of disinfection techniques on different tray materials.

The undergraduate should demonstrate an ability to carry out disinfection on impressions.

Prescription writing

The undergraduate should demonstrate knowledge of the rationale for prescription writing.

The undergraduate should demonstrate ability to:

- Write a laboratory prescription including:
  - the clinician's name
  - the clinician's address
  - the patient's name
  - the patient's address
  - the patient's age
  - the patient's gender
  - the name of the laboratory to which the work will be sent
  - date of dispatch
  - nature of laboratory work which may include:
    - stone to be used for models
    - type of prosthesis
    - type of articulator to be used
    - materials to be used in prosthesis
    - stage of prosthesis fabrication to be carried out
    - prosthesis design
    - tooth material, mould and size
    - shade(s), staining, special effects
  - date for return of laboratory work

- package impressions and laboratory work appropriately including:
  - master impression
  - opposing arch impression or model
  - photographic record.

Special impression techniques

The undergraduate should demonstrate knowledge of the rationale for specific impression techniques in the following clinical circumstances:

- Denture reline
- Denture rebase
- Free end saddle
- Flabby ridge
- Copy denture
- Obturators.

The undergraduate should demonstrate an ability to carry out impressions for the following clinical circumstances:

- Denture reline
- Denture rebase
- Free end saddle, including the altered cast technique
- Flabby ridge
- Copy denture.

Developments in impression-making

The undergraduate should demonstrate a familiarity with developments in impression techniques with specific reference to CAD CAM.

References and further reading

British Society for Restorative Dentistry (1999) *Guidelines for Crown and Bridge.* Available at http://www.derweb.co.uk/bsrd/bsrdgde.html and http://www.dpb.nhs.uk/download/digest/digest_2003.pdf

GDC (2002) *The First Five Years: a framework for undergraduate dental education*, 2nd edn. London, The General Dental Council.

Journal of Prosthetic Dentistry (1999) *The Glossary of Prosthodontic Terms.* Special Issue.

QAA (2002) *Dentistry: academic standards.* Subject benchmark statements. Gloucester, Quality Assurance Agency for Higher Education.

Wassell R. W., Barker D. and Walls A. W. G. (2002) Crowns and other extra-coronal restorations: impression materials and technique. *Br Dent J* 192, 679–90.

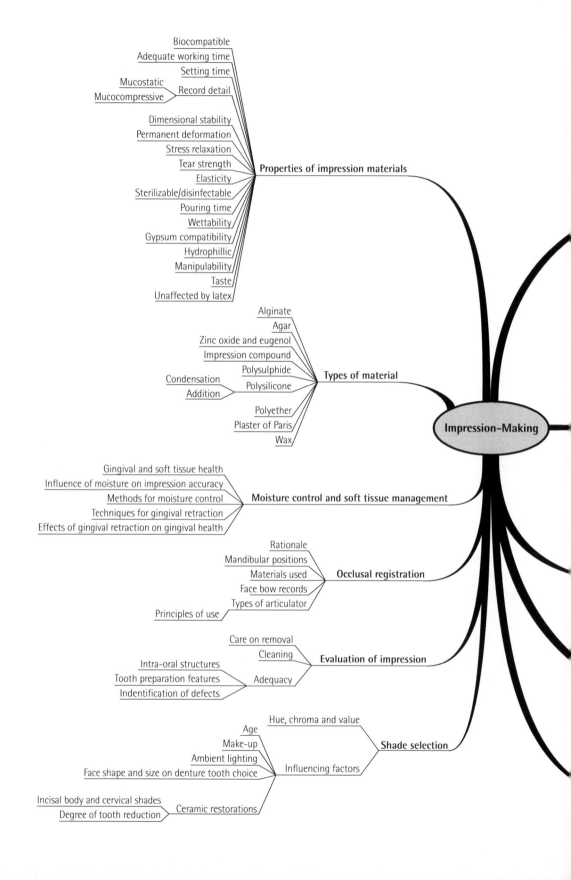

Properties of impression materials
- Biocompatible
- Adequate working time
- Setting time
- Record detail
  - Mucostatic
  - Mucocompressive
- Dimensional stability
- Permanent deformation
- Stress relaxation
- Tear strength
- Elasticity
- Sterilizable/disinfectable
- Pouring time
- Wettability
- Gypsum compatibility
- Hydrophillic
- Manipulability
- Taste
- Unaffected by latex

Types of material
- Alginate
- Agar
- Zinc oxide and eugenol
- Impression compound
- Polysulphide
- Polysilicone
  - Condensation
  - Addition
- Polyether
- Plaster of Paris
- Wax

Moisture control and soft tissue management
- Gingival and soft tissue health
- Influence of moisture on impression accuracy
- Methods for moisture control
- Techniques for gingival retraction
- Effects of gingival retraction on gingival health

Occlusal registration
- Rationale
- Mandibular positions
- Materials used
- Face bow records
- Types of articulator
  - Principles of use

Evaluation of impression
- Care on removal
- Cleaning
- Adequacy
  - Intra-oral structures
  - Tooth preparation features
  - Indentification of defects

Shade selection
- Hue, chroma and value
- Influencing factors
  - Age
  - Make-up
  - Ambient lighting
  - Face shape and size on denture tooth choice
- Ceramic restorations
  - Incisal body and cervical shades
  - Degree of tooth reduction

Impression-Making

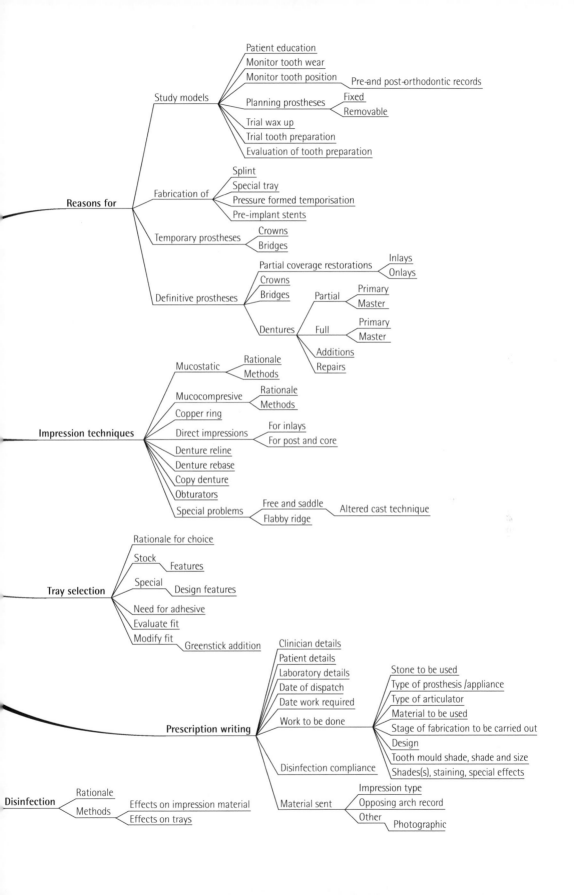

Reasons for

Study models
- Patient education
- Monitor tooth wear
- Monitor tooth position — Pre-and post-orthodontic records
- Planning prostheses
  - Fixed
  - Removable
- Trial wax up
- Trial tooth preparation
- Evaluation of tooth preparation

Fabrication of
- Splint
- Special tray
- Pressure formed temporisation
- Pre-implant stents

Temporary prostheses
- Crowns
- Bridges

Definitive prostheses
- Partial coverage restorations
  - Inlays
  - Onlays
- Crowns
- Bridges
- Dentures
  - Partial
    - Primary
    - Master
  - Full
    - Primary
    - Master
  - Additions
  - Repairs

Impression techniques
- Mucostatic
  - Rationale
  - Methods
- Mucocompresive
  - Rationale
  - Methods
- Copper ring
- Direct impressions
  - For inlays
  - For post and core
- Denture reline
- Denture rebase
- Copy denture
- Obturators
- Special problems
  - Free and saddle — Altered cast technique
  - Flabby ridge

Tray selection
- Rationale for choice
- Stock — Features
- Special — Design features
- Need for adhesive
- Evaluate fit
- Modify fit — Greenstick addition

Prescription writing
- Clinician details
- Patient details
- Laboratory details
- Date of dispatch
- Date work required
- Work to be done
  - Stone to be used
  - Type of prosthesis /appliance
  - Type of articulator
  - Material to be used
  - Stage of fabrication to be carried out
  - Design
  - Tooth mould shade, shade and size
  - Shades(s), staining, special effects
- Disinfection compliance
- Material sent
  - Impression type
  - Opposing arch record
  - Other
    - Photographic

Disinfection
- Rationale
- Methods
  - Effects on impression material
  - Effects on trays

1.16 Dental materials science
Garry Fleming

Key points

- Demonstrate the ability to assess the key differences in bonding, structure and properties of metals and alloys, polymers, ceramics and glasses.
- Recognize the three types of primary bonds: ionic, metallic and covalent.
- Identify the main groups of solids based on the primary bonds, namely ceramics and glasses, metals and polymers.
- Demonstrate how the microstructure and solidification of metals and alloys influence the properties following manufacturing processes.
- Recognize how the nature of ceramics and glasses facilitate the delivery of aesthetic restorative materials.
- Identify how the nature of polymers influence the final properties that can be achieved.

Introduction

Dental materials are essential to many areas of dentistry including restorative dentistry (Chapters 2.5, 2.6, 2.7), paediatric dentistry (Chapters 2.1a, 2.1b, 2.1.c), dental implants, orthodontics (Chapter 2.3) and reconstructive maxillofacial surgery (Chapter 2.7).

Paragraph 79 of the second edition of *The First Five Years* (GDC 2002) states that:

> Instruction in the properties, correct manipulation and the science under-pinning of the use of dental materials is needed to equip the student with the knowledge to select and handle those materials safely and effectively. Dental students need to understand how such materials, and the biological responses to them, are evaluated. This equips them to cope with future developments in this area. The GDC considers it is essential that staff teaching this part of the programme work in close collaboration with clinical colleagues.

The GDC elaborates further on communication with technical staff and states that:

Paragraph 76 Students will learn how to communicate effectively with a dental technician, so that indirect restorations and fixed and removable prosthesis can be constructed. Students should be aware of high standards in that work and have practical experiences of the processes involved. It is important that experience is gained in constructing indirect restorations and fixed and removable prosthesis. However, once that experience has been gained, students should be able to have the appliances and restorations required by their patients manufactured by dental technicians. The primary purpose of dental technology teaching should be to ensure that students have sufficient understanding of the clinical preparations and the laboratory processes so that they can appropriately evaluate their own clinical work and the work provided to and received from dental technicians. Students should appreciate the relevance of their preparations to the quality of technical work that can be produced.

In order to understand the key material properties of dental materials for specific clinical applications, it is important that the students recognize and understand the fundamental building blocks that make up the different materials, namely metals and alloys, polymers and ceramics and glasses.

Table 1.16.1 Intended learning outcomes in the area of restorative dentistry encompassing dental biomaterials and in the area of dental biomaterials

Be competent at	Have knowledge of	Be familiar with
Designing effective indirect restorations and complete and partial dentures	The design and laboratory procedures used in the production of crowns, bridges, partial and complete dentures and be able to make appropriate chair-side adjustment to these restorations	Those aspects of biomaterial safety that relate to dentistry
	The science that underpins the use of dental biomaterials	
	The limitations of dental materials	

Curriculum guidelines in undergraduate dental materials education

This section lists key areas that will be covered during an undergraduate course in dental materials. It is essential that the graduate have a good background knowledge in order to understand disease processes and how this may lead to the loss of tooth structure and as a result the need for restorative dentistry.

Materials

To address the learning objectives outlined in *The First Five Years* the student should be familiar with the different dental materials used in dentistry including:

- plastic restorations;
- extra coronal restorations;
- impression materials;
- luting and lining cements.

Plastic restorations

In the last ten years the demand for aesthetic restorative treatment of posterior teeth has focused dental materials research on identifying a direct posterior restorative material as a potential amalgam replacement. The driving forces behind this search include concerns regarding the safety of dental amalgam (Okamoto and Horibe 1991) and the possible adverse effects that might result from exposure to mercury from dental amalgam on both individuals and the environment.

The ideal posterior filling material

- Understand the material properties by which the performance of posterior filling materials is assessed:
  - Mechanical properties: compressive strength, hardness and wear resistance
  - Chemical properties: erosion, corrosion or dissolution in the mouth
  - Physical properties: dimensional stability
  - Biological properties: does not harm the patient or dentist
  - Adhesive properties: adhesive so there is no loss of sound tooth structure
  - Aesthetic properties: aesthetically pleasing, opacity/translucency, colour stability
  - Rheological properties: viscosity, tackiness, working characteristics.

Dental amalgam

- Understand the basic dental materials science, including the chemistry, to relate how the structure and composition of amalgam influence performance.

- Identify the composition and setting reaction for a traditional amalgam explaining why the γ^2 phase limits material properties such as creep and corrosion resistance. Describe how the addition of copper can minimize the γ^2 phase producing an improvement in properties.
- Understand the appropriate selection and correct manipulation of amalgam:
  - Explain how various parameters including powder particle size and shape, mercury amalgam alloy ratio and manipulation regime can influence the properties of the resultant alloy.
- Evaluate the performances of dental materials, including the biological response of the oral tissues:
  - Dental amalgam, despite being used as a restorative filling material for over 150 years, still has biocompatibility concerns and the presence of amalgams will increase the mercury levels in blood, urine and tissue. Awareness by dental students of the potential difficulties in the handling, placement and disposal of these materials is extremely important.

Resin-based composites

- Understand the basic dental materials science including the chemistry to relate how the structure and composition of resin-based composites (RBCs) influence performance:
  - Describe how the constituents of RBCs, namely the resin, filler particles and coupling agent, are combined to make a workable filling material. Explain how polymerization occurs through light irradiation and its implications in terms of depth of cure and polymerization shrinkage.
- Understand the appropriate selection and correct manipulation of RBCs:
  - Describe the nature of RBCs (traditional, microfilled and hybrid) explaining how particle size, particle volume and distribution influences the wear behaviour and other associated mechanical properties, including shrinkage of RBCs.
- Be familiar with dental laboratory materials, the technologies used in production of dental appliances and recognize limitations on accuracy and technical error:
  - RBCs are adhesively bonded to sound tooth structures a result of a complex procedure whereby the enamel and dentine are treated in accordance with the manufacturer's instructions for the chosen bonding agent.
- Evaluate the performances of dental materials, including the biological response of the oral tissues:
  - RBCs are known to cause little pulpal irritation once there is an adequate marginal seal present.

Glass-ionomer cement and its derivatives

◆ Understand the basic dental materials science including the chemistry to relate how the structure and composition of glass-ionimer cements (GICs) and their derivatives influence performance:

  ▪ Describe the acid-base setting reaction of a GIC and be able to discuss how the release of ions from the leachable glass phase controls the setting reaction. Discuss how and why a GIC bonds to both enamel and dentine.

◆ Understand the appropriate selection and correct manipulation of GICs:

  ▪ Explain how the setting reactions, mechanical properties and working characteristics of resin-modified GICs and compomers compare with the conventional GICs and composite materials from which they have evolved.

◆ Evaluate the performances of dental materials, including the biological response of the oral tissues:

  ▪ Explain how the pulpal response to GICs and their derivatives as restorative materials is favourable compared with other materials available.

Extra coronal restorations

Precious and non–precious metals for all metal–ceramic restorations

Since the first commercially successful dental gold alloy was patented in 1962 (Weinstein *et al.* 1962) attempts have been made to improve on the properties of the alloy and to develop technically superior alternatives.

◆ Understand the material properties by which the performance of precious or non-precious metal substructures are assessed:

  ▪ Adequate yield strength and modulus of elasticity allows the material to be used in thin sections.

  ▪ Easily castable and easy to reproduce the fine margins of the preparation.

  ▪ Adequate corrosion resistance in the oral environment and the metals utilized must be non-toxic in nature.

◆ Understand the basic dental materials science to relate the structure and composition of metals to their performance:

  ▪ The metal-ceramic restoration must withstand the thermal cycling regime, be able to support its own weight and maintain marginal integrity during porcelain firing.

◆ Understand the chemistry and structure of dental materials, and the interaction of such materials with their working environment:

  ▪ Success of metal-ceramic restorations is increased providing an intimate bond is achieved between the metal and the porcelain.

- ◆ Understand the appropriate selection and correct manipulation of clinical materials:
  - ▪ Since the first commercially successful dental gold alloy (84.1 per cent gold) in 1962 (Weinstein *et al.* 1962) attempts have always been made to improve on the properties of the alloy the majority of metal-ceramic restorations employed today are manufactured from non-precious alloys.
- ◆ Be familiar with dental laboratory materials, the technologies used in production of dental appliances and recognize limitations on accuracy and technical error the appropriate selection and correct manipulation of clinical materials. The production of a metal-ceramic crown is complex and involves several stages including casting the alloy, condensing and firing the porcelain.

Dental porcelains and aesthetic restorative dentistry

Dental porcelain is an ideal candidate material for many applications in restorative dentistry including jacket crowns, metal-ceramic restorations and veneers since dental porcelain has excellent aesthetics, resists wear extremely well and does not elicit a pulpal response from vital teeth.

- ◆ Understand the material properties by which the performance of the restoration is assessed:
  - ▪ There is poor correlation between the average fracture strength determined by conventional material science techniques and resultant clinical performance of all-ceramic restorations. It is imperative that the tooth restoration has adequate retention and resistance form (Shillingburg *et al.* 1987) rather than being constructed from the highest strength ceramic available.
- ◆ Understand the basic dental materials science including the chemistry to relate the structure and composition of dental porcelains to their performance:
  - ▪ Dental porcelains use the basic Si-O network as the glass forming matrix, but additional properties like improved aesthetics, adjustment of thermal expansion coefficient, low fusion temperature and high viscosity have to be built in by utilizing alkali ions (Na^+ and K^+) and intermediate oxides (Al_2O_3).
- ◆ Understand the appropriate selection and correct manipulation of clinical materials:
  - ▪ A variety of methods have been used to attempt to improve the strength of ceramic materials over the past four decades, including dispersion strengthening, glass infiltration, castable glasses and pressable and machinable ceramics. Brittle fracture in ceramics and glasses is often preceded by subcritical crack growth which is dependent on the rate of attack of moisture at the crack tip. The strength of ceramics are susceptible to an acidic environment and performance of cemented crowns can be influenced by cement type (Rosenstiel *et al.* 1993).
- ◆ Be familiar with dental laboratory materials, the technologies used in production of dental appliances and recognize limitations on accuracy and technical error the appropriate selection and correct manipulation of clinical materials:

■ The production of an all-ceramic crown is complex and involves several stages including condensing, firing and staining the porcelain.

Impression materials

Impression materials play a pivotal role in the accuracy of fabrication of dental devices from detailed crown and bridge work to orthodontic appliances. Material selection can be made following analysis of the key material properties required of the impression material.

◆ Understand the properties of the impression material by which performance is assessed.

◆ Prior to setting:

■ The viscosity determines the selection since mucostatic and mucocompressive impression materials are ideal for hard and soft tissue impressions, respectively.

◆ Properties of set impression materials:

■ Dimensional accuracy to ensure the appliance will be made to fit.

■ Adequate rigidity and elasticity when undercuts are present.

■ Tear resistance for the removal from the subgingival shoulders of a crown.

■ Hydrophilic so that a dry field of operation is not entirely essential.

■ Viscoelastic behaviour.

◆ Understand the basic dental materials science to relate the chemistry, structure and composition of flexible impression materials to their performance:

■ Identify the key differences between hydrocolloid and elastomeric impression materials by comparing and contrasting the basic setting reactions.

◆ Understand the appropriate selection and correct manipulation of clinical materials:

■ Discuss the factors that should be considered when deciding which type of impression material to be used for a particular clinical application. An example is given to illustrate the difficulties involved:

• Polysulphides or addition cured silicones for a full arch impression. The critical factors would be the key material properties of dimensional stability, high level of reproduction and high flexibility. The polysulphides have high flexibility which make them an ideal candidate material for the recognition of undercuts as they are easily removed. In contrast, the high rigidity of the addition cured silicones make them more difficult to remove the impression, especially from full arch impressions.

◆ Be familiar with dental laboratory materials, the technologies used in production of dental appliances and recognize limitations on accuracy and technical error:

■ Explain how variations in the chemistry of the different types of impression materials available may influence the accuracy of the dental stone casts.

Cavity linings, cavity bases and luting cements

Cavity linings and bases

Many types of cavity linings and bases are available, each with inherent advantages and disadvantages: however, the primary cavity linings and bases in current use must be appropriately selected since one type of cement is unlikely to perform adequately under all conditions.

Cavity linings

In the case of a cavity lining for placement under an amalgam restoration, the students should:

+ Understand the materials properties by which the performance of the cavity base is assessed:
  - Adequate compressive strength and increased modulus of elasticity during amalgam placement and subsequent service combined with reduced tooth sensitivity.
+ Understand basic dental materials science to relate the structure and composition of zinc oxide eugenol and calcium hydroxide to their performance:
  - If the cement type does not meet the criteria it must be applied as thin layers to minimize these effects.
+ Understand the chemistry and structure of dental materials, and the interaction of such materials with their working environment:
  - If the pulp is visible through the dentin will the cement stimulate secondary dentin formation, or if the dentin is not visible is one formulation known to be more tooth sensitive.
+ Understand the appropriate selection and correct manipulation of clinical materials:
  - Following appropriate selection the materials may set resulting in an exothermic reaction may require moderation of the heat of reaction through the incremental incorporation the cement powder constituent on a chilled glass-slab.

Cavity bases

In the case of a cavity base for placement under an amalgam restoration, the students should:

+ Understand the material properties by which the performance of the luting cement is assessed:
  - Adequate compressive strength and increased modulus of elasticity during amalgam placement and subsequent service combined with reduced tooth sensitivity.
+ Understand basic dental materials science to relate the structure and composition of zinc phosphate and glass-ionomer cements to their performance:
  - Both cement types have similar structure and composition, as they set by an acid-base reaction to enable them to encounter stresses of amalgam placement and the masticatory forces in service.

- ◆ Understand the chemistry and structure of dental materials, and the interaction of such materials with their working environment:

  - ■ A further consideration is the reason for the replacement, namely caries, and whether the cements offer the potential for fluoride release which is thought to reduce recurrent caries.

- ◆ Understand the appropriate selection and correct manipulation of clinical materials:

  - ■ Following appropriate selection the materials may set, resulting in an exothermic reaction that may require moderating.

Luting cements

The luting cements in current use include zinc phosphate, polycarboxylate, glass-ionomer, resin composite, compomer and resin modified glass-ionomer cements.

In the case of cementing a metal-ceramic or all-ceramic crown, the students should:

- ◆ Understand the materials properties by which the performance of the cavity linings is assessed:

  - ■ Adequate compressive strength, good marginal seal and reduced tooth sensitivity following crown placement.

- ◆ Understand basic dental materials science to relate the structure and composition of, say, the primary luting cements to their performance:

  - ■ Acid-base cements have been advocated for use in cementing all-ceramic crowns and metal–ceramic restorations, however the literature highlights the susceptibility of the strength of dental ceramics to an acidic environment (Rosenstiel *et al.* 1993).

- ◆ Understand the chemistry and structure of dental materials, and the interaction of such materials with their working environment:

  - ■ The product of the cement forming reaction between powder and acidic liquid for acid-base cements results in the initial cement mass reaching a pH level below 4.0 for up to 4 hours before approaching neutrality (Smith and Ruse 1986).

- ◆ Understand the appropriate selection and correct manipulation of clinical materials:

  - ■ Acid-base cements manipulated below the manufacturers' recommended mixing ratio for luting cements spend longer at lower pH levels and take longer during the course of the setting reaction to rise to a pH level approaching neutrality.

- ◆ Be familiar with dental laboratory materials, the technologies used in production of dental appliances and recognize limitations on accuracy and technical error:

  - ■ Non-precious metal alloys may have poor castability and potential biological concerns whilst the reproduction of fit of CAD-CAM all-ceramic restorations may not be accurate for some crown morphologies.

The range of dental materials that are routinely available to dentists are constantly changing with improved materials being developed, often being radically different to pre-existing products. To make full use of these developments the teaching of the appropriate elements of basic materials science is required. It is therefore important that we have a list of skills that every student must achieve in order successfully complete their course of study, i.e. the concept of key competencies. Therefore undergraduate courses in dental biomaterials science should test each of the skills listed below to ensure that a basic level of skill and knowledge has been achieved.

The dental undergraduate will be competent in:

◆ Knowing the chemistry and structure of clinical materials and how they are affected by interaction with their environment, including degradation and biological effects.

◆ Identifying the properties and parameters by which the performance of dental materials are assessed.

◆ Selecting and handling of materials in a safe and effective manner.

◆ Detailing the materials used at all stages of the production of items in laboratories by dental technicians, identifying the limitations on accuracy and potential errors to be encountered on manufacture.

Conclusions

The range of skills and knowledge that an undergraduate needs to acquire during the undergraduate dental materials course is extensive. It is important that the dental materials course reflects these and is constructed in such a way that the student has the opportunity to acquire the requisite knowledge and skills. The undergraduate dental materials course must also be able to assess the student in order to ensure that they have acquired the necessary skills that are set out at the start of this chapter. As with all dental education, the student must embrace the concept of continued professional development. Students must be aware that a number of areas where possibly they gained little or no experience at undergraduate level may need to be studied at postgraduate level.

References and further reading

GDC (2002) *The First Five Years: a framework for undergraduate dental education*, 2nd edn. London, The General Dental Council.

Okamoto Y. and Horibe T. (1991) Liquid gallium alloys for metallic plastic fillings. *Br Dent J* 5, 23–6.

QAA (2002) *Dentistry: academic standards*. Subject benchmark statements. Gloucester, Quality Assurance Agency for Higher Education.

Rosenstiel S. F., Gupta P. K., van der Sluys R. A. and Zimmerman M. H. (1993) Strength of a dental glass-ceramic after surface coating. *Dental Materials* 9, 274–9.

Shillingburg H. T., Jacobi R. and Brackett S. E. (1987) Biomechanical principles of preparations. In Shillingburg H. T., Jacobi R. and Brackett S. E. (eds) *Fundamentals of Tooth Preparations for Cast Metal and Porcelain Restorations*, Chapter 1. Chicago, IL, Quintessence Publishing Co.

Smith D. C. and Ruse N. D. (1986) Acidity of glass ionomer cements during setting and its relation to pulp sensitivity. *Journal of the American Dental Association* 112, 654–7.

Weinstein M., Katz S. and Weinstein A. B. (1962) Inventors; Permanent Manufacturing Corporation, assignee. Fused Porcelain-to-Metal Teeth. U.S. Patent No. 3,052,982, September, 11.

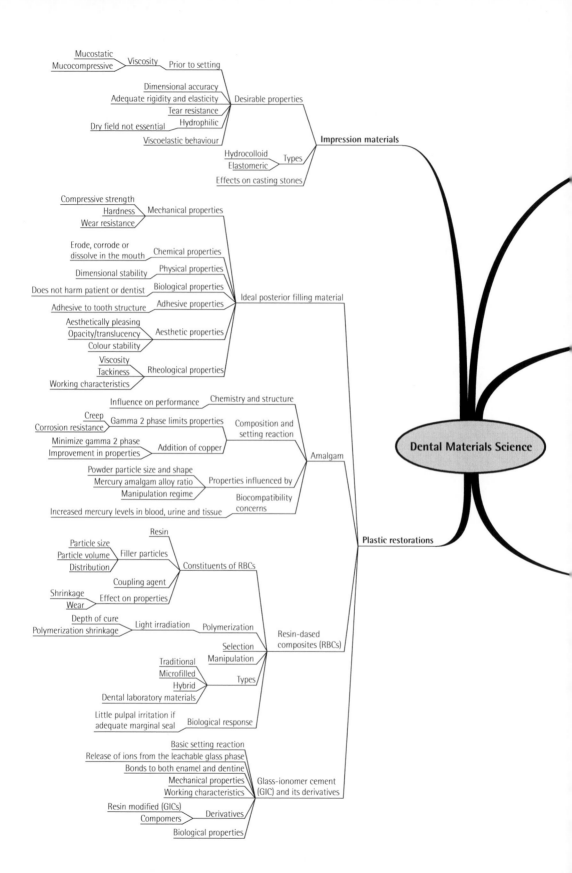

Dental Materials Science

Impression materials

Viscosity
- Mucostatic
- Mucocompressive
- Prior to setting

Desirable properties
- Dimensional accuracy
- Adequate rigidity and elasticity
- Tear resistance
- Hydrophilic — Dry field not essential
- Viscoelastic behaviour

Types
- Hydrocolloid
- Elastomeric

Effects on casting stones

Ideal posterior filling material

Mechanical properties
- Compressive strength
- Hardness
- Wear resistance

Chemical properties — Erode, corrode or dissolve in the mouth

Physical properties — Dimensional stability

Biological properties — Does not harm patient or dentist

Adhesive properties — Adhesive to tooth structure

Aesthetic properties
- Aesthetically pleasing
- Opacity/translucency
- Colour stability

Rheological properties
- Viscosity
- Tackiness
- Working characteristics

Amalgam

Chemistry and structure — Influence on performance

Composition and setting reaction
- Gamma 2 phase limits properties
  - Creep
  - Corrosion resistance
- Addition of copper
  - Minimize gamma 2 phase
  - Improvement in properties

Properties influenced by
- Powder particle size and shape
- Mercury amalgam alloy ratio
- Manipulation regime

Biocompatibility concerns — Increased mercury levels in blood, urine and tissue

Resin-dased composites (RBCs)

Constituents of RBCs
- Resin
- Filler particles
  - Particle size
  - Particle volume
  - Distribution
- Coupling agent
- Effect on properties
  - Shrinkage
  - Wear

Polymerization — Light irradiation
- Depth of cure
- Polymerization shrinkage

Selection

Manipulation

Types
- Traditional
- Microfilled
- Hybrid
- Dental laboratory materials

Biological response — Little pulpal irritation if adequate marginal seal

Glass-ionomer cement (GIC) and its derivatives

- Basic setting reaction
- Release of ions from the leachable glass phase
- Bonds to both enamel and dentine
- Mechanical properties
- Working characteristics
- Derivatives
  - Resin modified (GICs)
  - Compomers
- Biological properties

Plastic restorations

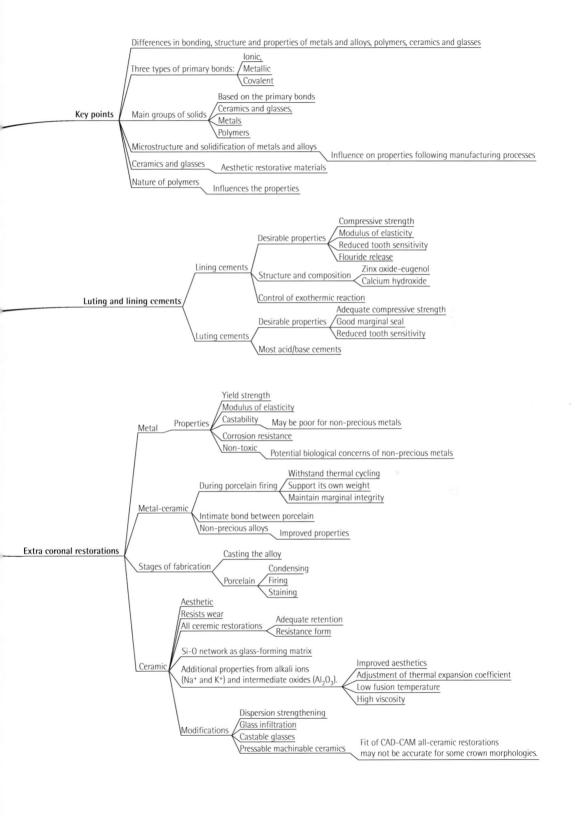

Key points
- Differences in bonding, structure and properties of metals and alloys, polymers, ceramics and glasses
- Three types of primary bonds:
  - Ionic,
  - Metallic
  - Covalent
- Main groups of solids
  - Based on the primary bonds
  - Ceramics and glasses,
  - Metals
  - Polymers
- Microstructure and solidification of metals and alloys — Influence on properties following manufacturing processes
- Ceramics and glasses — Aesthetic restorative materials
- Nature of polymers — Influences the properties

Luting and lining cements
- Lining cements
  - Desirable properties
    - Compressive strength
    - Modulus of elasticity
    - Reduced tooth sensitivity
    - Flouride release
  - Structure and composition
    - Zinx oxide-eugenol
    - Calcium hydroxide
  - Control of exothermic reaction
- Luting cements
  - Desirable properties
    - Adequate compressive strength
    - Good marginal seal
    - Reduced tooth sensitivity
  - Most acid/base cements

Extra coronal restorations
- Metal
  - Properties
    - Yield strength
    - Modulus of elasticity
    - Castability — May be poor for non-precious metals
    - Corrosion resistance
    - Non-toxic — Potential biological concerns of non-precious metals
- Metal-ceramic
  - During porcelain firing
    - Withstand thermal cycling
    - Support its own weight
    - Maintain marginal integrity
  - Intimate bond between porcelain
  - Non-precious alloys — Improved properties
- Stages of fabrication
  - Casting the alloy
  - Porcelain
    - Condensing
    - Firing
    - Staining
- Ceramic
  - Aesthetic
  - Resists wear
  - All ceremic restorations
    - Adequate retention
    - Resistance form
  - Si-O network as glass-forming matrix
  - Additional properties from alkali ions (Na^+ and K^+) and intermediate oxides (Al_2O_3).
    - Improved aesthetics
    - Adjustment of thermal expansion coefficient
    - Low fusion temperature
    - High viscosity
  - Modifications
    - Dispersion strengthening
    - Glass infiltration
    - Castable glasses
    - Pressable machinable ceramics — Fit of CAD-CAM all-ceramic restorations may not be accurate for some crown morphologies.

2.1a Paediatric dentistry
Treatment of primary and mixed dentition

Elizabeth Davenport and Patricia Baxter

Key points

- Prevention is the cornerstone of good management of dental caries in children
- History taking is fundamental to the execution of restorative care in the primary and mixed dentition.
- Communication skills are essential in obtaining a child's co-operation in completing treatment.
- Caries risk of a child patient provides markers for future preventive needs and restorative care.
- The recognition of dental caries and planning appropriate treatment related to disease activity and a child's age is key to restoring the primary and mixed dentition.
- The extent of dental caries will determine the cavity design and ultimate choice of restorative material.
- The selection and handling of dental materials is based on sound knowledge of their composition and physical properties.

Introduction

The 2003 survey of child dental health documented a reduction of 20 per cent in dental caries experience in the oldest children since the previous survey ten years earlier. This was not so for the five-year-olds with little improvement noted over the same time period (ONS 2003). Whilst considering the pattern of dental disease in children, there remains a significant proportion that is untreated. Hence the need to ensure that on graduation dentists have the basic skills to restore the primary and mixed dentition, and know when to appropriately refer a child for specialist advice and help with their management.

Fayle and colleagues (2001) have discussed the management of dental caries in the primary dentition on behalf of the British Society of Paediatric Dentistry (BSPD). Untreated dental caries in the deciduous dentition can lead to pain and infection, which may be detrimental to the general health of children. This may include interference with nutrition, loss of sleep, behaviour disturbance, and poor aesthetics. The ability to restore the primary dentition is therefore a requirement of a graduate.

In considering the treatment of the primary and mixed dentitions, it is also important to recognize the need for good relationships between the child patients, their family, and the dentist, as outlined in law and ethics, encompassing good communication skills (Chapters 1.2 and 1.3). Behaviour management (Chapter 1.10) and pain control (Chapter 1.9) should also be taken into account when planning treatment for children. Restorative treatment should be delivered to the highest standard possible. The requirements for the delivery of dental care in paediatric dentistry are outlined in the GDC's *The First Five Years. a framework for undergraduate dental education* (GCD 2002) and expressed in full below:

> **Paragraph 80** The study of child dental health should encompass the interrelationships between orthodontics and paediatric dentistry together with the general growth and development of the individual. It should be related to social and psychological factors and to the recognition, preventive treatment and operative management of the common disease processes.
>
> **Paragraph 81** Paediatric dentistry is concerned with the understanding of normal growth and development and the promotion and maintenance of oral health for children. In paediatric dentistry students should have a continuous responsibility for the care of a number of children in order to assess their overall needs, the efficacy of preventive measures, their behaviour, and management and restorative treatment. Students should also learn to manage children requiring emergency care, carry out diagnostic procedures in such circumstances, formulate treatment plans and relate them to comprehensive dental care for children. They should be made aware of the special dental needs of children with disabilities and have experience in the recognition and management of developmental dental abnormalities.

Paediatric dentistry is also listed in the Subject Benchmark for Dentistry (QAA 2002) as follows:

> Manage the oral health of children and adolescents and perform treatment for them in a manner that incorporates consideration for their expected growth and development, involving parents or guardians as required.

Intended learning outcomes

Table 2.1a.1 contains the intended learning outcomes incorporating those outlined in the GDC's *The First Five Years*, Subject Benchmark Statement for Dentistry, *Intended Learning Outcomes for Undergraduate Training in Paediatric Dentistry* (Maguire *et al.*

Table 2.1a.1 Intended learning outcomes for the restoration of the primary and mixed dentition

Be competent at	Have knowledge of	Be familiar with
Diagnosing active caries and planning appropriate non-operative care	Methods to assess quality of restorations	*Aesthetic management of non-vital permanent teeth*
Using rubber dam for the isolation of teeth	*Pre-formed stainless steel crown and pulp therapy in primary molars*	*Etch retained veneers*
Designing cavities in relation to tooth anatomy and the characteristics of the restorative material	*The management of trauma in both dentitions*	*The use of microabraision techniques*
Undertaking approximal and incisal tip restorations		*Vital and non-vital bleaching*
Performing aesthetic restorations using adhesive systems		
Analysing failures to minimize future complications		
The selection and handling of dental materials for restorative procedures based on a sound knowledge of their composition and physical properties and taking into account patient risk factors		

2004) (as devised by the BSPD Teacher's Branch) and the *Undergraduate Teaching Programme in Europe*: First draft of a 'Golden Standard' by European Academy of Paediatric Dentistry. Those in **_bold italics_** illustrate the interaction between other aspects of child patient care that are also essential skills for the restorative treatment of the primary and mixed dentition.

Preventive care is the cornerstone to good management of dental caries in children. The basic concepts for prevention are discussed in Chapter 1.12.

The treatment of the primary and mixed dentition is described in the following sequence (Gordon 2001; Blinkhorn 2001; Kilpatrick 2001; Page and Welbury 2001; Raadal *et al.* 2001).

History taking

♦ Be competent in obtaining, assessing and recording a medical, dental, family, social and, where appropriate, feeding, dietary, and developmental history from a child patient, parent or guardian.

History taking should include history of present complaint, past dental history, social and medical history – to assist in the overall management and treatment planning a judgement of the child's behaviour, the ability of the child to understand and co-operate, and the assessment of caries risk.

Clinical examination

♦ Be competent in performing a clinical examination of the patient (relevant to age group) that encompasses head and neck, facial, intra-oral, general and behavioural aspects of a child patient.

Clinical examination is performed once a history and examination has been completed; this should include intra-oral and extra-oral examination and where appropriate special investigations such as radiographs and study models.

The location and extent of disease, the stage of dental development and malocclusion development

♦ Be competent at diagnosing active caries and planning appropriate non-operative care and

♦ Be competent in identifying the type, location, extent and activity of dental caries.

The location and extent of disease, the stage of dental development and malocclusion development must be determined prior to making an informed choice about the extent of treatment in relation to the child's disease activity, age, and ability to cope with clinical procedures.

Treatment plans

♦ Be competent in developing comprehensive and integrated treatment and preventive plans, taking into account diagnosis, social, medical and psychological influencing factors for a child.

Treatment plans may be purely preventive in nature, for example placement of fissure sealant on the immature permanent molars on eruption, or more invasive using a preventive resin restoration (BSPD 2000; SIGN 2000). The requirement could also be one or two surface restoration with or without pulp involvement, or the repair of a fractured incisal tip. Where dental extractions are planned the long-term implications need to be carefully considered.

Restoration of the deciduous dentition

♦ Be competent at using rubber dam for the isolation of teeth

♦ Be competent at designing cavities in relation to tooth anatomy and the characteristics of the restorative material.

- Be competent at analysing failures to minimize future complications.

- Be competent in the selection and handling of dental materials for restorative procedures based on a sound knowledge of their composition and physical properties and taking into account patient risk factor.

- Have knowledge of methods to assess quality of restorations.

- Have knowledge of pre-formed stainless steel crown and pulp therapy in primary molar teeth.

Restoration of the deciduous dentition encompasses the recognition and determination of caries risk of the child patient; selection of the best method to restore the tooth including invasive and non-invasive procedures. The extent of dental caries determines the choice of restorative material. The hierarchy for the choice of restoration material for the deciduous dentition is that stainless steel crowns (SSC) are most suited to deciduous molars with more than two surfaces affected by dental caries (Roberts and Sheriff 1990), followed by amalgam, composite, compomer and glass ionomer (Welbury *et al.* 1991; Kilpatrick *et al.* 1995; Welbury *et al.* 2000). The adverse affects of amalgam must be borne in mind (Eley 1996). However, Rugg Gunn and colleagues (2001) considered that no restrictions should be placed on the use of amalgam to restore children's teeth at the present time and that rubber dam should be used where practicable to reduce mercury toxicity.

Restoration of immature permanent dentition

- Be competent at using rubber dam for the isolation of teeth.

- Be competent at designing cavities in relation to tooth anatomy and the characteristics of the restorative material.

- Be competent at undertaking approximal and incisal tip restorations.

- Be competent at performing aesthetic restorations using adhesive systems.

- Be competent in the selection and handling of dental materials for restorative procedures based on a sound knowledge of their composition and physical properties and taking into account patient risk factor.

- Have knowledge of the management of trauma in both dentitions.

- Have knowledge of the role of sedation in the management of young patients.

- Be familiar with the aesthetic management of non-vital permanent teeth.

- Be familiar with etch retained veneers.

- Be familiar with the use of microabrasion techniques.

- Be familiar with vital and non-vital bleaching.

Restoration of immature permanent dentition involves the philosophy of prevention of dental caries using a fissure sealant and if initial dental caries is detected in the occlusal surface a more invasive approach may be necessary using a preventive resin restoration.

Each of these will be considered in turn and where appropriate cross-referenced.

History taking including examination in paediatric dentistry

Standards

The student should:

◆ Appreciate the differences between taking a history and planning treatment for children as compared to adults.

◆ Understand the need to obtain consent and establish how child/parent relationships may affect the delivery of dental care for children.

◆ Demonstrate the ability to perform a thorough examination of the child patient that encompasses where necessary facial, intra-oral, head and neck, general, and behavioural aspects.

History taking in paediatric dentistry

Core clinical skills in the evaluation of the oral health of a child patient are not dissimilar to those described for taking a history of a child who is to undergo orthodontic treatment. History taking for children requiring dental treatment should have a greater emphasis in gaining the child's co-operation and getting to know each other.

See **Checklist 25** for history taking including examination in paediatric dentistry.

Underpinning knowledge

The student should be:

◆ Competent in making an assessment of the child's behaviour, relationship with parents/carers, child's risk for dental disease, especially dental caries.

◆ Competent in ascertaining the reason for attendance including pain, trauma history, or other worries for example the shape, size, and colour of teeth.

  ▪ Complaint

  ▪ Past dental history including previous treatment received

  ▪ Medical history

  ▪ Social history

◆ Competent at carrying out an examination of the hard and soft tissues of the head and neck, and associated extra-oral and intra-oral tissues.

◆ Demonstrate an understanding of primary, secondary and tertiary prevention.

◆ Have knowledge of children's growth and developmental stages.

◆ Competent at prescribing, taking and processing accurately a radiographic examination which is appropriate for the needs of the child.

◆ Competent in assessing intra- and extra-oral radiographs.

◆ Competent at making a diagnostic statement.

◆ Competent at record keeping.

- Competent to formulate an appropriate treatment plan for the child patient taking into account the longevity of the teeth.
- Competent at obtaining informed consent for the treatment to be provided.
- Have knowledge of the growth and development of children.
- Have knowledge of dental materials suitable for the restoration of primary and young permanent teeth.

Restoration of deciduous dentition

Core clinical skills in the restoration of the deciduous tooth

1. Diagnosis of dental caries in a tooth using visual, radiographic or other detection methodology.

2. Outline treatment objectives and discussion with child and their parent as to procedures required.

3. Administer appropriate topical gel application and local anaesthetic to ensure pain-free restorative treatment.

4. Placement of rubber dam or use of equivalent moisture control.

5. Cavity preparation related to the extent of the carious lesion:
   - Access to carious lesion.
   - Removal of dental caries, particularly at margins and walls of cavity.
   - Preparation of cavity relates to the extent of the lesion and subsequent choice of restorative material and retention.
     - SSC – minimal preparation of the tooth after caries removal and GIC for maximum retention on a molar tooth
     - Amalgam – shape cavity for retention or dual cure composite bonding of amalgam to the tooth
     - Composite – preparation of enamel bevel at the occlusal margins, enamel and dentine bonding and use incremental build up in the proximal box to reduce polymerization contraction problem
     - GIC – resistance to displacement may be required and hence small occlusal dovetail inserted or retention grooves in dentine
     - Compomer – bonding for retention
   - Treatment of pulpal–dentine complex – calcium hydroxide, GIC or bonded composite resin.
   - Restoration of tooth with appropriate material and use of matrix band and wedges for approximal surface contour.

6. Completion of restoration, occlusion and margins checked, reminder of anaesthetized soft tissues, reinforcement of good behaviour.

Underpinning knowledge

The student should be:

1. Competent at making an assessment of the caries risk of a child.

2. Competent at diagnosing active caries in the deciduous dentition.

3. Competent at giving a local anaesthetic to ensure pain-free dentistry for a child patient.

4. Competent in using rubber dam for the isolation of teeth.

5. Competent at carious tissue removal using rotary and hand instruments with consideration of the pulpal–dentine complex.

6. Competent in undertaking approximal restorations and designing cavities in relation to the tooth anatomy and the characteristics of the restorative material of choice.

7. Competent at making a choice of materials to restore the tooth in the most appropriate manner in view of the longevity of the tooth.

8. Have knowledge in carrying out extra-coronal restoration of primary teeth using preformed stainless steel crowns for molar teeth and bonded composite strip crowns for anterior teeth.

9. Have knowledge of the pulpal status from clinical signs and symptoms

   ◆ **One surface:** All dental materials available may be utilized in the restoration of deciduous molars. The extent of the caries, age of the child, caries risk and child's co-operation will influence the final choice of material. Alternatives to amalgam (the most durable material) can be chosen. GIC with fluoride-releasing and adhesive properties is ideal for a one-surface cavity. However, GIC is not strong enough to be used in large restorations with significant occlusal load. The choice of composite resin, compomer or GIC materials is disadvantaged by being technique sensitive and requires scrupulous moisture control during bonding and placement of the material which can be difficult to achieve in paediatric dentistry (Chapter 1.16).

   ◆ **Two surfaces:** A stainless steel crown should be used in preference for a molar tooth with more than one or two surfaces affected or if the tooth has had pulp therapy treatment. Alternative choices have lower survival rates over five years; amalgam 70–80 per cent, GIC between 60–75 per cent and composite may be as little as 40 per cent success rate. Adhesive restorative materials are constantly being developed to enhance their properties and to become more user friendly.

Treatment for primary teeth with symptoms of toothache or abscess

This aspect of treatment for the primary and mixed dentition will be primarily discussed under pulp therapy for the primary dentition (Chapter 2.1b and Chapter 2.6).

The student should:

1. Be competent in the management of dental emergencies.

2. Be competent in placement of appropriate temporary dressing (with or without initiating pulp therapy treatment) to relieve pain.

3. Be competent at extraction of primary teeth using local anaesthesia.

4. Have knowledge to perform pulp treatment of vital and non-vital primary teeth

5. Have knowledge of non-surgical endodontic treatment of immature permanent teeth.

6. Have knowledge of the difference between reversible and irreversible pulpitis and the symptoms experienced by the patient.

7. Have knowledge of controlling advanced carious lesions by stepwise excavation and temporization with hard setting CaOH and sealed with a dressing (Mejare 2001).

Immature permanent molar in the mixed dentition

Fissure sealants

The student should:

1. Appreciate that different materials exist and the need to utilize the most effective material in providing a fissure sealant in the occlusal surfaces of the permanent dentition.

2. Demonstrate ability to place a fissure sealant:

   • Diagnose absence of dental caries

   • Prepare tooth surface for etch (30 per cent phosphoric acid) until enamel surface is frosty after washing and drying

   • Place fissure sealant of choice and set

   • Test for adhesion and integrity of fissure sealant.

3. Monitor margins and retention of fissure sealant to cover all parts of the fissure.

   Checklist 26 outlines the requirements for fissure sealant or sealant restoration in first permanent molar.

Underpinning knowledge

   • Demonstrate the ability to perform accurate and appropriate clinical intra-oral examination.

   • Demonstrate the ability to perform accurate and appropriate radiographic examination.

   • Demonstrate the ability to assess radiographs.

   • Demonstrate the understanding of the technique employed in placing a fissure sealant and using most effective and commonly available materials.

   • Establish dental caries risk and implements a preventive regime.

Core skills in the restoration of early permanent dentition: occlusal enamel carious lesion, stained fissure or widening of the fissures or precavitated lesion
The student should have:

1. Discussion with child and parent prior to procedure undertaken

2. Established dental caries risk and implements a preventive regime

3. Obtained pain and anxiety control – i.e. topical gel application and local analgesia

4. Isolation using rubber dam or appropriate means

5. Access

6. Investigation of the fissure system

7. Remove incipient caries – with or without dentine involvement

8. Etch enamel surface in readiness for placement of composite resin and fissure sealant

9. Checked integrity of procedure, margins and occlusion

Checklist 27 outlines the requirements the restoration of early permanent dentition: occlusal enamel carious lesion.

If the carious lesion extends into dentine

1. Complete until stage 6

2. Extend cavity to remove caries

3. Consider the dentine – pulp complex

4. Choice of dental material appropriate in relation to extent of caries

5. Lining CaOH, GIC or bonded composite resin

6. Prepare tooth surface for restoration:

    ◆ etch enamel for 30 seconds, dentine for 15 seconds

    ◆ apply bonding agent

    ◆ place composite resin in increments and cure

    ◆ place fissure sealant over restoration and cover every fissure before curing

    ◆ or (remove unsupported enamel if using amalgam), place amalgam in increments and condense.

7. Check margin integrity and occlusion.

Underpinning knowledge

◆ Demonstrate the ability to identify the type, location, extent and activity of dental caries.

◆ Utilization of appropriate radiographs to aid diagnosis of dental caries.

Checklist 25 **History and examination of a child patient**

Clinical examination	Yes	No
History		
Clear statement of problem		
Past medical history		
Past dental history:		
• Dental caries		
• Trauma		
• Treatment		
• Preventive		
• Restorative		
• Extractions		
• Orthodontic		
• Other		
Social history		
Examination:		
• Communicates with patient		
• Communicates with parent/carer		
Carries out examination:		
• Extra oral		
• Intra oral (hard and soft tissues)		
• Chart (recognition caries/teeth)*		
• Oral hygiene status		
• Malocclusion		
Describes findings clearly		
Special tests		
• Appropriate discussion and interprets		
– Radiographs		
– Other		
Provides summary diagnosis		
Treatment plan and management		
Aetiology of disease		
Provides aims of overall treatment plan		
Obtains informed consent		

* Fail competency tests if fails to recognize caries or teeth!

Checklist 26 **Fissure sealant or sealant restoration in first permanent molar**

Task	Yes	No
Reasons for fissure sealant (BSPD Policy Document)		
• Patient		
• Mouth		
• Tooth		
Tooth preparation		
• Clean and dry		
• Etch, wash and dry (isolation is essential)		
• Choice material		
Placement of fissure sealant		
• Adheres		
• Position ~ to ½ cuspal incline		
• No ledges		
• No air blows		
• Occlusion		
Restoration		
• Materials use		
• Placement		
• Include unfilled resin		
Finish		
• Tooth surface and sealant – restoration flush		
• Occlusion		

- ◆ Demonstrate the ability to assess radiographs.
- ◆ Provide local analgesia to achieve comfort of child during treatment.
- ◆ Establish extent of dental caries lesion and removal of dental caries.
- ◆ Restore tooth to function using commonly available restorative materials.
- ◆ Demonstrate the ability to perform accurate and appropriate radiographic intra- and extra-oral examination.
- ◆ Understand the potential hazards of amalgam and the potential weakness of other plastic materials.

Checklist 27 **Restorative competency test**

Task	Yes	No
Presentation		
Patient:		
• Presenting complaint		
• Medical/social/ dental history		
Tooth:		
• Diagnosis*		
• Rationale for restoring		
* To include: extent of carious lesion, pulp involvement and adjacent teeth		
Treatment:		
• Preparation		
– Local analgesia		
– Rubber dam/moisture control		
– Infection control		
• Cavity preparation		
• Caries free		
• Management of pulp/dentine complex		
• Retention and placement of restoration		
– Occlusal and approximal preparation – material choice		
– Matrix or choice SSC		
• Restoration		
– Rationale for material choice		
– Placement of filling material		
– Placement/cementation SSC		
– Finish/occlusion		
Patient management:		
• Organization		
• Communication/consent		

If caries management is inadequate then competency is failed and a fail grade is awarded.

References and further reading

Blinkhorn A. S. (2001) Introduction to the dental surgery. In Welbury R. R. (ed.) *Paediatric Dentistry*, 2nd edn, pp. 17–36. Oxford, Oxford University Press.

Eley B. M. (1996) Have Germany and Sweden banned the use of amalgam? *Dental Update* 23, 313–14, 328; erratum *Dental Update* p996; 23: 432.

Fayle S. A., Welbury R. R. and Roberts J. (2001) Management of caries in the primary dentition. *Int J Paed Dent* 11, 153–57.

GDC (2002) *The First Five Years: a framework for undergraduate dental education*, 2nd edn. London, The General Dental Council.

Gordon P. H. (2001) Craniofacial growth and development. In Welbury R. R. (ed.) *Paediatric Dentistry*, 2nd edn, pp. 1–16. Oxford, Oxford University Press.

Kilpatrick N. (2001) History, examination and treatment planning. In Welbury R. R. (ed.) *Paediatric Dentistry*, 2nd edn, pp. 37–50. Oxford, Oxford University Press.

Kilpatrick N. M., Murray J. J. and McCabe J. F. (1995) The use of a reinforced glass–ionomer Cermet for the restoration of primary molars: a clinical trial. *Br Dent J* 179, 175–9.

Kilpatrick N., Page J. and Welbury R. R. (2001) Operative treatment of dental caries. In Welbury R. R. (ed.) *Paediatric Dentistry*, 2nd edn, pp. 133–56. Oxford, Oxford University Press.

Maguire A., Davenport E. S. and Craig S. A. (2004) Intended learning outcomes for undergraduate training in paediatric dentistry. *Int J Paed Dent* 14, 223–9.

Mejore I. (2001) Management of the advanced carious lesion in primary teeth. In Hugoson A., Falk M., and Johanson S. (eds) Caries in the Primary Dentition and its Clinical Management. Stockholm, Forlagshuset Gathia.

Nunn J. N., Murray J. J. and Smallridge J. (2000) A policy document on fissure sealants in paediatric dentistry. *Int J Paed Dent* 10, 174–7.

Office of National Statistics (2003) *UK Children's Dental Health Survey 2003*. Available at http://www.statistics.gov.uk/downloads/theme_health/Executive Summary-CDH.PDF. Accessed 8 November 2005.

QAA (2002) *Dentistry: academic standards*. Subject benchmark statements. Gloucester; Quality Assurance Agency for Higher Education.

Raadal M., Espelid I. and Mejare I. (2001) The caries lesion and its management in children and adolescents. In G. Koch and S. Poulsen (eds) *Paediatric dentistry a clinical approach*, pp. 173–212. Copenhagen, Munksgaard.

Roberts J. F. and Sheriff M. (1990) The fate and survival of amalgam and preformed restorations placed in a specialist paediatric dental practice. *Br Dent J* 169, 237–44.

Rugg Gunn A. J., Welbury R. R. and Tuomba J. (2001) A policy document on the use of amalgam in paediatric dentistry. *Int J Paed Dent* 11, 233–8.

SIGN (Scottish Intercollegiate Guidelines Network) (2000) *Preventing Dental Caries in Children at High Caries Risk*. Publication Number 47. pp. 12–15.

Welbury R. R., Walls A. W. G., Murray J. J. and McCabe J. F. (1991) The 5-year results of a clinical trial comparing glass polyalkenoate (ionomer) cement restoration with an amalgam restoration. *Br Dent J* 170, 177–81.

Welbury R. R., Shaw A. J., Murray J. J., Gordon P. H. and McCabe J. F. (2000) Clinical evaluation of paired compomer and glass ionomer restorations in primary molars: final results after 42 months. *Br Dent J* 189, 93–7.

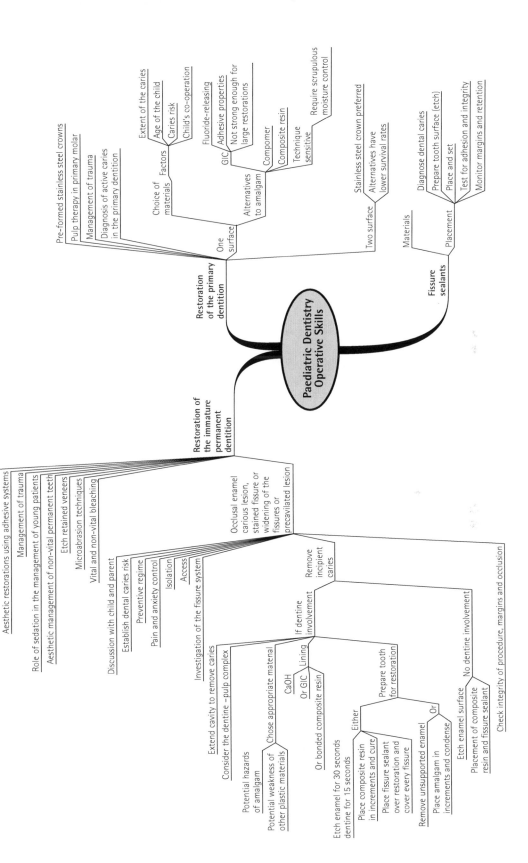

Paediatric Dentistry Operative Skills

Restoration of the primary dentition

- One surface
  - Pre-formed stainless steel crowns
  - Pulp therapy in primary molar
  - Management of trauma
  - Diagnosis of active caries in the primary dentition
  - Choice of materials — Factors
    - Extent of the caries
    - Age of the child
    - Caries risk
    - Child's co-operation
  - Alternatives to amalgam
    - GIC
      - Fluoride-releasing
      - Adhesive properties
      - Not strong enough for large restorations
    - Compomer
    - Composite resin
      - Technique sensitive
      - Require scrupulous moisture control
- Two surface
  - Stainless steel crown preferred
  - Alternatives have lower survival rates
- Materials
- Placement
  - Diagnose dental caries
  - Prepare tooth surface (etch)
  - Place and set
  - Test for adhesion and integrity
  - Monitor margins and retention

Fissure sealants

Restoration of the immature permanent dentition

- Approximal incisal tip restorations
- Aesthetic restorations using adhesive systems
- Management of trauma
- Role of sedation in the management of young patients
- Aesthetic management of non-vital permanent teeth
- Etch retained veneers
- Microabrasion techniques
- Vital and non-vital bleaching

- Discussion with child and parent
- Establish dental caries risk
- Preventive regime
- Pain and anxiety control
- Isolation
- Access
- Investigation of the fissure system
- Occlusal enamel carious lesion, stained fissure or widening of the fissures or precaviated lesion
- Remove incipient caries
  - If dentine involvement
    - Extend cavity to remove caries
      - Potential hazards of amalgam
      - Potential weakness of other plastic materials
      - Chose appropriate matenal
    - Consider the dentine –pulp complex
    - Lining
      - CaOH
      - Or GIC
      - Or bonded composite resin
    - Prepare tooth for restoration
      - Either
        - Etch enamel for 30 seconds dentine for 15 seconds
        - Place composite resin in increments and cure
        - Place fissure sealant over restoration and cover every fissure
      - Or
        - Remove unsupported enamel
        - Place amalgam in increments and condense
  - No dentine involvement
    - Etch enamel surface
    - Placement of composite resin and fissure sealant
- Check integrity of procedure, margins and occlusion

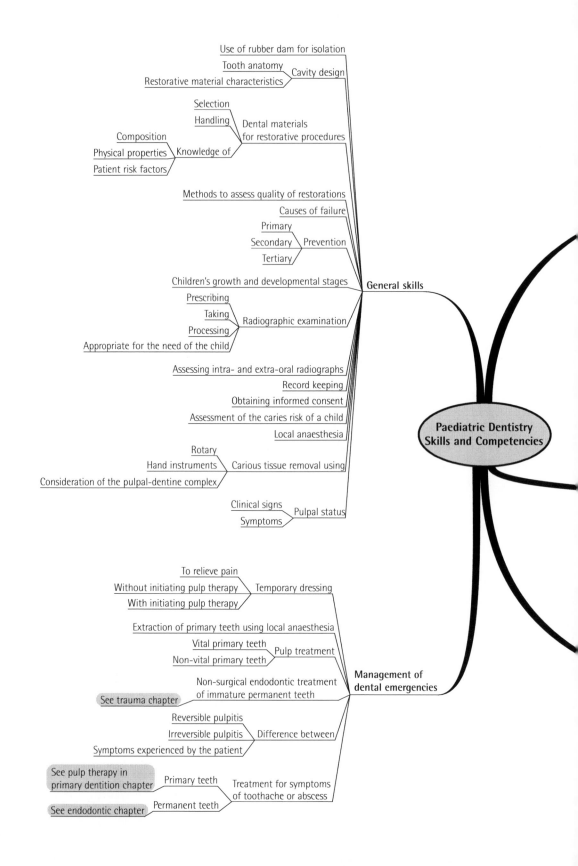

Paediatric Dentistry Skills and Competencies

General skills

Use of rubber dam for isolation

Cavity design
- Tooth anatomy
- Restorative material characteristics

Dental materials for restorative procedures
- Selection
- Handling

Knowledge of
- Composition
- Physical properties
- Patient risk factors

Methods to assess quality of restorations

Causes of failure

Prevention
- Primary
- Secondary
- Tertiary

Children's growth and developmental stages

Radiographic examination
- Prescribing
- Taking
- Processing
- Appropriate for the need of the child

Assessing intra- and extra-oral radiographs

Record keeping

Obtaining informed consent

Assessment of the caries risk of a child

Local anaesthesia

Carious tissue removal using
- Rotary
- Hand instruments
- Consideration of the pulpal-dentine complex

Pulpal status
- Clinical signs
- Symptoms

Management of dental emergencies

Temporary dressing
- To relieve pain
- Without initiating pulp therapy
- With initiating pulp therapy

Extraction of primary teeth using local anaesthesia

Pulp treatment
- Vital primary teeth
- Non-vital primary teeth

Non-surgical endodontic treatment of immature permanent teeth
- See trauma chapter

Difference between
- Reversible pulpitis
- Irreversible pulpitis
- Symptoms experienced by the patient

Treatment for symptoms of toothache or abscess
- Primary teeth — See pulp therapy in primary dentition chapter
- Permanent teeth — See endodontic chapter

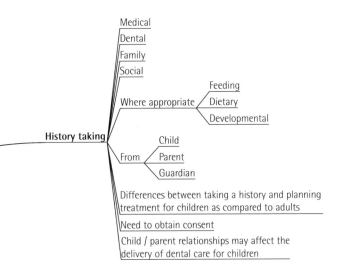

History taking
- Medical
- Dental
- Family
- Social
- Where appropriate
  - Feeding
  - Dietary
  - Developmental
- From
  - Child
  - Parent
  - Guardian
- Differences between taking a history and planning treatment for children as compared to adults
- Need to obtain consent
- Child / parent relationships may affect the delivery of dental care for children

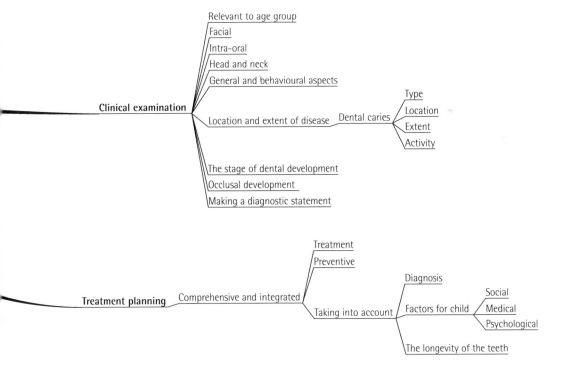

Clinical examination
- Relevant to age group
- Facial
- Intra-oral
- Head and neck
- General and behavioural aspects
- Location and extent of disease — Dental caries
  - Type
  - Location
  - Extent
  - Activity
- The stage of dental development
- Occlusal development
- Making a diagnostic statement

Treatment planning — Comprehensive and integrated
- Treatment
- Preventive
- Taking into account
  - Diagnosis
  - Factors for child
    - Social
    - Medical
    - Psychological
  - The longevity of the teeth

2.1b Pulp therapy in the primary dentition

Paula Jane Waterhouse

Key points

- Dental caries in primary molars remains widespread in the UK, and therefore restoration of carious primary molar teeth is an important part of paediatric dentistry.

- The primary aim of pulp therapy for carious primary molars is to conserve the damaged tooth, restore its function and avoid unplanned extraction.

- Extraction of deciduous teeth has a number of undesirable consequences, including reduced masticatory function, secondary crowding and malocclusion and the risks of mortality and morbidity associated with general anaesthesia and invasive surgery.

- The link between formaldehyde and carcinogenicity in humans has meant that Buckley's Formocresol is no longer an agent used for pulp therapy in carious primary molars. (Techniques discussed in this chapter might change or evolve in the light of more published evidence on their efficiency.)

- The General Dental Council recognizes that only limited clinical/practical experience of primary molar pulp therapy may be possible in the undergraduate dental curriculum, but a sound theoretical knowledge of the subject is necessary.

- Diagnosis of dental disease in primary teeth requires sound knowledge of special investigations such as vitality tests and radiographs; and subsequent interpretation before deciding whether it is appropriate to proceed with pulp therapy.

- Pulp treatment of carious primary molar teeth involves aspects of behaviour management, treatment planning, pain control, and restoration. Therefore there is significant interplay with other chapters of this book.

Introduction

Restoration of carious primary molar teeth is an important part of paediatric dentistry. Data derived from the UK Child Dental Health Survey (O'Brien 1994) showed that in the primary dentition, caries most frequently affected molars. Forty per cent of 5- year-olds and 50 per cent of 8-year-olds had dental caries in primary molars.

If a carious primary molar remains untreated or inadequately treated, bacterial invasion of the coronal pulp occurs by direct spread through dentinal tubules. In response to the microbial insult, the coronal pulp tissue lays down reactive, secondary dentine and mounts a defensive inflammatory response. At this stage the entire pulp is not moribund; if the irreversibly inflamed coronal pulp is removed and the radicular pulp treated with an appropriate agent, the remaining tissue possesses the ability to recover. However, if the infected coronal pulp remains, micro-organisms invade the radicular pulp, resulting in irreversible pulpitis. Control of infection can then only be secured by pulpectomy and root canal treatment, or extraction. If treatment is not undertaken, infection may spread from the pulp canal space to the periodontium through patent accessory, lateral, and apical foramina. The tooth may then become mobile and associated soft tissues may become painful and swollen.

The aims of pulp therapy for carious primary molars are to conserve the damaged tooth and restore its function. By successful treatment of pulp tissue, the paediatric dentist reduces the potential for unplanned extraction and the undesirable consequences that may follow. These include: loss of space for the successor tooth with crowding and a malocclusion; reduced masticatory function; and the risks of mortality and morbidity associated with general anaesthesia and invasive surgery (Waterhouse *et al.* 2000).

In the UK, up until the Summer of 2004 the main agent used for pulp treating carious primary molars was Buckley's Formocresol (Llewelyn 2000). However, the International Agency for Research on Cancer (IARC) published a press release confirming the link between formaldehyde and carcinogenicity in humans (International Agency for Research on Cancer 2004). This has resulted in a number of dental schools withdrawing Formocresol.

When considering the pulp treatment of carious primary molar teeth, it is important understand that the contents of this chapter have significant interplay with other chapters of this book, for example, behaviour management, treatment planning, pain and pain control, and treatment of primary and mixed dentition.

The requirements for the delivery of dental care in paediatric dentistry outlined in the General Dental Council's *The First Five Years, a framework for undergraduate dental education* (GDC 2002) are cited in Chapter 2.01a, Treatment of primary and mixed dentition.

Specifically with regard to pulp therapy in the primary dentition, the General Dental Council (GDC 2002) states within paragraph 111 (Specific learning outcomes) that the dental undergraduate should have: 'Knowledge of preformed stainless steel crown and pulp therapy in primary molar teeth.'

This means that dental undergraduates need 'a sound theoretical knowledge of the subject, but need have only a limited clinical/practical experience'.

The QAA Subject Benchmark Statement for Dentistry paragraph 3.14 states that: 'Graduating dentists should be able to manage diseases and conditions involving the periapical and periradicular tissues in both the primary and permanent teeth' (QAA 2002).

Intended learning outcomes

In order to undertake successful management of a pulpally involved primary molar tooth there are several intended learning outcomes that are relevant to the specific clinical skill. The range of intended learning outcomes are listed in Table 2.1b.1, and include those outlined by the GDC (2002), The Subject Benchmark Statement for Dentistry (QAA 2002) and the Teachers' Branch of the British Society of Paediatric Dentistry (Maguire *et al.* 2004).

Table 2.1b.1 Intended learning outcomes for pulp therapy in the primary dentition

Be competent at	Have knowledge of	Be familiar with
Obtaining a detailed history of the patient's dental state	The aetiology and processes of oral diseases	
Clinical examination and treatment planning	Obtaining informed consent	
Diagnosing active caries and planning operative care	Pulp treatment of vital and non-vital primary teeth	
The principles of radiographic interpretation and be able to write an accurate radiographic report	Preformed stainless steel crowns and pulp therapy in primary molars	
Using a rubber dam for the isolation of teeth	The appropriate special investigations and interpretation of their results	
Designing cavities in relation to tooth anatomy and the characteristics of the restorative material	The management of acute infection	
Analysing failures to minimize future complications		

Indications and contraindications for pulp therapy

The indications and contraindications for pulp treatment in the primary dentition are outlined below and are based upon those in the clinical guideline produced by the British Society of Paediatric Dentistry (Llewelyn 2000). However, modifications have been made to these techniques since the withdrawal of Buckley's Formocresol (IARC 2004).

General indications:

Pulp therapy in the primary dentition may be undertaken to:

◆ Maintain an intact arch in primary dentition

◆ Avoid extractions (e.g. in a patient with a bleeding disorder)

◆ Provide space maintenance in the mixed dentition

◆ Avoid physiological trauma of extraction

◆ Maintain a primary tooth if the permanent successor is absent.

Dental signs and symptoms, which may indicate that pulp therapy is required, are listed below.

Clinical and radiographic signs

◆ Caries involving, or very close to, pulp horns

◆ Occlusal caries greater than 4 mm in depth

◆ Approximal caries with greater than two-thirds marginal ridge breakdown

◆ Periradicular bony radiolucency

◆ Sinus formation

◆ Mobility of tooth

◆ Tenderness to percussion.

Symptoms

◆ Transient sharp pain from thermal stimuli (reversible pulpitis)

◆ Spontaneous throbbing pain (irreversible pulpitis)

◆ Pain from biting on the affected tooth (periapical periodontitis).

Before embarking on pulp therapy in the primary dentition, a paediatric dentist must take a holistic and pragmatic approach in treatment planning. In many instances, pulp treatment in the primary dentition can be a worthwhile undertaking. However, there are some instances when pulp therapy should not be considered and extraction should be favoured. These contraindications to pulp therapy are listed below.

Contraindications to pulp therapy

◆ Oral neglect – where 3 or 4 teeth are likely to require pulp therapy

◆ Lack of co-operation from child or carer

◆ Children at risk from bacteraemia (e.g. a cardiac anomaly where the child is at risk from endocarditis)

◆ Caries involving the root canal or pulp chamber

◆ A tooth that is unrestorable, this usually means that there is insufficient tooth tissue remaining to provide adequate restoration.

Criteria for successful pulp therapy in the primary dentition

These standards are specific for pulp therapy in the primary dentition. They will include:

+ The assessment of pulp status in the child patient.

+ The appropriate treatment planning and patient management for vital and non-vital carious pulpal exposures.

The following deals with statements taken from *Learning Outcomes for Undergraduate Training in Paediatric Dentistry*, as devised by the BSPD Teachers' Branch (Maguire *et al.* 2004) which, in turn, are based on both the GDC (2002) and QAA (2002) documents.

History taking

'Be competent in obtaining, assessing and recording a medical, dental, family, social and, where appropriate, feeding, dietary, and developmental history from a child, parent or guardian.'

The student should:

+ Be aware that taking accurate histories from young patients can be difficult. Young children are poor historians.

+ Be aware that a child's carer also has a key role in providing this information.

+ Demonstrate the ability to communicate with young patients and their carers in order to acquire appropriate details for diagnosis and treatment planning involving pulp therapy for the primary dentition.

For example:
Assess the motivation of the child and carer towards restorative treatment.
Obtain a concise social history – distances travelled, ability to attend for treatment.
Obtain an accurate, relevant medical history with special reference to conditions, which would have bearing upon future pulp therapy such as:

+ Cardiac anomalies

+ Bleeding disorders

+ Immunosupression.

Obtain a pain history, where possible, to aid diagnosis of pulpal status (see Chapter 1.1 for generic aspects):

+ Short-lived, sharp pain stimulated by cold

+ Dull ache of longer duration

+ Continual throbbing pain causing insomnia.

Obtain an accurate dental history:

+ Previous extractions

+ Previous restorations

- Level of cooperation
- Experience of local anaesthesia
- Ability to sit for long appointments.

Underpinning knowledge:
- Demonstrate knowledge of the importance of cooperation in pulp therapy.
- Be aware how symptoms relate to the type of pulp therapy that may be required.
- Be aware a how medical history may have bearing up on the indications/contraindications for pulp therapy.

Clinical examination (of relevance to pulp therapy)

'Be competent in performing a clinical examination of the patient (relevant to age group) that encompasses facial, interiorly, head and neck, general and behavioural aspects of a child patient.'

Extra-oral examination (see Chapter 1.1 for generic aspects)

The student should be able to assess the soft tissues of the head and neck for signs of:

- The presence of facial swelling associated with spread of infection from dento alveolar sources.
- The presence of lymph node enlargement as a response to dento-alveolar infection.

Intra-oral examination

The student should:

1. Be able to recognize the possible sequelae to pulp necrosis manifest in the soft tissues:
    - Gingival swelling and erythema
    - Sinus formation
    - Tenderness to percussion
    - Understand the significance of such clinical signs.
2. Be able to diagnose caries in the primary dentition.
3. Be able to assess the likelihood of pulpal involvement in a cariously exposed tooth with reference to the:
    - Identification of deep occlusal caries deeper than 4 mm
    - The significance of greater than two-thirds marginal ridge breakdown.
4. Be able to assess whether a satisfactory coronal restoration could be placed post-pulpotomy and understand the significance of good coronal seal to successful treatment outcome.

Underpinning knowledge

Demonstrate knowledge of the possible signs and symptoms of reversible and irreversible pulpitis.

◆ Demonstrate knowledge of the possible signs and symptoms of pulp necrosis and infection.

◆ Understand the importance of the need for good coronal restoration if pulp therapy is undertaken upon a successful outcome.

Special investigations

Share with patients provisional assessment of their problems and formulate plans for their further investigation and management.

Have knowledge of appropriate special investigations and the interpretation of their results.

Be competent at the principles of radiographic interpretation and be able to write an accurate radiographic report.

The student should:

◆ Be able (with assistance) to prescribe the most relevant radiographic examination for a child with carious primary dentition.

◆ Accurately diagnose caries involving dentine.

◆ Accurately diagnose the probable extent of the carious lesion.

◆ Be able (with assistance) to assess the possible extent of pulpal involvement from the radiograph.

◆ Accurately identify the features of periapical pathology.

◆ Accurately identify the features of furcation pathology.

◆ Identify pathological resorption.

◆ Assess the radiographs set in the context of the clinical picture.

◆ Effectively communicate these findings to the child and carer.

Underpinning knowledge

◆ Able to prescribe the most appropriate radiographic examination for (a) caries diagnosis, and (b) the child's level of co-operation.

◆ Ability to identify the radiographic features of a carious lesion in a primary tooth

◆ Ability to identify the radiographic features of the sequelae to dental caries.

Checklist 28 Special investigations as a means of provisional diagnosis of pulpal involvement.

	Yes	No
Demonstrate knowledge of why the radiographs are required		
Radiographic examination		
Remove dental caries		
Identification of potential carious exposures in primary teeth		
Assess the extent of pulpal involvement		
Identify signs of periradicular pathology		
Identify signs of pathological resorption		

Provisional diagnosis of pulp status

Have knowledge of the aetiology and processes of oral diseases.

Have knowledge of management of acute infection.

Share with patients provisional assessment of their problems and formulate plans for their further investigation and management.

From the preceding information (the clinical signs and symptoms and radiographic signs) the student should:

◆ Be able to formulate a provisional diagnosis of the following pulpal conditions:

■ Asymptomatic tooth with a cariously exposed but vital pulp

■ A reversibly inflamed pulp

■ An irreversibly inflamed pulp

■ A non-vital pulp +/– infective sequelae.

◆ Demonstrate their understanding that such diagnoses are often subject to gathering additional information once caries is removed and the pulp chamber entered.

◆ Demonstrate their understanding that a pulp may still be partially vital despite, for example, one root canal having associated periapical pathology.

Underpinning knowledge

◆ Understand the need to merge information from clinical and radiographic sources.

◆ Understand the concepts of pulpal exposure, reversible inflammation, irreversible inflammation and pulp death.

◆ Understand that accurate diagnosis of pulp status may be difficult and that additional information can be acquired after pulp exposure.

Treatment planning

Be competent at clinical examination and treatment planning.
Have knowledge to be able to explain and discuss treatments with patients and their parents.

From a provisional diagnosis the student should:

◆ Be able to provisionally assess whether a patient is able to tolerate pulp therapy.

◆ Be able to indicate which carious teeth are likely to require pulp therapy.

◆ Be aware that the stage of physiological root resorption has bearing on the suitability for pulp therapy.

◆ Identify the probable type of pulp therapy required.

◆ Stage the treatment involving pulp therapy at the most appropriate time for the patient.

◆ Discuss and explain the process of pulp therapy to the patient/carer.

Underpinning knowledge

◆ Understand the need to superimpose the patient's motivation, co-operation and stage of development upon the treatment planning process.

◆ Understand the principles of treatment planning for paediatric patients (see Chapter 2.1a).

Management of primary teeth requiring pulp therapy

Have knowledge of preformed stainless steel crown and pulp therapy in primary molar teeth.

The student should:

◆ Be able to demonstrate knowledge of the following techniques in vital and non-vital pulp therapy, in view of the profession moving away from the use of Formocresol.

Vital pulp therapy

1. Indirect pulp therapy (Farooq *et al.* 2000; Falster *et al.* 2002).

2. Single visit ferric sulphate pulpotomy (Ibricevic and Al-Jame 2003).

3. Managing a carious pulpal exposure in an unco-operative child or hyperalgaesic pulp.

Non-vital pulp therapy

1. Pulpectomy (Mortazavi and Mesbahi 2004).

Vital pulp therapy

Indirect pulp therapy

This procedure is undertaken if there is deep dentinal caries in a primary tooth. The tooth should be symptom free. Stained dentine is left at the floor of the cavity. A lining such as glass-ionomer cement or setting calcium hydroxide, facilitating reparative dentine formation, is placed at the pulpal aspect of the cavity floor.

Technique:

1. Remove caries from cavity walls.

2. Carefully excavate the cavity floor, removing softened dentine, but leaving hard, stained dentine.

3. Place a glass-ionomer cement or setting calcium hydroxide lining material at the base of the cavity.

4. Place a well-sealed coronal restoration, such as a preformed metal crown or bonded resin based restoration:

   ♦ The tooth must be symptom free before treatment.

   ♦ Following removal of softened dentine, there must be no frank exposure of pulp.

   ♦ The intra-coronal restoration must be well sealed, for example a preformed stainless steel crown or a bonded resin/compomer restoration.

   ♦ Regular clinical and radiographic reviews are essential.

Underpinning knowledge

The student should understand that:

♦ This technique is used to maintain vital pulp tissue, eliminate microbial flora and stimulate reparative dentine formation beneath the deep dentine caries.

♦ The direct pulp cap is *not* advocated for use in carious exposures in the primary dentition.

Checklist 29 **Indirect pulp cap**

	Yes	No
Explanation of technique to parent/carer and child • Demonstrate knowledge		
Appropriate materials available		
Pain control		
Removal of caries at cavity walls		
Excavation of cavity floor		
Accurate placement of indirect pulp capping agent		
Placement of an appropriate coronal restoration		
Effective cross-infection control		

- The restoration must be well sealed to prevent microleakage.
- If successful, it is no longer thought appropriate to remove the restoration in order to then remove the stained dentine.

The single visit ferric sulphate pulpotomy

The student should:

- Be familiar with the clinical procedure of vital pulpotomy.
- Show an understanding of the term pulpotomy.
- Be able to assess the patient for suitability for pulp therapy.
- Be able to assess the tooth for suitability for pulp therapy:
  - the amount of coronal breakdown,
  - the stage of exfoliation,
  - the probability of a carious exposure.

Technique

1. Administer topical and local anaesthesia. (See Chapter 1.9)
2. Obtain adequate isolation, ideally by placing dental dam. If this is not possible a saliva ejector, cotton wool rolls and dry guards should be used.
3. Cavity outline should be established with diamond burs in a high-speed handpiece. Carious dentine should be removed with steel burs in a slow handpiece.
4. A carious exposure of pulp tissue may be seen or detected with gentle exploration with a straight probe. If a carious exposure has occurred, if the tooth has vital pulp tissue, the exposed pulp will bleed.
5. Prepare good access to pulp chamber by removing the roof of pulp chamber using a non-end-cutting bur.
6. The whole roof should be removed to facilitate full removal of the pulp occupying the coronal pulp chamber.
7. Amputate the coronal pulp using a sterile excavator or slowly rotating round steel bur. Extreme care should be exercised in order to avoid perforating the thin pulpal floor.
8. Irrigate with sterile saline (0.9%) or sterile water to remove debris and blood. Apply pressure with saline-moist cotton wool for 3 minutes.
9. Remove cotton wool and assess for presence of bleeding from the radicular pulp stumps. If the bleeding has stopped, one can assume the radicular pulp is not irreversibly inflamed and so it is appropriate to proceed with vital pulpotomy.

10. Soak a small pledget of cotton wool in 15.5% solution of ferric sulphate solution, blot the cotton wool on fresh, dry cotton wool (to remove the excess liquid) and apply the moist cotton wool pledget to the radicular pulp stumps for 15 seconds. Cap the cotton wool with fresh, dry cotton wool to prevent leakage of ferric sulphate onto soft tissues. Ferric sulphate may also be applied with a dento-infuser tip supplied by the manufacturers.

11. Remove the cotton wool and restore the pulp chamber with fast setting zinc oxide-eugenol cement.

12. Restore the tooth using a preformed metal crown. (See Chapter 2.1a.)

Underpinning knowledge

The student should understand that:

- ◆ Pulpotomy involves amputation of the coronal pulp leaving the radicular pulp *in situ*.

- ◆ The scientific basis to the technique is to remove irreversibly inflamed (coronal) pulp, leaving reversibly inflamed or healthy pulp behind.

- ◆ Assessment of the inflammatory status of the pulp is very difficult clinically. It is achieved by subjective assessment of the amount of bleeding from the radicular pulp stumps after coronal pulp amputation. The type of pulp therapy required can be decided at this stage.

- ◆ An irreversibly inflamed radicular pulp will bleed copiously and be difficult to arrest with moist cotton wool applied for three minutes. A reversibly inflamed or healthy pulp should stop bleeding after three minutes.

- ◆ A one-fifth dilution of Buckley's formocresol solution is no longer advocated.

- ◆ Ferric sulphate is haemostatic in its actions. Ferric ions bind with blood proteins to produce mechanical blockage of severed blood vessels. It does not possess the fixative properties of formocresol, therefore should not be applied to an irreversibly inflamed radicular pulp.

- ◆ In recent reviews of pulp therapy, ferric sulphate was as effective as formocresol in the short term (Nadin *et al.* 2003; Loy *et al.* 2004). Alternatives to formocresol have not yet shown equivalent longitudinal clinical success rates.

The student should understand that a successful outcome is dependent upon:

- ◆ Accurate of assessment of pulp status

- ◆ Effective isolation

- ◆ Appropriate use of ferric sulphate solution

- ◆ Removal of whole coronal pulp

- ◆ Safe use of burs, particularly at the floor of the pulp chamber

- ◆ Effective coronal seal post-pulpotomy.

Checklist 30 **Vital pulp therapy on a cariously exposed primary molar tooth**

	Yes	No
Explanation of procedure to patient/carer		
• Demonstrates knowledge		
Appropriate equipment available		
Satisfactory analysis of radiographs		
Pain control		
Moisture control		
Cross-infection control		
Access to pulp chamber		
Coronal pulp amputation		
Safe placement of ferric sulphate solution for 15 seconds		
• Achieve haemostasis		
Restoration of pulp chamber		
Coronal restoration		

Managing a carious exposure in an uncooperative child or where the pulp is hyperalgaesic

The student should be familiar with the clinical procedure of placing a sedative dressing over an exposed, bleeding pulp. It is used if local anaesthesia cannot be administered or if LA has been ineffective.

Technique

This treatment takes a minimum of two visits.

Visit 1

1. Irrigate exposure site with sterile saline and dry with cotton wool.

2. Place Ledermix™ on cotton wool directly over exposure

3. Anchor the cotton wool with setting calcium hydroxide cement.

4. Place a well-sealed temporary restoration, such as glass ionomer cement, for 7–14 days.

5. If co-operation poor, arrange extraction.

Visit 2

1. LA must now be obtained.

2. Proceed with ferric sulphate pulpotomy.

3. If the pulp is still sensitive despite LA, extraction may be indicated.

Underpinning knowledge

The student should understand that:

◆ A Ledermix™ dressing may be placed in a primary tooth with a carious exposure of vital pulp tissue, because a single visit ferric sulphate cannot be undertaken as either the child will not accept local anaesthesia or pain control has not been fully achieved by local anaesthesia already administered.

◆ Ledermix™ paste contains steroid triamcinolone acetonide and the broad spectrum antimicrobial clemethyl chlortetracycline. When applied to inflamed pulp tissue it is thought to be anti inflammatory (Seow and Thong 1993).

◆ Placement of Ledermix™ paste can be difficult. A small cotton wool pledget dipped in the paste should be placed over the amputation site and 'anchored' into position with a fast setting calcium hydroxide cement.

◆ Clinical experience shows that the cotton wool should be placed in a gentle manner since excess pressure can cause pulpal pain.

◆ This technique has been suggested in order to 'calm' an inflamed pulp either prior to extraction or before progressing on to a Ferric Sulphate pulpotomy under LA. It is not advocated as a long term pulpotomy dressing.

Checklist 31 **Placing an interim dressing on a sensitive cariously exposed primary molar tooth**

	Yes	No
Explanation of procedure to patient/carer		
• Demonstrates knowledge		
Infection control		
Appropriate equipment available		
Satisfactory analysis of radiographs		
Moisture control		
Management of the pulpal exposure site		
Placement of Ledermix™ paste		
Review 7–10 days post-placement of Ledermix™		
Complete coronal restoration		

Non-vital pulp therapy

Pulpectomy

Traditionally in the UK pulpectomy has not been performed routinely in the primary dentition because of several perceived problems:

♦ The close proximity of the developing tooth germ to the apices of the primary tooth may pose a relative risk of damaging the successor tooth.

♦ Physiological apical root resorption results in wide-open apical regions. This may result in an increased risk of damaging a developing tooth germ with careless use of files.

♦ Lateral and furcal communications make cleaning and obturation difficult.

♦ Ribbon-shaped root canals are thought to be difficult to instrument.

♦ Thin walls to canals may pose a relative risk of perforation.

The student should be able to:

♦ Identify irreversibly inflamed radicular pulp post-amputation by the presence of persistent, copious bleeding.

♦ Identify a non-vital radicular pulp and any signs of associated periradicular pathology.

♦ Demonstrate that they are familiar with the clinical procedures/techniques of pulpectomy in the primary dentition, bearing in mind the special considerations listed in the previous paragraph.

♦ Understand that the decision on the type of pulpectomy to be used should only be made after coronal pulp amputation.

♦ If a radicular pulp bleeds persistently (indicative of an irreversibly inflamed radicular pulp), a one-visit pulpectomy can be undertaken.

♦ If a radicular pulp is necrotic or periapical pathology is present, a two-visit pulpectomy is indicated.

The one visit pulpectomy (irreversible inflammation)

1. Place dental dam.

2. Remove caries and establish cavity outline.

3. Identify the carious exposure.

4. Remove the roof of the pulp chamber using a non-end cutting bur (Batt bur or Endo-Z bur)

5. Remove the coronal pulp with sterile excavators and slowly rotating steel burs.

6. Identify the openings of the root canals.

7. Attempt to arrest bleeding if present (see section on vital pulpotomy).

8. If the radicular pulp is necrotic a two-stage technique should be used (see later).

9. Irrigate with sodium hypochlorite solution (0.5–1%) or chlorhexidine solution (0.4%) to clear debris.

10. Place small files (≤ size 30) into the canals keeping 2 mm short of the radiographic apex.

11. Wherever possible take a periapical radiograph of the file(s) in place to establish working lengths.

12. Record the working lengths.

13. Gently clean the walls of each canal, do not shape the canals, as this will remove too much dentine and risk perforation.

14. Dry canals with measured paper points.

15. Obturate each canal with a resorbable, slow-setting paste such as pure zinc oxide powder mixed with eugenol or calcium hydroxide – iodoform paste such as Vitapex. This can be spun down with spiral paste fillers or packed down (if of a firm consistency) with paper points.

16. Take a radiograph to check the obturation.

17. Place a well-sealed definitive restoration such as a preformed metal crown.

The two visit pulpectomy (necrotic pulps with or without peri radicular infection)

Visit 1

◆ Same as above (steps 1–13).

◆ Dress with non-setting calcium hydroxide, or a calcium hydroxide–iodoform paste for 7–14 days.

◆ Place a well-sealed temporary restoration such as glass-ionomer.

Visit 2

◆ If at the subsequent visit, the tooth has been symptom-free and there are signs of healing:

◆ Remove all dressings from the tooth.

◆ Follow the steps described in 15–17 in the previous section.

Underpinning knowledge

The student should have an understanding of:

◆ The two different approaches to pulpectomy depend on the radicular pulp status.

◆ The need for preoperative radiographs to estimate working lengths.

◆ The importance of endodontic files remaining 2 mm from the radiographic apex to safeguard the underlying tooth germ.

◆ The reasons for using small endodontic files.

◆ The need for radiographs to confirm the position of the file in the root canal.

◆ The importance of gently cleaning the canal walls via instrumentation and that no shaping is attempted.

◆ The benefits of using (0.5–1% sodium hypochlorite solution) as a canal irrigant.

◆ The importance of obturating with a material that will resorb as the root undergoes physiological resorption e.g. slow-setting pure zinc oxide powder mixed with eugenol liquid, or a calcium hydroxide–iodoform paste.

◆ The need to provide regular clinical and radiographic review.

Monitoring

Be competent at analysing failures to minimize future complications.

Clinical and radiographic review following pulp therapy is essential. The student should be able to:

◆ Undertake regular clinical and radiographic review of teeth that have been treated with some form of pulp therapy.

◆ Accurately assess the status of the tooth and its surrounding structures.

◆ Be familiar with documented possible unwanted sequelae to pulpotomy/pulpectomy:
  ■ Delayed exfoliation
  ■ Early exfoliation
  ■ Pathological resorption of primary tooth
  ■ Developmental enamel defects in permanent successor
  ■ Ectopic eruption defects in permanent successor.

Recognize a successful treatment by the absence of:

◆ Soft tissue pathology:
  ■ Tenderness
  ■ Swelling
  ■ Sinus formation.

◆ Periradicular pathology:
  ■ Periapical radiolucency
  ■ Furcal radiolucency
  ■ Pathological resorption (internal and external).

◆ Leaking coronal restoration.

References and further reading

Falster C. A., Araujo F. B., Straffon L. H. and Nor J. E. (2002) Indirect pulp treatment: *in vivo* outcomes of an adhesive resin system vs calcium hydroxide for protection of the dentin-pulp complex. *Pediatric Dentistry* 24, 241–8.

Farooq N. S., Coll J. A., Kuwabara A. and Shelton P. (2000) Success rates of formocresol pulpotomy and indirect pulp treatment in the treatment of deep dentinal caries in primary teeth. *Pediatric Dentistry* 22, 278–86.

GDC (2002) *The First Five Years: a framework for undergraduate dental education*, 2nd edn. London, The General Dental Council.

Ibricevic H. and Al-Jame Q. (2003) Ferric sulphate and formocresol in pulpotomy of primary molars: long term follow-up study. *European Journal of Paediatric Dentistry* 4, 28–32.

International Agency for Research on cancer. Press Release no. 153 15 June 2004. Available at http://www.iarc.fr.pageroot/PRELEASES/pr153a. html accessed on 27 August 2004.

Llewelyn D. R. (2000) The Pulp of the Primary Dentition – UK National Clinical Guidelines in Paediatric Dentistry. *Int J Paed Dent* 10, 248–52.

Loh A., O'Hoy P., Tran X., Charles R., Hughes A., Kubo K. and Messer L. B. (2004) Evidence-based assessment: evaluation of the formocresol versus ferric sulfate primary molar pulpotomy. *Pediatric Dentistry* 26, 401–9.

Maguire A., Davenport E. S. and Craig S. A. (2004) Intended learning outcomes for undergraduate training in paediatric dentistry. *Int J Paed Dent* 14, 223–9.

Mortazavi M. and Mesbahi M. (2004) Comparison of zinc oxide and eugenol, and Vitapex for root canal treatment of necrotic primary teeth. *Int J Paed Dent* 14, 417–24.

Nadin G., Goel B. R., Yeung C. A. and Gleny A. M. (2003) Pulp treatment for extensive decay in primary teeth. *Cochrane Database Systematic Review* (1) CD003220.

O'Brien M. (1994) *Children's Dental Health in the United Kingdom 1993*. London, HMSO.

QAA (2002) *Dentistry: academic standards*. Subject benchmark statements. Gloucester; Quality Assurance Agency for Higher Education.

Seow W. K. and Thong Y. H. (1993) Evaluation of the anti-inflammatory agent tetrandine as a pulpotomy medicament in a canine model. *Pediatric Dentistry* 15, 259–66.

Waterhouse P. J., Nunn J. H. and Whitworth J. M. (2000) An investigation of the relative efficacy of Buckley's Formocresol and calcium hydroxide in primary molar vital pulp therapy. *Br Dent J* 188, 32–6.

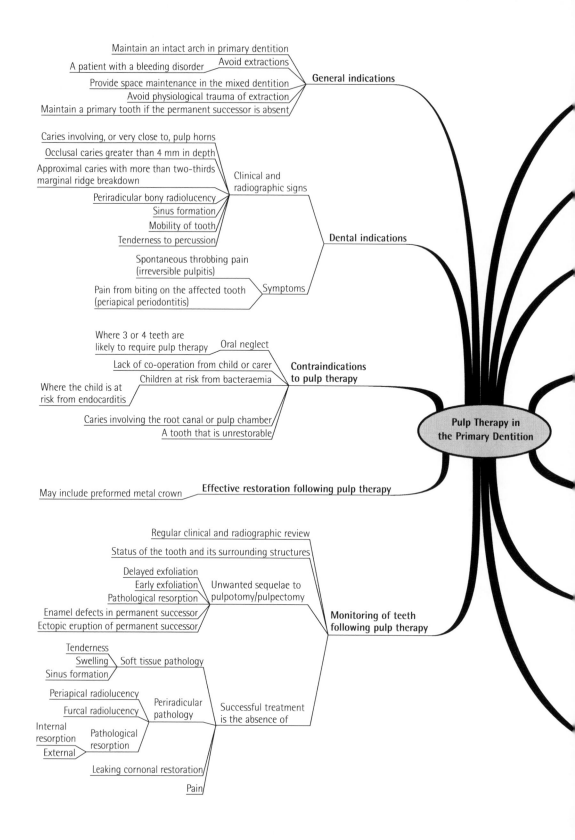

Maintain an intact arch in primary dentition
A patient with a bleeding disorder — Avoid extractions
Provide space maintenance in the mixed dentition
Avoid physiological trauma of extraction
Maintain a primary tooth if the permanent successor is absent

General indications

Caries involving, or very close to, pulp horns
Occlusal caries greater than 4 mm in depth
Approximal caries with more than two-thirds marginal ridge breakdown — Clinical and radiographic signs
Periradicular bony radiolucency
Sinus formation
Mobility of tooth
Tenderness to percussion

Dental indications

Spontaneous throbbing pain (irreversible pulpitis)
Pain from biting on the affected tooth (periapical periodontitis) — Symptoms

Where 3 or 4 teeth are likely to require pulp therapy — Oral neglect
Lack of co-operation from child or carer
Children at risk from bacteraemia
Where the child is at risk from endocarditis
Caries involving the root canal or pulp chamber
A tooth that is unrestorable

Contraindications to pulp therapy

May include preformed metal crown — **Effective restoration following pulp therapy**

Pulp Therapy in the Primary Dentition

Regular clinical and radiographic review
Status of the tooth and its surrounding structures
Delayed exfoliation
Early exfoliation
Pathological resorption — Unwanted sequelae to pulpotomy/pulpectomy
Enamel defects in permanent successor
Ectopic eruption of permanent successor

Monitoring of teeth following pulp therapy

Tenderness
Swelling — Soft tissue pathology
Sinus formation
Periapical radiolucency
Furcal radiolucency — Periradicular pathology
Internal resorption — Pathological resorption
External — Successful treatment is the absence of
Leaking cornonal restoration
Pain

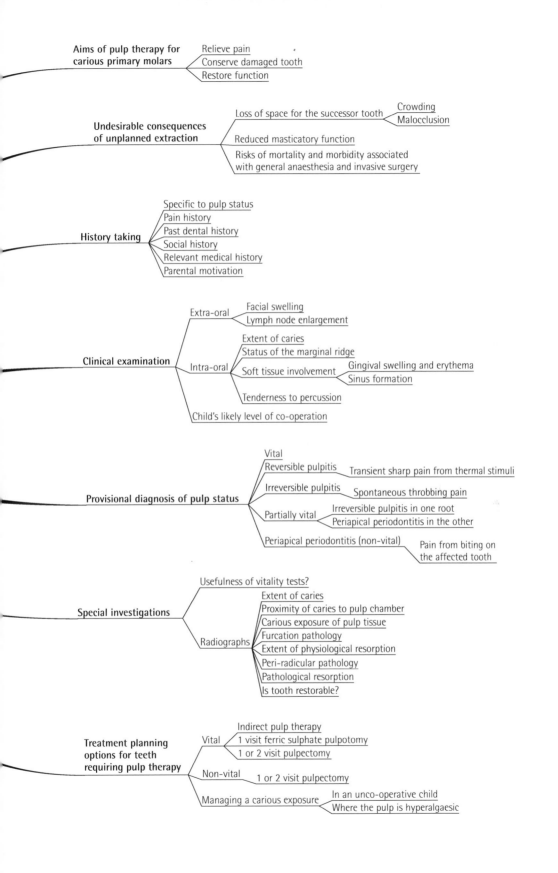

Aims of pulp therapy for carious primary molars
- Relieve pain
- Conserve damaged tooth
- Restore function

Undesirable consequences of unplanned extraction
- Loss of space for the successor tooth
  - Crowding
  - Malocclusion
- Reduced masticatory function
- Risks of mortality and morbidity associated with general anaesthesia and invasive surgery

History taking
- Specific to pulp status
- Pain history
- Past dental history
- Social history
- Relevant medical history
- Parental motivation

Clinical examination
- Extra-oral
  - Facial swelling
  - Lymph node enlargement
- Intra-oral
  - Extent of caries
  - Status of the marginal ridge
  - Soft tissue involvement
    - Gingival swelling and erythema
    - Sinus formation
  - Tenderness to percussion
- Child's likely level of co-operation

Provisional diagnosis of pulp status
- Vital
- Reversible pulpitis — Transient sharp pain from thermal stimuli
- Irreversible pulpitis — Spontaneous throbbing pain
- Partially vital
  - Irreversible pulpitis in one root
  - Periapical periodontitis in the other
- Periapical periodontitis (non-vital) — Pain from biting on the affected tooth

Special investigations
- Usefulness of vitality tests?
- Radiographs
  - Extent of caries
  - Proximity of caries to pulp chamber
  - Carious exposure of pulp tissue
  - Furcation pathology
  - Extent of physiological resorption
  - Peri-radicular pathology
  - Pathological resorption
  - Is tooth restorable?

Treatment planning options for teeth requiring pulp therapy
- Vital
  - Indirect pulp therapy
  - 1 visit ferric sulphate pulpotomy
  - 1 or 2 visit pulpectomy
- Non-vital
  - 1 or 2 visit pulpectomy
- Managing a carious exposure
  - In an unco-operative child
  - Where the pulp is hyperalgaesic

2.1c Paediatric dentistry
Dental trauma
Dafydd Evans

Key points

- The graduating dentist should demonstrate a knowledge base of dental trauma and its management sufficient to ensure that, when combined with competency in basic generic skills, patients attending with dental trauma will receive appropriate treatment.

- These basic generic skills will include taking a history, conducting an examination (including dental pulp vitality assessment), basic dento-alveolar surgical techniques, and the clinical application of composite materials and removable prosthodontics.

- The graduating dentist should also demonstrate a broad knowledge base of the long-term management of patients who have had dental trauma, including appropriate timing of endodontic procedures, and the restorative and orthodontic options for managing a traumatized dentition.

Introduction

Dental trauma in childhood is common, with around 16 per cent of 15-year-old boys and 10 per cent of 15-year-old girls showing some evidence of traumatic injury of their anterior teeth (Office for National Statistics 2004). The consequences of traumatic injury can range from being insignificant through to the loss of the tooth, as either an immediate or delayed effect of the trauma. In fact, trauma is the most common cause of loss of permanent anterior teeth in childhood.

Effective immediate management of dental injuries can significantly improve the prognosis of the teeth affected. However, although the prevalence of dental injuries is high, their relatively low incidence means that it is unlikely the average dental student will manage sufficient cases of dental trauma to achieve competence while an undergraduate. *The First Five Years* (GDC 2002) limits the specific learning outcomes for the management of dental trauma to aknowledge base. However, the competentices relating to this area that might be expected of the dental graduate are elaborated on below, according to the GDC's terminology of competence at, knowlede of and familiraity with.

> ... have knowledge of the management of trauma in both dentitions
>
> General Dental Council (2002, Paragraph 90)

The Dentistry Benchmarking Statement (QAA, 2002), however, does refer to competencies. It states that the dental graduate must have the competency to:

> ... identify and manage dental emergencies and appropriately refer those that are beyond the scope of management by a primary care dentist.
>
> QAA for Higher Education (2002, Paragraph 3.12)

Nevertheless, patients have the right to expect competent initial management of dental trauma by their general practitioners, and appropriate referral facilities for secondary care might not always be available. Fortunately, most of the skills required to manage dental trauma are generic, and will already be included within the skill mix of most clinicians. A well-founded knowledge base should, therefore, be sufficient for most clinicians to manage most dental trauma competently.

Intended learning outcomes

The intended learning outcomes for management of dental trauma in *The First Five Years* (GDC 2002, paragraph 111, states are summarized in Table 2.1c.1).

The competencies that are expected of the dental graduate (outlined in Table 2.1c.1) are elaborated on below, according to the GDC's terminology of competence at, knowledge of and familiarity with specific areas.

The graduate should be competent at

1. History taking and examination of the patient, with specific reference to consideration of the following:
   - the ordering and interpretation of appropriate radiographs
   - investigation of the possibility of
     - cerebral trauma
     - fractures of the facial bones
     - soft tissue inclusions
     - non-accidental injury (Welbury 2005).
2. Fabricating a splint to retain displaced teeth using orthodontic wire. Students should be competent in bending up a passive labial arch wire extending from 3–3. (See **Checklist 32**)

Table 2.1c.1 Intended learning outcomes for dental trauma

Be competent at	Have knowledge of	Be familiar with
History taking and examination of the patient with dental trauma	The diagnosis and management, both immediate and follow-up, of dental injuries involving enamel, dentine or root	Restorative options for the traumatized or missing incisor, including tooth bleaching and implants
The ordering and interpretation of appropriate radiographs	The diagnosis and management, both immediate and follow-up, of dento-alveolar injuries	
Investigation of the possibility of cerebral trauma, fractures of the facial bones, soft tissue inclusions, non-accidental injury	How the management may differ depending on dental medical and patient factors	
Fabricating a splint to retain displaced teeth using orthodontic wire	The rationale and methodology of the pulpotomy procedure for a traumatized permanent incisor with pulpal exposure	
The vitality assessment of anterior teeth	The indications for root canal therapy in the traumatized incisor	
Placement of an acid-etched retained composite restoration involving the incisal edge of an anterior tooth	The management of the non-vital incisor with immature root formation	

3. The vitality assessment of anterior teeth (see **Checklist 33**). Students should be able to apply, interpret and understand the limitations of the following vitality tests:

   ◆ History of symptoms

   ◆ Colour

   ◆ Transillumination

   ◆ Tenderness to percussion

   ◆ Mobility

- Ethyl chloride
- Electric pulp test
- Assessment of alveolus for a) sinus b) erythema/ tenderness
- Radiographic assessment for a) periapical area b) arrested root growth c) inflammatory root resorption.

4. The placement of an acid-etched retained composite restoration involving the incisal edge of an anterior tooth (**Checklist 34**).

The graduate should have knowledge of

1. The diagnosis and management, both immediate and follow-up, of the four main categories of dental injuries:
   - enamel fracture
   - enamel/dentine fracture
   - enamel/dentine fracture with pulp exposure
   - root fracture.

2. The diagnosis and management, both immediate and follow-up, of the four main categories of dento-alveolar injuries:
   - concussion
   - loosening (subluxation)
   - displacement (luxation)
   - avulsion.

3. How the management may differ depending on (a) whether the primary or permanent dentition is affected, (b) the medical history, (c) the patient's ability to accept treatment.

4. The rationale and methodology of the pulpotomy procedure for a traumatized permanent incisor with pulpal exposure.

5. The appropriate storage and subsequent management of an avulsed permanent incisor, including methods of space maintenance if the tooth cannot be replanted.

6. The indications for root canal therapy in the traumatized incisor.

7. The management of the non-vital incisor with immature root formation

The graduate should be familiar with

1. Restorative options for the traumatized or missing incisor, including tooth bleaching and implants.

Checklist 32 **Splinting of anterior teeth**

The student is asked to select an appropriate wire, and bend up a splint extending from upper 3 to 3, using a colleague as a patient.

	Yes	No
Student explains to patient what they will be doing		
Patient is placed in appropriate position; supine, with safety glasses and a bib		
Student maintains optimum position while carrying out procedure; spine straight, feet on floor, elbows by side		
Student observes infection control protocol throughout procedure		
Student selects correct wire		
Bends archwire so that it extends to cover the teeth indicated		
Archwire is passive		
Archwire is contoured so that it is no more than 2 mm above the labial surface of the tooth		
Archwire is safe ended		
Student advises patient on plaque control, and prescribes chlorhexidene mouthwash		
Student offers to make patient appointment in two weeks' time for splint removal		
Student disposes of offcuts of wire in sharps bin		

Checklist 33 **Vitality assessment of anterior teeth**

	Yes	No
Student explains to patient what they will be doing		
Patient is placed in appropriate position; supine, with safety glasses and a bib		
Student maintains optimum position while carrying out procedure; spine straight, feet on floor, elbows by side		
Student observes infection control protocol throughout procedure		
Asks the patient if they have had any pain or discomfort from their anterior teeth		

Checklist 33 **Vitality assessment of anterior teeth** – *continued*

The student is asked to assess the vitality of the anterior teeth of a patient, or a colleague, and to record the results. The student should be observed providing the following tests.

	Yes	No
Assesses labial alveolus visually for sinus		
Manually palpates labial alveolus for tenderness		
Checks mobility of teeth digitally using their finger and the handle of an instrument		
Checks all anterior teeth for tenderness to percussion, using appropriate force, and giving patient appropriate information as to what the test involves and what their required response is		
Tests anterior teeth using ethyl chloride, taking care that the gingivae are not included in the test, and giving patient appropriate information as to what the test involves and what their required response is		
Tests anterior teeth using an electric pulp tester, drying the teeth, and placing the probe on the incisal edge of the tooth, and giving patient appropriate information as to what the test involves and what their required response is		
Assesses the colour of the crowns directly		
Uses transillumination to assess the colour of the crowns, placing the mirror at the back of the mouth and using the overhead light		
Records the information appropriately		

Adjunctive assessment of radiographs

The student is shown six radiographs, three of which are pathology-free, and one case each of: periapical area, arrested root growth and inflammatory root resorption.

	Yes	No
Student identifies periapical area		
Student identifies arrested root growth		
Student identifies inflammatory root resorption		

Checklist 34 **Placing an acid-etched retained composite tip on an anterior tooth**

The student is asked to place an acid etch retained composite restoration to restore the incisal edge of a traumatized permanent incisor. The student should be observed providing the following:

	Yes	No
Student explains to patient what they will be doing		
Patient is placed in appropriate position; supine, with safety glasses and a bib		
Student maintains optimum position while carrying out procedure; spine straight, feet on floor, elbows by side		
Student observes infection control protocol throughout procedure		
Local anaesthesia given, if necessary		
Tooth cleaned with pumice		
Tooth isolation, with rubber dam or cotton wool rolls as appropriate		
Lining material placed, if necessary		
Etchant applied appropriately (not passed over patient's face; applied just to tooth being restored; applied for correct length of time; rinsed off with consideration)		
Tooth dried appropriately, with relevant areas clearly dry and frosty in appearance		
Bonding agent applied and cured (with no excessive pooling in gingival sulcus)		
Composite applied and cured as appropriate for restorative system		
Final restoration is satisfactory in:		
• Shape (length, width and contours match patients dentition)		
• Colour		
• Surface (no air blows, margins from incremental additions, acceptable polish)		
• Margins (checks for overhangs with floss, correcting if necessary)		
• Occlusion (occlusion checked, and adjusted if necessary)		

References and further reading

GDC (2002) *The First Five Years: a framework for undergraduate dental education*, 2nd edn. London, The General Dental Council.

Lader I. D. *et al.* (2004) *Children's Dental Health in the United Kingdom 2003*. London, Office for National Statistics. Available at:
http://www.statistics.gov.uk/CHILDREN/dentalhealth/downloads/cdh_non-carious_dental_decay.pdf

QAA (2002) *Dentistry: academic standards.* Subject benchmark statements. Gloucester, Quality Assurance Agency for Higher Education.

Welbury R. R. (ed.) (2005) *Paediatric Dentistry*, 3rd edn. Oxford, Oxford University Press.

In cases of suspected child abuse:

What To Do If You're Worried A Child Is Being Abused (31553), Department of Health Publications, PO Box 777, London SE1 6XH, E-mail: doh@prolog.uk.com

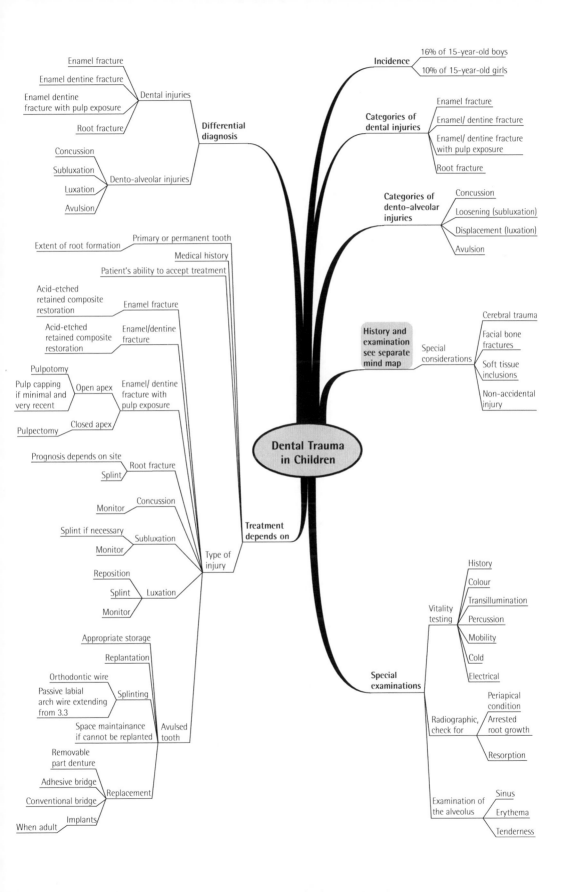

Dental Trauma in Children

Differential diagnosis

Dental injuries
- Enamel fracture
- Enamel dentine fracture
- Enamel dentine fracture with pulp exposure
- Root fracture

Dento-alveolar injuries
- Concussion
- Subluxation
- Luxation
- Avulsion

Incidence
- 16% of 15-year-old boys
- 10% of 15-year-old girls

Categories of dental injuries
- Enamel fracture
- Enamel/ dentine fracture
- Enamel/ dentine fracture with pulp exposure
- Root fracture

Categories of dento-alveolar injuries
- Concussion
- Loosening (subluxation)
- Displacement (luxation)
- Avulsion

History and examination see separate mind map

Special considerations
- Cerebral trauma
- Facial bone fractures
- Soft tissue inclusions
- Non-accidental injury

Treatment depends on

- Primary or permanent tooth
- Extent of root formation
- Medical history
- Patient's ability to accept treatment

Type of injury
- Enamel fracture — Acid-etched retained composite restoration
- Enamel/dentine fracture — Acid-etched retained composite restoration
- Enamel/ dentine fracture with pulp exposure
  - Open apex
    - Pulpotomy
    - Pulp capping if minimal and very recent
  - Closed apex — Pulpectomy
- Root fracture
  - Prognosis depends on site
  - Splint
- Concussion — Monitor
- Subluxation
  - Splint if necessary
  - Monitor
- Luxation
  - Reposition
  - Splint
  - Monitor
- Avulsed tooth
  - Replantation — Appropriate storage
  - Splinting
    - Orthodontic wire
    - Passive labial arch wire extending from 3.3
  - Space maintainance if cannot be replanted
  - Replacement
    - Removable part denture
    - Adhesive bridge
    - Conventional bridge
    - Implants
    - When adult

Special examinations

Vitality testing
- History
- Colour
- Transillumination
- Percussion
- Mobility
- Cold
- Electrical

Radiographic, check for
- Periapical condition
- Arrested root growth
- Resorption

Examination of the alveolus
- Sinus
- Erythema
- Tenderness

2.2 Special care dentistry

June Nunn

Key points

Dental graduates:

- Should recognize their duty of care to manage the oral health of the patient with special needs.

- Understand that this may include management of the dental health care needs of those who have impairments or disabilities and those who may be socially excluded.

- Must be able to identify and distinguish patients who can be treated within the practice setting and those who require referral.

- Should be familiar with the legislative and biopsychosocial issues allowing the qualifying dentist to have an understanding appropriate to patients' needs.

- Should be aware of the multidisciplinary care considerations within and outside the dental team and involve the patient's carer where appropriate.

Introduction

Special care dentistry is the branch of dentistry that aims to secure and maintain the oral and dental health of, and enhance the quality of life for, people with impairments where an inter-professional approach, supported by appropriate behaviour management techniques, is required to deliver efficacious and effective care in a holistic way.

To define what is meant by impairment and disability is important:

- *Impairment*: is the functional limitation within the individual caused by physical, mental or sensory impairment.

- *Disability*: is the loss or limitation of opportunities to take part in the normal life of the community on an equal level with others due to physical, social and attitudinal barriers.

At its simplest, not being able to walk is an impairment but not being able to get into a dental surgery because of the steps up into the building is a disability (Watson 2000).

The General Dental Council's document *The First Five Years* (GDC 2002) does not make any specific reference to dental care in special needs patients, but this is implied in many generic statements referring to the duty of care, awareness of physical, medical, social and psychological aspects of dental care.

People who may come within the remit of special care dentistry include, for example, those:

- with moderate to profound learning disabilities
- who have physical impairments such as cerebral palsy, spina bifida
- who have Parkinson's disease, rheumatoid arthritis, multiple sclerosis
- who have significant medical compromise, perhaps in addition to a physical or learning impairment, for example autoimmune disease, heart defects, poorly controlled systemic disease like epilepsy
- with sensory impairments, alone or in addition to other impairments
- who are marginalized for oral and dental care because of lifestyle factors like addiction, homelessness, alone or in combination.

The Dentistry Benchmarking Statements (QAA 2002) stated that qualifying dentists must have:

1. Knowledge and understanding of:
   - The oral health needs of different sections of the community, such as those with special needs (paragraph 2.18).

2. Skills and attributes to:
   - Analyse and resolve problems, deal with uncertainty and make decisions based on sound ethical, moral and scientific principles (paragraph 3.1).

3. Through a professional approach, be able to:
   - Provide empathetic care for all patients, including members of diverse and vulnerable populations and respect the principle of patient autonomy (paragraph 3.2).

4. And specifically, under establishment and maintenance of a healthy oral environment, to:
   - recognize their duty of care to manage the oral health of the patient with special needs (including the additional considerations for the dental team) and involve the patient's carer where appropriate; and
   - manage the dental health care needs of those who may be considered to be 'socially excluded' (paragraph 3.22).

People with impairments fall broadly into two groups: those for whom oral and dental disease and/or its treatment may impose a significant disability; for example, the person with brain injury who is profoundly intellectually and physically impaired. A second group, whose oral and dental status as a consequence of an underlying defect, is different and dentally challenging; for example, the person with a syndrome that encompasses a dental defect, such as people with epidermolysis bullosa or the young person with a cleft palate.

In the former group, the oral and dental needs of the person may be relatively routine, but the barriers faced in accessing and receiving care may be such as to have precluded that person from regular dental care, largely because of lack of knowledge and experience on the part of the primary dental care team. However, such persons should be seen as a priority since dental disease, or indeed its treatment, may impose further impairments.

The second group of people have significant dental anomalies, often in addition to an underlying defect, which require multi-professional help with good co-ordination to ensure that appropriate and timely care is delivered.

For a proportion of people with impairments, oral and dental care will need to be provided within a hospital setting, so-called secondary or tertiary care, depending on the level of sophistication of services required. However, much of the basic dental needs of many people with impairments can be effectively and efficiently delivered by practitioners within the community, within primary care.

An essential skill for the dental graduate therefore should be as follows:

Be able to recognize their duty of care in the attainment of achievable treatment outcomes for patients with specific medical, physical or mental health problems and to know the appropriate pathways for referral of patients whom they are unable to treat or who require further assessment.

(Thompson et al. 2001)

Unlike most other branches of dentistry, with the exception of paediatric dentistry, the role of, and reliance on, family and carers in delivering dental care, as well as support at home, is vital.

Competencies, knowledge and familiarity

In the context of special care dentistry, these are presented in a sequence appropriate to the gradual acquisition of knowledge and skills by the student:

- Disability awareness, for example, recognize person first, impairment second; communication; teamworking; empathy; managing a complaint;

- Ethics – aspects of consent; confidentiality; giving bad news; awareness of potential for abuse (see Chapter 1.2);

- Legislation principally the Disability Discrimination Act (DDA); Human Rights Act; health and safety legislation; General Dental Council and Department of Health Guidance on conscious sedation and general anaesthesia; safe handling and moving, clinical governance; audit; evidence-based care, critical appraisal, teamwork, professionalism; life-long learning;

- Public health aspects, which centre on provision of services; domiciliary care; other agencies; health economics; health promotion, risk management (see Chapter 1.6);

- Eliciting a history and undertaking an examination to decide a diagnosis, treatment plan and appropriate care pathway for a person with an impairment (see Chapter 1.1);
- Types of impairments including general considerations, dental implications, how to access information, patient support groups;
- Management of specific issues arising out of impairment such as cooperation, communication, physical limitations, clinical – disease risk, feeding problems, drooling and xerostomia, self-mutilation. Prevention of oral and dental disease in conjunction with dieticians, speech therapists and other relevant professionals.

Those aspects not dealt with in the Section 1 Chapters referred to above are detailed below. Using and integrating information from *The First Five Years* (GDC 2002) and the QAA benchmarking documents (QAA 2002), the intended learning outcomes for identification and treatment of patients with special needs are summarized below.

Learning outcome 1: disability awareness

The dental graduate should:

- Be able to acknowledge the person first and the impairment second
- Demonstrate skills in empathetic listening
- Demonstrate positive attitudes towards diversity
- Be able to recognize barriers to communication and how to manage these
- Have the knowledge to make referrals to other professional and support groups
- Demonstrate leadership qualities for team management
- Be a role model in terms of attitudes towards people with disabilities
- Show initiative in involving other agencies
- Respond positively to stress
- Be able to deal with complaints/unreasonable expectations from patients and/or carers.

Learning outcome 2: legislation

The dental graduate should:

- Be familiar with the principles of the Disability Discrimination Act, Human Rights Act and associated legislation
- Be able to interpret the meaning of the Acts as they apply to dental practice
- Know what benefits a person is entitled
- Have an awareness of the way in which the Equal Opportunities legislation affects dental practice

Table 2.2.1 Essential skills with regard to disability awareness

Subject matter	Be competent at	Have knowledge of	Be familiar with
People first, impairment later	Greeting the person; sensitivity towards the wishes of the person	Impaired people's wishes to be recognized; acknowledging difference; range in presentation of disability	Psychological impact of impairment
Communication	Recognizing communication needs and organizing appropriate help Recognizing the role of the carer	Different communication aids e.g. Makaton	Sophisticated methods of communicating with people with impairments
Barriers	Methods to reduce physical barriers; ability to recognize and counter discrimination	Recognition of physical and attitudinal barriers; ways in which society makes an impairment a disability	Political imperatives to remove barriers
Demonstrate empathy	Recognition of need for empathetic approach	Skills required to be empathetic	Managing a situation requiring empathy
Managing a complaint/ different expectations	Recognize complaint for what it is; acknowledge complainant's distress and upset; gather facts	Techniques to diffuse a difficult situation	Sensitivity required to manage unrealistic expectations and dealing with frustrations
Role of team work	Role of team members in providing care for people with disabilities	Roles of the extended interprofessional team	Agencies and support groups involved in disabilities

Checklist 35 **For disability awareness**

Disability awareness	Yes	No
Introduces him/herself as well as team member(s) to patient and carer		
Positions him/herself to facilitate communication with the patient		
Speaks with patient first, carers involved later and with consent of patient		
Ascertain reason(s) for visit and any problems encountered		
Acknowledge anxieties about care with constructive reassurance		
Deal with unrealistic expectations sensitively and make positive alternative suggestions		
Be willing to refer for second opinion if indicated and if this will be an appropriate use of resources		
Ascertain other relevant people to be involved in decision-making (e.g. social workers, parents)		
Gather facts of a complaint with empathy and detail action to be taken to manage the investigation of the complaint		
Document the interview, concisely and legibly in the patient's record		

Assessment: Direct observation of interview with person with a disability and a carer.

- ◆ Know how to recognize and manage discrimination and prejudice in relation to disability
- ◆ Be able to identify barriers – physical and attitudinal – to disability and the way in which they can be avoided, minimized, prevented
- ◆ Know how to access information and update themselves on current, relevant legislation.

Safe handling and moving

The dental graduate should:
- ◆ Be able to carry out a risk assessment prior to care of a disabled patient
- ◆ Be familiar with safe moving and handling techniques of compromised patients
- ◆ Know of their responsibilities towards training in manual handling skills of members of the dental team
- ◆ Be aware of the aids to facilitate patient movement and comfort whilst under dental care

Table 2.2.2 Essential skills with regard to legislation

Subject matter	Be competent at	Have knowledge of	Be familiar with
Disability Discrimination Act	Recognizing the way in which the dentist has to address the requirements of the legislation	Relevant sections of the legislation for dental practice; know how to access information on relevant legislation;	The DDA and Human Rights Acts
Human Rights Act			
Health and safety legislation		Know how to access information on relevant disability benefits	
Equal opportunities			
State disability benefits			
Safe handling and moving	Safe handling of patients as part of a team; positioning the disabled patient, with appropriate aids, to ensure comfort during treatment	Safe movement of compromised patients; ergonomic design features for a dental clinic/domiciliary care; resources for facilitating disabled patient care	Manual Handling Regulations 1994; how to access training for dental team; the need to set up protocols for safe handling

Checklist 36 **For safe handling and moving**

Safe handling and moving	Yes	No
Complete a checklist for a risk assessment in a similar manner to non-disabled people but to include consideration of:		
• Safe access to treatment facility		
• Appropriate physical accommodation for people with disabilities		
• Safety of patient, staff and other patients in relation to cross-infection control issues e.g. MRSA status		
• Safe moving and handling of patients		
• Need for physical intervention ('restraints')		
• Risks of adjuncts, for example, sedation and patient's ASA grade		
• Interactions between prescribed drugs and patient's medication, for example, warfarin and anti-microbial therapy		

Checklist 36 **For safe handling and moving** – *continued*

Safe handling and moving	Yes	No
Describe aids and adjuncts to facilitate dental care for a patient with a disability:		
• learning disability		
• physically impaired		
• wheelchair aided		
• visual/hearing impairment		
• aged patient after a CVA		
• communication (speech) impaired		

Assessment: discussion with student after observation of a video of patient treatment scenario

Learning outcome 3: understanding of impairments

Impairments – general

The dental graduate should:

♦ Demonstrate a positive attitude to the person with an impairment

♦ Know about the commoner impairments seen in primary dental care

♦ Be knowledgeable about the impairment in general terms.

Information retrieval

The dental graduate should:

♦ Know where to obtain further information about different impairment types

♦ Be able to locate resources, including patient support groups, equipment, materials.

Impairments – dental

The dental graduate should:

♦ Be able to predict the dental conditions and anomalies associated with the commonly presenting impairments for example, delayed eruption, periodontal disease, microdontia/hypodontia in Down syndrome

♦ Be able to discuss the management of such dental conditions with patients and/or carers

♦ Be able to write a succinct, pertinent letter of referral (see Chapter 1.13).

Understanding impairment and oral/dental aspects

Table 2.2.3 Essential skills with regard to understanding of impairments

Subject matter	Be competent at	Have knowledge of	Be familiar with
Impairments: general	Displaying positive attitude towards person with impairment; distinguishing the features of more common impairments; relating the impairment with relevant oral/dental features	A range of impairments; the potential for impairments to be multiple; the way in which beliefs and attitudes impose/reduce barriers	Epidemiology of commoner impairments, likely to be seen in dental practice; discrimination legislation
Information retrieval	Searching out relevant information on impairment and disability; setting up a database of patients with impairments under care for audit and research purposes	Resources and electronic databases for information on impairments and services	Local resources and support groups for the different disability groups
Impairments: dental	Referring to secondary care when unfamiliar oral/dental conditions and/or anomalies encountered; writing a letter of referral	Conditions, habits or specific oral/dental features seen in the commoner impairments	Management of more complex oral/dental features seen specifically with some types of impairments for example, drooling in cerebral palsy

Checklist 37 **For understanding impairment**

Understanding impairment	Yes	No
Able to itemize main features of impairments found in patients from clinical portfolio case load		
Able to discuss patient abilities and barriers faced		

Checklist 37 **For understanding impairment** *– continued*

Understanding impairment	Yes	No
Able to discuss related oral/dental features, where relevant, of the impairment for example, tooth anomalies, ectopic eruption in young people with a cleft palate		
Able to describe and demonstrate suitable sources of information e.g. websites, companies for oral hygiene aids		
Write a letter of referral to a specialist/consultant		

Assessment: Interview with clinical portfolio

Write a referral letter (Chapter 1.13)

Learning outcome 4: management of oral/dental conditions seen with impairments

Oral and dental disease

The dental graduate should:

♦ Know the differing prevalence of oral diseases and conditions in people with disabilities and the reasons for these differences

♦ Be able to provide basic dental care for all non-challenging people with disabilities, for example, people with well-controlled epilepsy, patients with congenital heart defects requiring standard antibiotic prophylaxis

♦ Know where to refer patients' whose needs are beyond their experience and skills.

Co-operation and behaviour management

The dental graduate should:

♦ Be familiar with adjuncts to enable the safe and effective delivery of care

♦ Have some hands-on experience of providing dental care under conscious sedation as operator-sedationist under supervision

♦ Be aware of the need for additional training in order to employ such adjuncts in primary care

♦ Know the responsibilities of the dental team in providing care under conscious sedation

♦ Be practised in basic life support and regularly updated.

Preventive dental care

The dental graduate should:

♦ Be able to undertake a risk assessment, and be able to decide the most appropriate preventive protocol for a patient with a disability (see Chapter 1.12).

Table 2.2.4 Essential skills with regard to management of oral/dental conditions seen with impairments

Subject matter	Be competent at	Have knowledge of	Be familiar with
Dental conditions	Diagnosing and managing caries in people with disabilities, by routine methods	Novel methods of caries management; aids and techniques to help with caries treatment and oral hygiene; indices to monitor oral/dental health	Epidemiology of dental caries and periodontal disease in disabled people; investigations required for rapid, advanced toothwear
	Managing periodontal disease in non-challenging patients and instructing carers in oral hygiene options for home care	Need for interprofessional care for some conditions	
	Discriminate between different types of toothwear and relate to aetiology, for example GORD in patients with cerebral palsy, in order to manage appropriately		
Self-inflicted trauma	Recognize the condition, its aetiology and refer appropriately for management	Treatment options; role of primary dental care practitioner in reviews	Outcomes of treatment and sequelae
Drooling and xerostomia	Recognize the conditions and be able to discuss, in outline, the options for management; referral for specialist help	Treatment options, sequelae of treatment; facilities for secondary care	Evidence base for management; best evidence; management protocols

Table 2.2.4 Essential skills with regard to management of oral/dental conditions seen with impairments – *continued*

Subject matter	Be competent at	Have knowledge of	Be familiar with
Malocclusion	Recognition of need for treatment; discussing in outline the options for care and organizing interceptive care as required with advice on assistance with oral hygiene if patient has physical impairment	Appliances used in treatment; timescale of active care, retention; managing orthodontic emergencies; adjuncts required during treatment.	Appliance philosophy and rationales; practical mechanics of fixed appliances
Co-operation and behaviour management	Basic behaviour management skills; recognize limitation of skills and patient's need for adjuncts; obtaining valid and appropriate consent for procedures under conscious sedation and GA for people with disabilities	Options available to manage poor co-operation and other behavioural problems; scope and limitations of conscious sedation; practical application of IV and inhalation sedation; need for additional training and experience in conscious sedation techniques	Familiar with the role of general anaesthesia (GA) as an adjunct to care for disabled people; roles of the dental team in providing care under conscious sedation for people with disabilities
Preventive care	Prescribing appropriate preventive care plans for high-risk patients; writing a prescription	Protocols for preventive care for people with disabilities; risk assessment; toxic doses of fluoride agents Sources for dental health education material dependant on disability type	Arguments pro and con fluoridation; setting priorities in terms of patient groups

Table 2.2.4 Essential skills with regard to management of oral/dental conditions seen with impairments – *continued*

Subject matter	Be competent at	Have knowledge of	Be familiar with
Dental trauma	Provide emergency care and make arrangements for appropriate follow-up mindful of the patient's underlying condition, for example, a Down syndrome patient with complex cyanotic heart disease	Knowledge of factors affecting prognosis and medium to long-term treatment options	Ethical, moral and pragmatic treatment planning issues for family/carers in relation to prostheses, for example, in a patient with uncontrolled seizures

References and further reading

British Society for Disability and Oral health Guidelines are available on the website: www.bsdh.org.uk

GDC (2002) *The First Five Years: a framework for undergraduate dental education*, 2nd edn. London, The General Dental Council.

Griffiths, J. (2005) At risk groups: people with special needs. In J. Griffiths and S. Boyle (eds) *Holistic Oral Care. A guide for health professionals.* London, Stephen Hancocks Limited.

QAA (2002) *Dentistry: academic standards.* Subject benchmark statements. Gloucester; Quality Assurance Agency for Higher Education.

Thompson S., Griffiths J., Hunter L., Jagger R., Korszun A. and McLaughlin W. (2001) Development of an undergraduate curriculum in special care dentistry. *Journal of Disability and Oral Health* **2**(2), 71–7.

Watson N. (2000) Barriers, discrimination and prejudice. In J. H. Nunn (ed.) *Disability and Oral Care.* London, FDI World Dental Press Ltd.

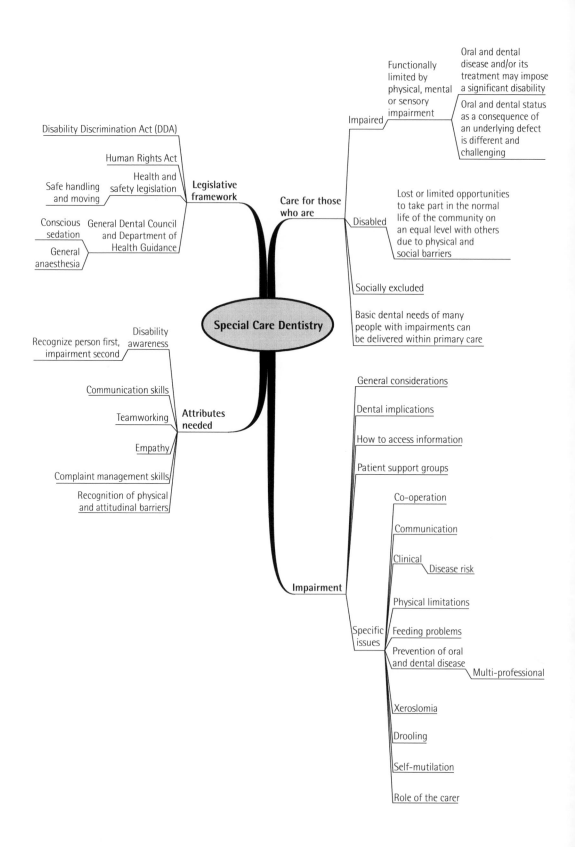

Special Care Dentistry

Care for those who are

Impaired
- Functionally limited by physical, mental or sensory impairment
  - Oral and dental disease and/or its treatment may impose a significant disability
  - Oral and dental status as a consequence of an underlying defect is different and challenging

Disabled
- Lost or limited opportunities to take part in the normal life of the community on an equal level with others due to physical and social barriers

Socially excluded

Basic dental needs of many people with impairments can be delivered within primary care

Legislative framework
- Disability Discrimination Act (DDA)
- Human Rights Act
- Health and safety legislation
  - Safe handling and moving
- General Dental Council and Department of Health Guidance
  - Conscious sedation
  - General anaesthesia

Attributes needed
- Disability awareness
  - Recognize person first, impairment second
- Communication skills
- Teamworking
- Empathy
- Complaint management skills
- Recognition of physical and attitudinal barriers

Impairment
- General considerations
- Dental implications
- How to access information
- Patient support groups
- Specific issues
  - Co-operation
  - Communication
  - Clinical
    - Disease risk
  - Physical limitations
  - Feeding problems
  - Prevention of oral and dental disease
    - Multi-professional
  - Xeroslomia
  - Drooling
  - Self-mutilation
  - Role of the carer

2.3 Orthodontics

Peter Mossey and David Stirrups

Key points

+ The general dental practitioner has an important role as 'gatekeeper' to ortho-dontic care and should have sufficient orthodontic knowledge to enable them to know when to intervene or refer.

+ An understanding of orthodontics includes many aspects of the scientific basis of dentistry, including oral and dental anatomy, growth of the dento-facial complex, tooth morphogenesis, eruption of teeth and development of occlusion.'

+ Orthodontics, like many other dental specialties, is a complex blend between an art and a science, and a range of generic skills are brought to bear during clinical orthodontic treatment.

+ The technical aspects of orthodontics are concerned with the use of various types of orthodontic appliances in the treatment of dental irregularities and dento-facial abnormalities.

+ Orthodontic treatment is designed to benefit dental health, function and aes-thetics, but there is also a complex balance between benefit and risk – and both aspects must be appreciated by the dentist and the patient.

+ Core skills in orthodontics are essential for the understanding of the scope for interdisciplinary treatment with pediatric dentistry, oral and maxillofacial surgery, restorative dentistry and periodontology.

Introduction

Orthodontics is often perceived to be a post-graduate specialty. General dental practi-tioners will, however, have patients who present with problems in the developing occlusion, and others who are undergoing orthodontic treatment, whether or not this has been carried out in their own practise. It is therefore essential that the dental graduate has attained core skills in orthodontics.

In paragraph 82 of *The First Five Years* (GDC 2002) the General Dental Council describes the relevant study of orthodontics:

Paragraph 82 Orthodontics is concerned with the development and growth of the face and occlusion, the extent of normal variation in the form and function of both the hard and soft tissues of the mouth and face, and particularly the ways in which such variation produces differences in occlusion. The study of these factors should emphasize their interrelationship with the general and psychosocial development of the individual. Changing patterns of orthodontic care have been influenced by changes in the perception of simple orthodontic treatment by both patients and practitioners. Most orthodontic treatment is now delivered by specialists. Students should be able to:

- carry out orthodontic assessment;
- identify treatment needs;
- understand the role of orthodontics in overall patient care;
- recognize and describe developing and manifest malocclusions;
- understand the appropriate timing of interventions and what these interventions are likely to be;
- know when and how to refer for specialist advice;
- make safe all types of orthodontic appliance;
- know when and how to refer for specialist advice;
- recognize and manage those problems of the mixed dentition where interceptive treatment is indicated, including space maintenance.

Table 2.3.1 Intended learning outcomes for orthodontics

Be competent at	Have knowledge of	Be familiar with
Carrying out an orthodontic assessment including an indication of treatment need	The management of problems in the mixed dentition where interceptive treatment is indicated, including space maintenance	The principles of treatment of dento-facial anomalies including the common orthodontic/maxillofacial procedures involved
Managing appropriately all forms of orthodontic emergency including referral when necessary	The design, insertion and adjustment of space maintainers	The role of orthodontics in overall patient care

Table 2.3.1 Intended learning outcomes for orthodontics – *continued*

Be competent at	Have knowledge of	Be familiar with
Making appropriate referrals based on assessment.	The design, fitting and adjustment of active removable appliances to move a single tooth or correct a crossbite	The limitations of orthodontic treatment
Radiographic interpretation and be able to write an accurate radiographic report	Biomedical sciences, oral physiology and craniofacial, oral and dental anatomy in the management of patients	Contemporary treatment techniques
Communicating effectively with patients, their families and associates and with other health care professionals involved in their care	The scope of orthodontic treatment, sufficient to explain and discuss treatment with patients and their parents	

Evaluation of malocclusion in orthodontics

The essential clinical skills in orthodontics will be described below under the following headings:

1. History taking: obtain and record a comprehensive history, perform an appropriate physical examination, interpret the findings and organize appropriate further investigations.

2. Clinical examination – intra-oral and extra-oral

   ◆ Extra-oral:

     ▪ Anterio-posterior skeletal pattern

     ▪ Vertical skeletal pattern/face height proportions

     ▪ Asymmetry

     ▪ Lip morphology/competence/position

     ▪ Aesthetic component of index of orthodontic treatment need (IOTN)

   ◆ Intra-oral:

     ▪ Overjet, overbite and centre lines

     ▪ Molar and canine relationship

     ▪ Cross-bite and scissors bite

  - Local irregularities, including rotations, vertical and horizontal displacements
  - Angulations of teeth, mesio-distally and bucco-lingualy
  - Space analysis: spacing/crowding assessment
  - IOTN dental health component
 ♦ Functional occlusal assessment: Recognition of displacing contacts on closing

3. Special investigations
 ♦ Radiographs: Which? When? Why? How?
 ♦ Reporting: systematic description of dentopantogram (DPT)
 ♦ Radiographic localization of unerupted teeth (parallax)
 ♦ Interpretation of lateral cephalometric tracing
 ♦ Vitality tests as appropriate

4. Diagnosis and recording problems in a 'diagnostic statement'
5. Treatment objectives (treatment plan not required)
6. Interceptive orthodontics
7. Making appropriate referral
8. Use of IOTN
9. Explain and discuss orthodontic treatments with patients and their parents
10. Explain and discuss multidisciplinary treatments with patients and their parents
11. Know how to design, insert and adjust space maintainers
12. Know how to design, insert and adjust active removable appliances
13. Managing orthodontic emergencies.

History taking in orthodontics

Standards

The student should:
  Appreciate that history taking is the first part of a sequence as follows:
  History taking ⇒ examination, ⇒ diagnosis, ⇒ treatment
 ♦ Demonstrate ability to communicate with patients in order to elicit appropriate details as follows:

  1. Patient's name, date of birth and age
  2. Reason for attendance
  3. Assess the patients motivation for orthodontic treatment
  4. Describe in appropriate detail and appropriate language (non-jargonized) what orthodontic treatment might entail

5. Medical history: demonstrate a knowledge of aspects of history which are particularly relevant to orthodontics such as the following:

  ◆ infective endocarditis

  ◆ asthma

  ◆ allergies

  ◆ bleeding problems

  ◆ diabetes and epilepsy.

6. Dental history: demonstrate a knowledge of aspects of history which are particularly relevant to orthodontics such as the following:

  ◆ caries/restorations/extractions experience

  ◆ home dental care

  ◆ previous experience of orthodontics

  ◆ anaesthesia (LA or GA).

7. Social history:

  ◆ Factors affecting ability to attend on a regular basis over a prolonged time period.

8. Record dated, accurate, concise and legible entries in the hospital notes.

Underpinning knowledge

The student should:

◆ Demonstrate knowledge about the importance of good record keeping

◆ Demonstrate knowledge of which orthodontic procedures may pose a risk, and particularly those in relation to a particular medical history.

History taking in orthodontics

The checklist should include:

◆ Introduction and explanation of procedure to patient

◆ Records basic identification/demographic details

◆ Establishes reason for attendance

◆ Asks questions regarding internal motivation

◆ Takes history of patient's presenting complaint, using appropriate questions and answers

◆ Systematic and appropriate medical history details

◆ Takes a dental history with specific mention of:

  ▪ previous orthodontic experience

  ▪ anaesthetic experience

◆ Makes enquiries about social history and ability to attend

◆ Records the above concisely and legibly in patients notes.

Clinical examination

Extra-oral examination

The student should:

◆ Demonstrate the ability to assess the skeletal pattern in three dimensions, antero-posterior, vertical and transverse

◆ Demonstrate a clinical examination following the sequence:

  ▪ prior explanation of procedure

  ▪ patient positioning with Frankfort plane horizontal

  ▪ assessment of antero-posterior and vertical skeletal pattern

  ▪ examination of transverse skeletal pattern with patient prone palpitating the temporomandibular joint (TMJ) observing symmetry of face and mandibular opening and examination of lymph nodes

  ▪ identify and appreciate the significance of mandibular deviation on closure – either forward or transverse

  ▪ elicit and demonstrate a knowledge of the significance of a clicking TMJ, or muscular tenderness, limited opening or lymphadenopathy

  ▪ examination of soft tissues in orthodontics:

    • examination of lip morphology at rest and in function, describe lip competence, level and activity

    • appreciate reasons for incompetent lips and implications for orthodontic treatment instability

    • recognize lip trap and its significance

    • observe tongue behaviour in relation to lip morphology, and identify tongue thrust.

Intra-oral clinical examination

Evaluation of occlusion

The student should:

◆ Be able to classify incisor relationship into Class 1, Class 2 division 1, Class 2 division 2, and Class 3

◆ Measure the overjet, overbite and midline discrepancy (if any) and identify a midline shift in the maxillary and mandibular arches

◆ Be able to evaluate buccal segment occlusion

◆ Classify first permanent molar relationship into angles Class 1, 2, and 3 and quantify the degree of discrepancy

- Appreciate the significance of Class 1 occlusion in the molars, pre-molars and canines and the concept of functional occlusion
- Recognize the dental features in a patient with a digit sucking habit
- Recognize the significance of cessation of a digit sucking habit and the consequences for the occlusion of a failure to cease the habit
- Carry out the above with due regard to cross infection procedures.
- Communicate effectively with the patient and parent(s) in the course of this examination.

Local irregularities

The student should:

- Be able to recognize local irregularities such as crowding with displacement of contact points, rotations (and describe with appropriate terminology) axial inclination of teeth, in particular canines, proclination and retroclination of incisors
- Cross bite (buccal or incisor cross-bite with or without mandibular deviation):
  - Appreciate the significance of cross-bite with deviation and appropriate methods of management
- Crowding/spacing:
  - Appreciate the degree of crowding and be able to carry out a space analysis in the deciduous or permanent dentition
  - Recognize significant tooth size discrepancy and its implications
  - Appreciate that malocclusions may be treated on an extraction or non-extraction basis
  - Appreciate the methods of obtaining space for relief of crowding in orthodontics.

Special investigations

The student should demonstrate the ability to systematically describe the features of a DPT radiograph along the following lines:

1. Identify the field being visualized from the orbits, TMJs, and maxillary/mandibular structures
2. Count and account for all the teeth
3. Identify any pathological features in the hard tissues, identify normal physiological radiolucencies and pathological radiolucencies
4. Identify soft tissue shadows
5. Identify the normal developmental features and be able to accurately estimate chronological age from the stage of development of the teeth, by calcification and root development
6. Identify features that are likely to compromise the long term prognosis of the teeth

7. Identify critical stages of development relevant to orthodontic intervention such as bifurcation formation in the second molars when first permanent molars are to be extracted

8. The principles of interceptive orthodontics e.g. missing 35, 45 etc. (see Treatment objectives).

The student should demonstrate the ability to systematically describe the features of a lateral cephalogram along the following lines:

1. Appreciation of indications for lateral cephalogram and the value of a cephalometric analysis in orthodontic treatment planning

2. Knowledge of the following landmarks, Sella, Nasion, A point, B point, ANS, PNS, upper incisor apex and tip, lower incisor apex and tip, pogonion, gonion and articulare

3. Appreciate the significance of the following planes and angles: SN plane, maxillary plane and mandibular plane

4. Angles Sella-Nasion A-point (SNA), Sella-Nasion B-point (SNB), maxillary-mandibular planes angle (MMPA), upper incisor to maxillary plane, lower incisor to mandibular plane

5. Knowledge of the normal values and ranges for the angles recorded above, and appreciation of the clinical significance of abnormal values in a cephalometric analysis.

Other special investigations

Use of paragraphllax for localization of unerupted or supernumerary teeth.

The student should appreciate the need for other special investigations such as additional radiographs, vitality tests and other diagnostic tests.

Diagnosis and recording problems in a 'diagnostic statement'

The student should:

♦ Be able to formulate a diagnostic statement or problem list in the light of all the information collected during the history taking and examination

♦ Should appreciate that the diagnostic statement draws together the salient features in a particular malocclusion in a holistic context, a diagnostic statement should include the following features:

▪ classification of the malocclusion with incisor and molar classification, the antero-posterior and vertical skeletal pattern and whether there is any transverse discrepancy, the complicating factors with regard to crowding/spacing, rotations, unerupted or missing teeth and any other irregularities

▪ the overbite, overjet and midline relationship and relationship of the buccal segments on right and left sides

▪ a brief summary of any radiographic findings of significance to the orthodontic treatment plan and whether any teeth are of limited prognosis

- the patients attitude to treatment, oral hygiene and ability to attend regularly over a prolonged period must be mentioned

- Any aspect of the medical or dental history that has an impact on the treatment plan is also required.

Treatment objectives

The student should:

- Appreciate the difference between recording the treatment objectives and a definitive treatment plan.

- Demonstrate the ability to record the objectives in the context of the diagnosis and the patient's motivation, history and individual circumstances.

- The treatment objectives should always include mention of oral hygiene, desirable changes to the occlusion, incisor and buccal segment relationships indicate whether treatment will require relief of crowding.

- Indicate whether the treatment plan should be a definitive, intermediate or compromise treatment plan.

- Recognize when interceptive orthodontics is indicated.

Interceptive orthodontics

The student should:

- Appreciate the role of interceptive orthodontics in overall treatment planning

- Appreciate that interceptive orthodontics is confined mainly to the developing dentition and, ordinarily in the mixed dentition, be aware of the implications of the following:

  - early eruption of teeth (neonatal teeth)
  - delayed eruption of teeth
  - physiological spacing
  - cross bite in the mixed dentition
  - digit sucking habit
  - crowding of the erupting anterior teeth
  - impaction of first permanent molars
  - super numerary or supplemental teeth
  - hypodontia
  - ectopic eruption
  - transposition
  - abnormal tooth morphology
  - failure to palpate upper 13, 23 (at age 9–10).

Ethical/legal implications of orthodontic treatment (see Chapter 1.2)

♦ Orthodontic treatment is designed to benefit dental health, function and aesthetics, but there is also a complex balance between benefit and risk – and both aspects must be appreciated by the dentist and the patient. This has significant implications for informed consent.

♦ The dentist must appreciate the ethical and legal guidelines surrounding orthodontic care in terms of diagnosis, consent, confidentiality and access to medical records.

♦ They should also be aware of the ethical and legal guidelines surrounding record collection and management, in particular with regard to ionizing radiation and the legal requirement for storage of records

Making appropriate referral

The student should have a good understanding of the limits of his own competence and be willing to refer cases that are outside his level of competence.

Letter of referral

The referrer should be aware of the secondary care services and be able to refer appropriately. In addition to the generic aspects (see Chapter 1.13), a letter of referral for orthodontic advice should contain:

♦ background information on the patient and the particular problem for which they are being referred, including the patient's perception of this problem

♦ medical, dental and social history relevant to orthodontic or dental treatment

♦ a brief description of the malocclusion/orthodontic problem (see problem list)

♦ a clear statement of whether the patient is being referred for advice or for treatment. Indicate what treatment the practitioner is able and willing to provide.

♦ relevant records enclosed such as study models and particularly radiographs (dated), and/or a statement of when radiographs were last taken

♦ signature and practice stamp (where applicable).

Use an index of orthodontic treatment need (IOTN)

The student should:

♦ Appreciate the concept of an IOTN and that the two components of this index are:

  ▪ aesthetic

  ▪ dental health.

IOTN dental health component

The student should:

♦ Demonstrate the ability to allocate an IOTN score to any malocclusion according to the single worst feature

◆ Use of the 'MOCDO' system for systematic analysis. (MOCDO refers to the hierarchy of occlusal problems identified using the dental health component of the Index of Orthodontic Treatment [IOTN] which are: missing, overjet, cross-bite, displacement and overbite.)

◆ Demonstrate the ability to use the IOTN appropriately in the interpretation of dental health problems and to specifically identify the following features:

■ Hypodontia with two or more teeth per quadrant missing or an unerupted tooth which is impeded or impacted as indicators of a score of 5

■ Overjet of greater than 9 mm or reverse overjet greater than −3.5 mm (Class III) both score 5

■ Scissors bite and buccal cross bite, and differentiate between those that have an associated mandibular displacement and those which do not, and to score appropriately

■ Displacement of contact points and measure these accurately to determine the IOTN score

■ Deep overbite and differentiate between traumatic and non-traumatic overbite in the scoring of IOTN

◆ Recognize the significance of the IOTN dental health and aesthetic components with respect to treatment need in borderline cases, and the impact this may have on patient well-being and clinical practice.

Explain and discuss orthodontic treatments with patients and their parents

Prerequisites:

1. Knowledge of normal and abnormal development

2. Knowledge of use and limitations of active removable appliances

3. Knowledge of use and limitations of functional appliances

4. Knowledge of use and limitations of fixed appliances

5. Familiar with the scope of multidisciplinary interventions.

Explain and discuss multidisciplinary treatments with patients and their parents

Prerequisites:

1. Knowledge of the risks/ benefits of orthodontic treatment

2. Familiar with orofacial clefts

3. Familiar with adult orthodontics

4. Familiar with TMJ and ortho.

Know how to design, insert and adjust space maintainers

Competent use of space maintainers will require knowledge of:

◆ Indications and contraindications

◆ Designs (removable or fixed)

◆ Fitting if removable, and referral if fixed

◆ Maintenance

◆ When to stop.

Checklist 38 **Clinical orthodontic examination**

Extra-oral	✔, X or N/A
1 Prior explanation of procedure	
2 Patient positioning with Frankfort plane horizontal	
3 Assessment of antero-posterior and vertical skeletal pattern	
4 Examination of transverse skeletal pattern with patient prone palpitating the TMJ observing symmetry of face and mandibular opening and palpation of lymph nodes	
5 Identify and appreciate the significance of mandibular deviation on closure – either forward or transverse	
Examination of soft tissues	
6 Examination of lip morphology at rest and in function, describe lip competence, level and activity	
7 Recognize lip trap and its significance	
8 Tongue behaviour in relation to lip morphology, and identify tongue thrust	
9 Recognize the dental features in a patient with a digit sucking habit	
Evaluation of occlusion	
10 Be able to classify incisor relationship into Class 1, Class 2.1, Class 2.2 and Class 3	
11 Measure the overjet, overbite and midline discrepancy (if any) and identify a midline shift in the maxillary and mandibular arches	
12 Be able to evaluate buccal segment occlusion (molar and canine)	
13 Record inclination of incisors and identify if canines are distally or mesially inclined	
14 Recognize crossbite and when this is accompanied by a mandibular deviation	
15 Carry out the above with due regard to cross infection procedures	
16 Communicate effectively with the patient and parent(s) in the course of this examination	

Know how to design, insert and adjust active removable appliances

Appliance design requires a consideration of (a) active components, (b) retention, (c) anchorage and (d) baseplate modifications.

Managing orthodontic emergencies

- Making safe broken fixed appliances
- Making safe problems with extra-oral appliances.

Checklist 39 **Removable appliance adjustment**

		✔, X or N/A
1	Checks with patient for experience since last visit	
2	Checks appliance in mouth for appropriate wear/spring positions	
3	Checks appliance for damage	
4	Assessment of tooth movement since last visit	
5	Carries out any necessary adjustments to active components	
6	Checks fit of appliance and retention	
7	Adjusts cribs as needed using appropriate pliers	
8	Checks final fit of appliance	
9	Instructions to patient on insertion and removal	
10	Check patient can insert and remove appliance correctly	
11	Home care and emergency instructions given	
12	Organizes next appointment	
13	Repeats 11 and 12 with parent if appropriate	
14	Appropriate cross-infection control procedures used	
15	Appropriate general communication with patient	

Checklist 40 **Functional appliance occlusal record**

		✔, X or N/A
1	Collects appropriate materials	
2	Explanation to patient	
3	Practices required jaw position with patient	
4	Assessment of required inter-occlusal space and chooses appropriate spacer	
5	Practice required jaw position with patient using spacer	
6	Records jaw position	
7	Check records for accuracy (including midlines)	
8	Check recorded jaw position is as planned	
9	Record washed, disinfected and covered	
10	Organizes next appointment	
11	Explanation of next visit, with parent if appropriate	
12	Appropriate cross-infection control procedures used	
13	Appropriate general communication with patient	

References and further reading

GDC (2002) *The First Five Years: a framework for undergraduate dental education*, 2nd edn. London, The General Dental Council.

Houston W. J. B., Stephens C. and Tulley W. J. (1992) *A Textbook of Orthodontics*, 2nd edn. London, John Wright.

Isaacson K. G., Muir J. D. and Reed R. T. (2002) *Removable Orthodontic Appliances*. London, Wright.

Jones M. L. and Oliver R. G. (2000) *Walther and Houston's Orthodontic Notes*, 6th edn. London, Wright.

Mitchell L. (2001) *An Introduction to Orthodontics*, 2nd edn. Oxford, Oxford University Press.

QAA (2002) *Dentistry: academic standards*. Subject benchmark statements. Gloucester, Quality Assurance Agency for Higher Education.

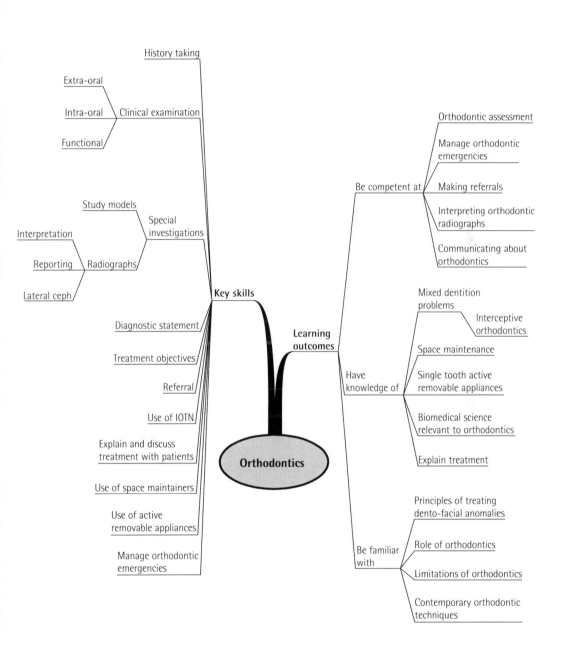

History taking

Extra-oral

Intra-oral — Clinical examination

Functional

Study models

Interpretation — Special investigations

Reporting — Radiographs

Lateral ceph

Diagnostic statement

Treatment objectives

Referral

Use of IOTN

Explain and discuss treatment with patients

Use of space maintainers

Use of active removable appliances

Manage orthodontic emergencies

Key skills

Orthodontics

Learning outcomes

Be competent at

Orthodontic assessment

Manage orthodontic emergencies

Making referrals

Interpreting orthodontic radiographs

Communicating about orthodontics

Have knowledge of

Mixed dentition problems — Interceptive orthodontics

Space maintenance

Single tooth active removable appliances

Biomedical science relevant to orthodontics

Explain treatment

Be familiar with

Principles of treating dento-facial anomalies

Role of orthodontics

Limitations of orthodontics

Contemporary orthodontic techniques

2.4 Periodontology

Mike Milward and Iain Chapple

Key points

- Periodontal diseases are becoming increasingly important to oral and systemic health, given their prevalence in children and adults in the UK, and in particular in older patients who are retaining their teeth for much longer than ever before.

- The undergraduate curriculum must provide students with the core basic skills and knowledge necessary for competent management of a range of common periodontal conditions.

- The core skills and knowledge gained must be measurable using a variety of assessment methods which examine defined outcomes.

- Knowledge of a range of basic and applied biological and health care sciences is essential to underpin the competent practice of this clinical discipline.

- The graduate must understand the biological basis for common periodontal problems; be able to extract a relevant history from a patient; to examine, perform specific investigations, diagnose, plan and execute non-surgical treatment and design appropriate maintenance programmes for patients with common periodontal problems.

- The graduate must be capable of safe and effective use of a range of instrumentation appropriate for the non-surgical management of supra- and subgingival deposits on tooth surfaces, and understand the indications for, and principles of, a range of surgical periodontal therapies.

- The graduate should understand the legal framework within which dental care professionals DCPs operate and their role in the management of the periodontal patient. They should also have some practical experience of how such a team-based approach benefits patients.

- The graduate should be fully aware of the importance of continuing medical education (CME) and life-long learning in relation to the periodontal diseases and their management.

> ## Key points – *continued*
>
> ◆ The graduate must appreciate their personal limitations in the management of more complex periodontal problems, as well as when and how to refer for specialist advice/management.
>
> ◆ Assessing competence alone is not sufficient for the safe management of periodontal patients and there must be some assessment of proficiency in the application of key clinical skills.

Introduction

Periodontal diseases are common. The 1998 UK Adult Dental Health Survey reported that 95 per cent of the adult population had gingival inflammation, 8 per cent had severe periodontitis, and 85 per cent of over-65-year-olds had periodontitis (Morris *et al.* 2001). It is, therefore, essential that the dental graduate has a comprehensive knowledge of periodontal diseases and their management, in order to offer a high level of care to patients.

The graduate must be able to screen patients and identify those with periodontal disease, and be able to diagnose, treat, monitor, and maintain patients with common periodontal conditions. It is also essential that the graduate is aware of their limitations, and is able to recognize aggressive periodontal diseases that require prompt referral to a specialist in periodontology. As can be seen, the range of skills and knowledge that a student needs to acquire during the undergraduate course is extensive. It is important that the course reflects these and is constructed in such a way that the student has the opportunity to acquire the requisite knowledge and skills. The course should also be able to assess the student in order to ensure that they have acquired the necessary skills that are set out in this chapter.

The undergraduate dental course needs to deliver the education and experience as outlined in the General Dental Council (GDC) document *The First Five Years* (GDC 2002). This document states the following in regard to restorative dentistry:

> **Paragraph 74** Restorative dentistry is concerned with the management of the plaque-related diseases (dental caries and periodontal diseases), tooth wear and tooth loss. Management includes preventive, non-operative care as well as the restoration of teeth using the well-established techniques of conservative dentistry, including crowns and endodontics, the replacement of teeth by means of prostheses, and the treatment and maintenance of the supporting structures of the teeth by the procedures of periodontology. In restorative dentistry students should have continuous responsibility for the care of a number of adults in order to assess their overall needs, the efficacy of preventive measures, their behaviour, management and long-term success or failure of restorative treat-

Paragraph 74 – *continued*

ment. Students should learn to manage adults requiring emergency care, carry out diagnostic procedures in such circumstances, formulate treatment plans and relate them to comprehensive dental care. All aspects of restorative dentistry may be required for medically compromised patients and those with other special needs. In its advanced forms restorative dentistry can involve extensive occlusal rehabilitation, sometimes requiring the use of dental implants. Students should appreciate that these forms of treatment may be delivered by specialists as secondary or tertiary care. They should be aware of when to refer such cases, understand the principles involved in their management and observe such treatment being carried out.

Paragraph 75 All restorative techniques can be invasive in nature, and some are irreversible. The GDC considers that dental students on graduation must be competent in procedures of restorative dentistry including non-surgical treatment of single and multi-rooted teeth, crowns and simple bridges, removable partial and complete dentures and periodontal therapy. They should be fully aware of when patients should be directed to specialists for advice and treatment.

The European Federation of Periodontology has produced another important publication—*Curricular Guidelines in Undergraduate Periodontal Education* (1996)—and this document sets out a number of global objectives.

Both these documents will help in the design of appropriate undergraduate courses in periodontology, but a more detailed breakdown of the key skills that are required will be highlighted in this chapter

Whilst the paragraphs quoted above from the GDC's undergraduate document relate directly to periodontology, requirements from other clinical disciplines that impact on periodontology, for example local anaesthesia, history taking, occlusion, management of the medically compromised patient, injection control etc., and these are discussed elsewhere in this book.

This chapter outlines the learning outcomes for periodontology that are deemed appropriate for dental undergraduates, as well as taking a more detailed look at the skills dental students will need to develop during their undergraduate course in periodontology in order to offer comprehensive care for their patients upon graduation.

Intended learning outcomes

This section contains an additional list of learning outcomes (see Table 2.4.1) that are felt appropriate for the undergraduate in periodontology. Each of the outcomes should be tested during a student's training. Satisfying a particular learning outcome can be assessed using a variety of methods including competency tests, written examinations, viva voce examinations, clinical assessments, continuous assessment etc. Methods of assessment will be discussed later in this chapter.

Table 2.4.1 Intended learning outcomes for periodontology

Be competent at	Have knowledge of	Be familiar with
Completing a basic periodontal examination (BPE) and detailed periodontal charting where indicated, and interpreting and reporting on radiographs of the periodontal tissues	The basic biological sciences which underpin the study of periodontology and the practice of periodontics	The legal requirements underpinning the practice of dental hygiene and therapy
Assessing presenting signs and symptoms and diagnosing, treatment planning and managing in their broadest sense, the most common mild and moderate forms of chronic periodontal disease	Clinical medicine and surgery, in regards to periodontal/gingival manifestations of systemic diseases and the periodontal management of the medically compromised patient	Different types of periodontal surgery available and when they might be advised
The assessment and diagnosis of severe chronic and aggressive forms of periodontal disease	Periodontal epidemiology and the role of periodontology in public health dentistry	The importance of periodontal health/disease to implantology.
Educating patients about their disease and their role in its management, including provision and prescription of specific forms of oral hygiene instruction, as appropriate to individual patient needs	The impact of periodontal diseases and their management upon the practices of other dental and medical/surgical specialties (e.g. orthodontics, oral medicine, restorative dentistry)	The principles of managing patients with osseo-integrated implants
Supra- and subgingival scaling and root surface debridement, using both powered and manual instrumentation, and in stain removal and prophylaxis	The range of medical and surgical therapeutic options for managing common periodontal problems i.e. clinical periodontics.	
Knowing when and how to prescribe appropriate anti-microbial therapy in the management of plaque-related diseases	The causes of and risk factors for periodontal diseases enabling their prevention, diagnosis and management	

Table 2.4.1 Intended learning outcomes for periodontology – *continued*

Be competent at	Have knowledge of	Be familiar with
Preparing and making appropriate referrals for primary care (special interests practitioners within PCTs) or specialist (secondary) care	The effects of periodontal diseases and expected outcomes of therapy and how to prepare/manage the outcomes of treatment plans for dental hygienists	
Designing and implementing periodontal supportive care programmes for chronic periodontal diseases and be able to implement a prescribed regime for cases returning to their practice after specialist care	Their limitations in managing periodontal disorders	
	The impact of smoking on periodontitis and how to counsel patients on smoking cessation	

Curriculum guidelines in undergraduate periodontal education

This section lists the key areas that should be covered during an undergraduate course in periodontology (GDC 2002; European Federation of Periodontology 1996).

Background knowledge

It is essential that graduates have sound background knowledge in order to understand the disease process, relate this to their patients, and provide a high level of care.

Basic and applied sciences

A solid foundation in, and understanding of, the basic and applied sciences is essential to the practice of periodontology. Key areas and examples of their importance are listed below.

Anatomy

Comprehensive knowledge of applied anatomy can only be built upon a solid foundation in the gross and micro-anatomy of the head, neck and oral/dental tissues. For example, the safe placement of local anaesthesia or examination of regional lymph nodes to determine the routes of spread of infection, require knowledge of gross anatomy; forming a list of differential diagnoses for a gingival swelling requires micro-anatomical knowledge of the tissues and cells within that region; the basic principles of periodontal surgery cannot be appreciated without knowledge of tissue planes and vital structures that may be damaged if their location is not known; the reasons for failure of non-surgical therapy at local sites requires knowledge of potential defects in root anatomy or variations in normal tooth anatomy. In addition, an understanding of the concept of attachment loss and its relationship to probing prockel depth and recession is essential.

Microbiology

Students require a broad understanding of the principles of microbial colonization, ecology and behaviour to enable the safe management of local infections by drainage, or to appreciate when it is acceptable or necessary to prescribe systemic anti-micro-bial drugs. The potential risks involved with anti-microbial prescription, such as drug resistance and hypersensitivity reactions, are vital concepts for the safe management of oral infections. Basic diagnosis and treatment planning for conditions such as necro-tizing ulcerative gingivitis (NUG) and necrotizing ulcerative periodontitis (NUP) require a sound knowledge of the causative pathogens.

Physiology

Knowledge and understanding of broad aspects of oral physiology, such as saliva flow, dynamics and composition are important when attempting to understand or manage the effects of xerostomia on gingival and periodontal health. The impact of environmental risk factors such as smoking on oral physiology (e.g. gingival blood supply and crevicular fluid – GCF flow) underpin the understanding of such risk factors and provide part of the evidence base for smoking cessation advice as a strategy for improving oral health. The dynamics of GCF flow place therapeutic limitations on the value of using chlorhex-idine or other subgingival irrigants for managing periodontitis.

Immunology

A thorough understanding of immunology, both innate and acquired, is essential for the graduate to appreciate why some patients develop periodontitis and others do not. The safe and appropriate prescription of novel host-modulating drugs already in the *British National Formulary* (e.g. low dose doxycycline) requires thorough appreciation of how such drugs modulate inflammatory responses and for which groups of patients they may be therapeutic.

Pathology

It is important that the graduate has a firm foundation in the basic pathological processes that underlie human disease and how these translate to clinical oral pathology. Correct management of a vascular epulis or central giant cell granuloma requires a knowledge of the histopathology of the lesion and its likely association with underlying bone or even parathyroid disease. If the correct treatments are to be implemented in the appropriate sequence, the management of tooth mobility caused by occlusal forces acting on a compromised periodontium requires understanding of the relative roles of both pathologies. This is also the case for periodontal–endodontic lesions,

Natural history

A comprehensive understanding of the natural history of periodontal diseases is essential to the dental graduate's understanding of patient-specific treatment protocols and why some patients require closer maintenance support than others. Such knowledge also helps identify patients who fall outside the diagnostic criteria for less aggressive diseases and therefore may require a combined mechanical and chemotherapeutic approach to their initial management.

Epidemiology

Understanding disease prevalence from a national and international public health perspective helps the graduate plan for the most appropriate and efficient resource management strategies for periodontal diseases in their specific demographic area. This is key to helping the graduate provide the most they can for the majority of their patients and also enables them to formulate their own views on when referral for secondary care is necessary, for which patients, and at which stages of each patient's management.

Systemic diseases

Many systemic diseases present with gingival or periodontal manifestations and these may often be the presenting sign of that disease/disorder. Conditions such as cicatricial pemphigoid may often present orally as a desquamative gingivitis before dermal or ocular lesions develop. Similarly, rare conditions such as Papillon-Lefevre syndrome or systemic lupus erythematosis may present with signs that alert the graduate to early specialist referral, thereby improving the prognosis and quality of life for the individual patient. Conditions such as Crohn's disease, sarcoidosis and even tuberculosis present more commonly with oral and gingival manifestations. Whilst definitive diagnosis cannot be expected from the graduate without further postgraduate training, it is important that the graduate recognizes the potential for systemic disease underlying the periodontal pathology, to ensure appropriate referral and subsequent patient management within defined care pathways.

Pharmacology and therapeutics

It is entirely inappropriate and unethical for any dental graduate to prescribe a drug without a thorough foundation and understanding of how the drug functions, which organs are involved in its metabolism and what its side-effects and drug interactions may be. It is also important that the dental graduate is aware of the issues regarding bacterial resistance, and where possible to avoid inappropriate use of broad-spectrum systemic antibiotics.

Some recommended outcomes from the basic and applied sciences are listed in Table 2.4.2.

Instrumentation

It is not appropriate to be prescriptive with respect to specific forms of instrumentation the graduate should be competent at using. However, knowledge of the range of automated and manual instruments available for supra- and subgingival instrumentation of the tooth surface is essential, alongside the advantages and disadvantages of each.

Table 2.4.2 Intended learning outcomes of basic biological science courses

Basic/Applied science	Intended learning outcomes
Anatomy	Be aware of the anatomy (and applied anatomy) of the periodontium and how this relates to its function, to periodontal diseases and their management
Microbiology	Be aware of the microflora of the periodontal pocket and of dental plaque biofilms, both in health and disease, as well as the micro-organisms implicated in various periodontal diseases
	Be aware of the importance of the bacterial insult on the immune system
Physiology	Have a basic understanding of the physiology and biochemistry of saliva and gingival crevicular fluid in health and disease
Immunology	Have an understanding of inflammation and specific immunity in relation to periodontal disease and how these impact on patient management
Pathology	Have a broad understanding of common pathological processes and their features at a microscopic level
	Understand the features and mechanisms involved in a broad range of oral pathologies pertinent to the oral and periodontal tissues
Natural history	Be aware of the natural history of periodontal diseases and patterns of disease progression
Epidemiology	Have an understanding of the epidemiology of periodontal diseases
Systemic diseases/medical science	Be aware of the links between periodontal and systemic disease and how systemic diseases can present in the periodontal tissues
Pharmacology and therapeutics	Have knowledge of the types and uses of antimicrobial and anti-inflammatory drugs in the management of periodontal disease, along with the basic pharmacology of these agents
	Have knowledge of systemic drugs that have a potential impact on the periodontium

Specifically, the graduate should specifically be able to identify, describe and use the following instruments:

- WHO probe
- Graduated pocket measuring probe
- Ultrasonic and/or sonic scaler

- Universal curettes

- Area specific curettes

- Hoes (if preferred to area-specific curettes)

- Root surface explorers.

Mouthrinses/toothpastes

Mouthrinses and dentifrices have an important role to play in the prevention and management of a range of periodontal diseases. Such local antiseptic/antimicrobial agents also have limitations (e.g. subgingival access), interactions (e.g. chlorhexidine with sodium lauryl sulphate [SLS] in toothpastes) and advantages for certain groups of patients. As a minimum, the graduate should:

- Be aware of the active constituents of mouthrinses and toothpastes

- Have a detailed knowledge of the uses, side-effects and actions of chlorhexidine.

Clinical skills

The development of clinical skills is essential to the practice of dentistry, and this applies equally to periodontology. The graduate needs to be able to diagnose and manage common periodontal diseases, and to this end a variety of clinical skills is required. In this section a number of core skills are highlighted with emphasis on how they specifically relate to periodontology.

History taking

- To be able to ask questions that have particular relevance to periodontal disease, e.g. family history, oral hygiene regime, smoking history (including frequency, type, duration), diet history, history of stress and coping strategies, and interpret the impact of such information.

- To take a thorough medical history and be aware of the relevance in relation to periodontal disease and its management.

Examination

Be able to examine the patient extra-orally and note any abnormality associated with lymph nodes (this may indicate spreading oral infection, including periodontal infections), muscles of mastication, temporomandibular joints (which may impact on periodontal disease in the form of secondary occlusal trauma) etc. It is also important to be aware of the significance of any findings, and manage such findings, (e.g. facial asymmetry) in an appropriate manner.

- Be able to carry out a thorough intra-oral examination including:

  - The oral soft tissues, and be able to identify any abnormal lesions.

  - An assessment of oral hygiene in relation to plaque and calculus deposits.

- The identification of gingival inflammation, bleeding on probing and suppuration along with an understanding of the clinical significance of each.

- The identification of mobile teeth and classify them using a mobility index.

- The detection of abnormal dental anatomy (root grooves, deficient restoration margins, exposed furcations, crowding/rotated teeth) and be aware of their implications with regard to the periodontium.

- The identification and measurement of gingival recession.

- The identification and classification of furcation lesions

- The ability to perform a six-point detailed pocket chart as part of a baseline and follow-up examination.

- An ability to recognize and record evidence of parafunctional activity.

- An assessment of the occlusion, (both static and dynamic), with regard to premature contacts, patterns of guidance, interferences, and relate these to periodontal disease experience.

- The ability to carry out a basic periodontal examination as described by the British Society of Periodontology, and be aware of the implications and limitations of the results.

Special tests
Radiographs

- To be able to determine what radiographs are appropriate for each individual periodontal case.

- To have knowledge of the limitations and advantages of each appropriate type of radiograph in relation to periodontal disease (long cone paralleling periapicals, vertical bitewings, horizontal bitewings and orthopantomogram).

- To be able to interpret radiographs in relation to type, quality and quantity of bone loss, apical pathology and periodontal-endodontic lesions.

- To be able to document in the patient records a concise and accurate report of the radiographic features in relation to periodontal disease.

Vitality testing

To be able to test the viability of a tooth using ethyl chloride, electric pulp testers and test cavities in order to diagnose periodontal–endodontic lesions. Also to be able to interpret the results of such pulp tests and appreciate their limitations.

Study models

To appreciate the indications for the recording of study models in periodontology (e.g. to monitor recession or examine occlusal dysharmonies).

Diagnosis

It is, obviously, essential that a correct diagnosis is arrived at, so that the disease can be appropriately managed.

- To be able (using the findings above) to arrive at an accurate diagnosis of periodontal conditions along with any modifying factors.

- If a diagnosis is unclear, to be able to produce a differential diagnosis.

- To be able to classify the type of periodontal disease in relation to current classification schemes.

Treatment planning

Following on from diagnosis, a treatment plan needs to be formulated for the management of common periodontal diseases. The key skills are listed below.

- To be able to formulate an appropriate treatment plan for managing the periodontal condition. To be able to integrate this plan with any other specialty treatment needs.

- To be aware that treatment plans are flexible, and dependent upon patient compliance.

- To be able to decide which teeth are saveable and which teeth require extraction i.e. assess prognosis.

- To ensure that the treatment plan involves regular reassessment and reinforcement of oral hygiene.

- To discuss the aetiology, findings and treatment options with the patient in order to enable the acquisition of informed consent for treatment.

Oral hygiene instruction

Be able to provide verbally, and by demonstration, comprehensive oral hygiene instruction that is targeted to a particular patient's needs including:

- The importance of oral hygiene in relation to periodontal disease.

- The use of plaque and bleeding scores as feedback for patient motivation.

- The selection of appropriate oral hygiene aids (e.g. powered vs. manual brushes, interdental cleaning aids etc).

- The methods and frequency of brushing (e.g. modified Bass technique).

- The methods for interproximal cleaning (interproximal/interdental brushes, floss).

- Patient self-assessment using disclosing tablets.

- Oral hygiene instruction for patients with manual dexterity problems.

Dietary analysis and advice

To be able to perform dietary analysis, and offer advice in relation to the management of erosion and dentine sensitivity.

Smoking cessation advice

- ◆ To be able to discuss the general systemic problems associated with smoking.
- ◆ To discuss the impact of smoking on the periodontium.
- ◆ To offer support and information on smoking cessation, and if appropriate to give the patient information as to where further support/advice can be obtained.
- ◆ To review a patient's smoking habits in relation to their periodontal health and offer further support if required.
- ◆ To refer to specialist smoking cessation services.

Monitoring oral hygiene

- ◆ To be able to monitor patient's oral hygiene using plaque and bleeding scores.
- ◆ To be able to reinforce the oral hygiene message when and where appropriate.

Scaling and prophylaxis

- ◆ To be competent in supra- and subgingival calculus and stain removal using both hand and ultrasonic/sonic instruments and be able to do so without causing unnecessary soft tissue trauma.
- ◆ To be able to remove soft deposits and pellicle by prophylaxis.

Note: subgingival calculus removal is also integral to the procedure of root surface debridemement (see below).

Detailed pocket charting

- ◆ To know when a detailed pocket chart should be performed.
- ◆ To be able to perform a detailed and accurate six-point pocket chart; noting areas of bleeding, suppuration, furcation exposure, and recession.
- ◆ To be able to interpret the subsequent results, alone and in conjunction with previous detailed pocket charts.

Identification of sites requiring further treatment

- ◆ From detailed pocket charts, clinical signs (e.g. bleeding on probing) and supporting radiographs.
- ◆ From the exploration of root surfaces for subgingival deposits or relevant anatomy.

Non-surgical root surface debridement

- ◆ To be able to use appropriate local anaesthesia (when indicated).
- ◆ To be able to instrument root surfaces in order to achieve a calculus-free surface, without causing excessive gingival trauma.

◆ Be able to use area-specific curettes, and ultrasonic/sonic scalers with appropriate inserts.

◆ Be aware of the complications of root surface debridement and be able to discuss these with the patient, prior to embarking on a course of treatment.

Monitoring treatment outcome

◆ To appreciate the need to allow sufficient time for healing (e.g. after root surface debridement).

◆ To repeat the detailed pocket chart, assessing probing pocket depth reduction and reduction in the number of sites of bleeding/suppuration.

◆ To appreciate that the BPE is not suitable as an outcome measure for treatment of periodontitis.

◆ Monitoring of oral hygiene.

◆ To be able to observe and record any reduction in mobility.

◆ To be able to observe improvements in inflammation.

◆ To be able to assess remaining attachment levels where necessary and where changes in attachment level have resulted from therapy

Indications for using adjunctive systemic antimicrobial therapy

◆ Be aware of the systemic antimicrobial drugs that can be used.

◆ Be aware of the situations in which their use should be considered.

◆ Be aware of the metabolism, interactions and basic pharmacology of such agents.

◆ Be aware of the dosage and regimes used in systemic antimicrobial therapy.

◆ Be aware of the indications and contraindications to systemic antimicrobials.

Indications for using local antimicrobial delivery systems

◆ Be aware of the systems available and the advantages/disadvantages compared with systemic delivery.

◆ Be aware of the situations where their use may be considered or is contraindicated.

Indications for use of open root surface debridement (surgery)

◆ Be able to discuss the situations when periodontal surgery should be considered (indications and contraindications).

◆ Have knowledge of the basic principals underlying periodontal surgery (aims and objectives).

◆ Be able to briefly outline some of the techniques used and communicate these to patients.

- ◆ Be able to communicate complications of periodontal surgery to patients.
- ◆ Be aware of surgical principles.

Indications to repeat treatment

- ◆ Be able to decide when treatment should be repeated and when sites should simply be monitored.

When to refer a patient

See British Society of Periodontology (2001, 2002).

- ◆ Be aware of their limitations in treating periodontal disease.
- ◆ Be aware of the periodontal diseases that should be referred to a specialist periodontologist (see the British Society of Periodontology 2002; European Federation of Periodontology 1996).

Writing a referral letter

- ◆ Be able to write a suitable referral letter to a specialist in periodontology, giving the salient points required to allow for expedient patient management by the clinician receiving the referral (see Chapter 1.13).

The dental hygienist

- ◆ To understand the legal requirements related to the practice of dental hygienists, and other dental care professionals (e.g. dental therapists).
- ◆ Be able to write a detailed treatment plan for a dental hygienist.
- ◆ To take overall responsibility for the treatment plan implemented by the dental hygienist, by delegation rather than abdication.

To be able to implement a supportive care programme

- ◆ Once a patient has undergone a course of periodontal treatment, the graduate should be able to design a supportive care (maintenance) programme appropriate to individual patient needs.
- ◆ Undertake regular detailed monitoring of the patient's periodontal condition through detailed periodontal charting and identify when further treatment or re-referral may be necessary, and be able to implement any necessary remedial care.

Management of patients who fail to maintain an adequate level of oral hygiene

- ◆ To be aware that some patients will fail to respond to the hygiene phase of therapy and will continue to have inadequate oral hygiene, and are thus not suitable for more advanced treatment. In such a case disease progression should be anticipated and the management of such patients should take this into account. Periodontal treatment should remain limited to regular professional deposit removal, i.e. palliative care, rather than more involved root surface therapies, for chronic periodontitis.

- To be familiar with the classification of *periodontal–endodontic lesions*
- To have knowledge that endodontic treatment has priority over periodontal treatment in such cases.
- To manage the primary care of such lesions.

Be aware of the issues relating to the management of patients with complex medical histories

- Be able to manage the periodontal needs of patients requiring oral antimicrobial prophylaxis, those on Warfarin, or those who have had organ transplantation (or who are immunocompromised due to other causes).

Be able to integrate periodontal therapy with other specialties (orthodontics, restorative dentistry, oral surgery, oral medicine etc.) in order to formulate a coherent treatment plan

- Be able to place periodontal disease in context in relation to other dental specialties.
- Be aware of how other treatments impinge on periodontal health.
- Be able to design restorations that minimize any effect on the periodontal tissues.
- Be aware of the basic concepts of implantology and be aware that implants should
  - not be used in patients with active periodontal disease, and be aware of the increased
  - failure rate of implants in smokers.

Be aware that the undergraduate course, although comprehensive, needs to be reinforced at regular intervals by continued professional education (life-long learning)

Areas which are covered in the undergraduate curriculum but where clinical experience is limited, and where further postgraduate education will be required are:

- Periodontal resective surgery, access, regenerative and plastic surgery
- Implantology
- Treatment of aggressive disease
- Use of adjunctive periodontal therapies (e.g. local antimicrobial delivery systems)
- Recurrent disease and its management
- Periodontal management of certain 'medically complex cases'
- Managing patients who present with periodontal manifestations of systemic diseases
- Managing of patients with complex restorative problems, where periodontal diseases are part of the aetiology
- Orthodontic therapy in patients with a reduced but healthy periodontium.

Table 2.4.3 Example of competency test for root surface debridement

THE PERIODONTAL UNIT CLINICAL COMPETENCY ASSESSMENT	
STUDENT .... SUPERVISOR	
TASK: Root surface instrumentation – root surface debridement	
OBJECTIVE: To debride the root surface safely, efficiently and effectively	
ASSESSMENT	
Detailed pocket chart done/available	Yes / No
Recognises correct sites to be debrided	Yes / No
Check PMH	Yes / No
Correctly locates deposits	Yes / No
Explores root morphology	Yes / No
Appropriate analgesia	Yes / No
Selects correct instruments	Yes / No
Interaction with chairside assistant	Yes / No
Demonstrates correct technique for instruments	Yes / No
Complete removal of subgingival deposits	Yes / No
Absence of soft tissue trauma	Yes / No
Absence of root surface trauma	Yes / No
Management of haemorrhage	Yes / No
Good posture	Yes / No
Correct discharge advice to patient	Yes / No
COMPETENT	Yes / No
Staff signature	
	Date:
STUDENT COMMENTS:	
Student signature	
	Date:

Competency tests

The previous sections have attempted to build a comprehensive picture of the knowledge and skills a dental undergraduate should have gained during their course in periodontology. It is however, not practical to test everyone to ensure that every student has gained each of these skills. Moreover, as some of the skills outlined are more important than others, it is important that we have a list of skills that every student must achieve in order to successfully complete their course of study, i.e. the concept of 'key competencies'.

Therefore, undergraduate courses in periodontology should test each of the skills listed in Table 2.4.1 to ensure that a basic level of skill and knowledge has been achieved.

Assessing competency

If a student is said to be 'competent' in a certain skill, then he or she will need to achieve a certain level of skill and this will need to be assessed using a competency test. The outcome of this test can be either pass, (and they are competent in the particular skill), or fail (not competent in the particular skill).

Therefore, when a number of key skills (see previous section and Table 2.4.1) have been identified which a student must achieve during their course of study, then these will need to be individually assessed to ensure competency.

Competency can be assessed in a number of ways, including competency tests, continuous assessment, written examinations, viva, spotters etc, but the vast majority of assessments in periodontology will be clinically based (as the key competencies mainly relate to practical skills). An example of a competency test used for root surface debridement is shown in Table 2.4.3.

Conclusions

As with all dental education, students must embrace the concept of continued professional development, and be aware that a number of areas exist where, as undergraduates, they gain little or no experience and, if appropriate, these will need to be studied at the a postgraduate level. In the case of periodontology, this for example, would include periodontal surgery, management of aggressive or advanced diseases, implant surgery etc.

It is essential to recognize that in clinical practice, competence in a given procedure or skill relates to an individual's performance on a designated occasion, satisfying the criteria set for that procedure. It does not mean that the next time that individual performs the same procedure, but in a different setting or context, they will do so to the required standard. Consistency of competence is termed 'proficiency' and proficiency results from experience gained by repetition of a procedure or skill so as to fine-tune cognitive and practical skills in any given situation.

With a contribution from Dr Sarah Manton.

Acknowledgements

We would like to thank the members of The British Society of Periodontology, Professor P. Heasman, Dr V. Booth, Professor V. Clerehugh, Dr A. Tugnait, Miss H. Pontefract, Dr P. Hodge, Professor R. M. Palmer, Mr R. Mc Andrew, for their constructive comments on this chapter.

References and further reading

ADHS (2000) *Adult dental health survey: oral health in the United Kingdom 1998*. London, The Stationery Office.

British Society of Periodontology (2002) *Referral Policy and Parameters of Care*. The British Society of Periodontology October 2002. Available at: http://www.bsperio.org.uk/members/referral.htm

British Society of Periodontology (2001) *Periodontology in General Dental Practice in the United Kingdom; A policy statement*. Available at: http://www.bsperio.org.uk/members/policy.pdf

European Federation of Periodontology (1996) *Curricular Guidelines in Undergraduate Periodontal Education*. Available at: http://www.efp.net/periodontal/edu_undergrad.asp

Morris A. J., Steele J. and White D. A. (2001) The oral cleanliness and periodontal health of adults in 1998. *British Dental Journal* 191, 186–92.

GDC (2002) *The First Five Years: a framework for undergraduate dental education*, 2nd edn. London, The General Dental Council.

QAA (2002) *Dentistry: academic standards*. Subject benchmark statements. Gloucester, Quality Assurance Agency for Higher Education.

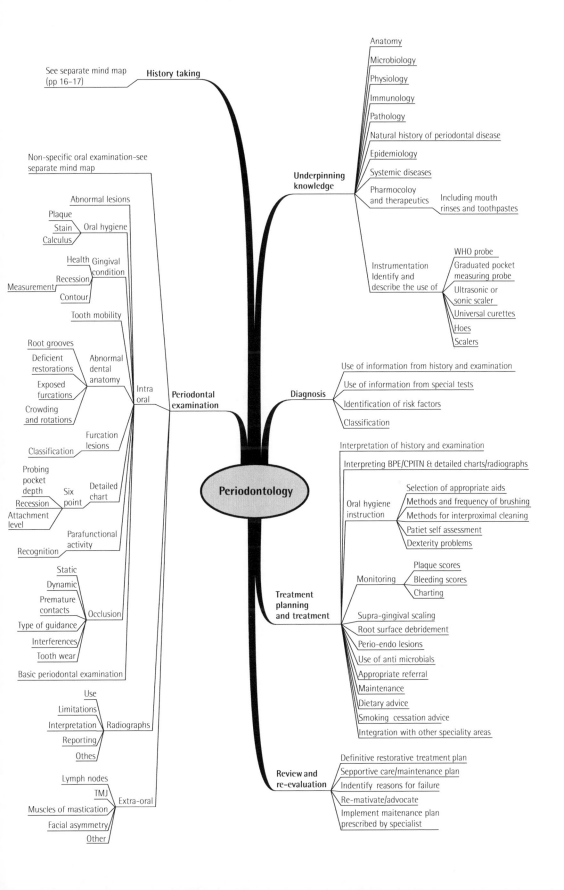

Periodontology

History taking
- See separate mind map (pp 16–17)

Underpinning knowledge
- Anatomy
- Microbiology
- Physiology
- Immunology
- Pathology
- Natural history of periodontal disease
- Epidemiology
- Systemic diseases
- Pharmocoloy and therapeutics
  - Including mouth rinses and toothpastes
- Instrumentation Identify and describe the use of
  - WHO probe
  - Graduated pocket measuring probe
  - Ultrasonic or sonic scaler
  - Universal curettes
  - Hoes
  - Scalers

Periodontal examination
- Intra oral
  - Non-specific oral examination-see separate mind map
  - Oral hygiene
    - Abnormal lesions
    - Plaque
    - Stain
    - Calculus
  - Gingival condition
    - Health
    - Recession
    - Contour
    - Measurement
  - Tooth mobility
  - Abnormal dental anatomy
    - Root grooves
    - Deficient restorations
    - Exposed furcations
    - Crowding and rotations
  - Furcation lesions
    - Classification
  - Detailed chart
    - Six point
      - Probing pocket depth
      - Recession
      - Attachment level
  - Parafunctional activity
    - Recognition
  - Occlusion
    - Static
    - Dynamic
    - Premature contacts
    - Type of guidance
    - Interferences
    - Tooth wear
  - Basic periodontal examination
- Radiographs
  - Use
  - Limitations
  - Interpretation
  - Reporting
  - Othes
- Extra-oral
  - Lymph nodes
  - TMJ
  - Muscles of mastication
  - Facial asymmetry
  - Other

Diagnosis
- Use of information from history and examination
- Use of information from special tests
- Identification of risk factors
- Classification

Treatment planning and treatment
- Interpretation of history and examination
- Interpreting BPE/CPITN & detailed charts/radiographs
- Oral hygiene instruction
  - Selection of appropriate aids
  - Methods and frequency of brushing
  - Methods for interproximal cleaning
  - Patiet self assessment
  - Dexterity problems
- Monitoring
  - Plaque scores
  - Bleeding scores
  - Charting
- Supra-gingival scaling
- Root surface debridement
- Perio-endo lesions
- Use of anti microbials
- Appropriate referral
- Maintenance
- Dietary advice
- Smoking cessation advice
- Integration with other speciality areas

Review and re-evaluation
- Definitive restorative treatment plan
- Sepportive care/maintenance plan
- Indentify reasons for failure
- Re-mativate/advocate
- Implement maitenance plan prescribed by specialist

2.5 Restorative dentistry

Francis Burke and Finbarr Allen

Key points

♦ Prevention is essential for the management of dental caries and tooth wear.

♦ The selection and handling of dental materials is based on sound knowledge of their composition and physical properties.

♦ The extent of dental decay or tooth wear will determine the cavity design and ultimate choice of restorative material.

♦ All operative treatment should seek to minimize loss of dental tissues.

♦ Precise communication with dental technicians is necessary for optimal results in indirect restorations.

♦ The ageing population together with changes in their oral health will present the profession with a fresh range of challenges.

Introduction

The 1998 Adult Dental Health Survey documented an increase in the population who are retaining their teeth. Eighty-seven per cent of the population was dentate compared to 68 per cent in 1968. It is projected that 96 per cent of the population will be dentate by 2028 (Nuttall *et al.* 2001).

The average number of sound teeth has increased and untreated decay has decreased. However, half of the 16–24-year-old age group had untreated decay and 11 per cent of adults had wear of their anterior teeth. Over half the population experienced oral problems in the previous year with pain being the most common problem. Tooth decay is still the most commonly cited reason for tooth loss, with toothache/abscess or broken or decaying teeth being the most immediate problem prior to tooth loss.

Ninety per cent of the population had at least one filled tooth with an average of seven fillings per patient. A third of the population had at least one crown. In 2002–2003 the Dental Practice Board for England and Wales reported that 16 million fillings, four million crowns and 750,000 bridges were placed. This accounted for almost 40 per cent of the cost of adult treatment (DPB 2003).

A specific cohort whose oral health is changing is the elderly. In the Adult Dental Health Survey the proportion of the elderly who were dentate was 54 per cent with 64 per cent of the young elderly, 65–74 years old, being dentate. Older age groups had higher levels of tooth wear, and root caries as well as a higher proportion of recurrent caries than the general population. Increasing polypharmacy and resultant xerostomia are likely to contribute to increased levels of caries in the future in this population group. Furthermore, older patients are more likely to have their teeth filled or crowned. Almost five million claims for treatment were made for the elderly in 2002–2003 accounting for 16.5 per cent of all adult treatments.

The ability to provide restorative care is likely to continue to play an essential role in the undergraduate curriculum. Provision of such care will also need to encompass an understanding of behaviour management (Chapter 1.10), cross-infection control (Chapter 1.5), law and ethics (Chapter 1.2), radiology (Chapter 1.11), dental materials (Chapter 1.16), removable prostheses (Chapter 2.7), impression-making (Chapter 1.15) and isolation and moisture control (Chapter 1.14).

The requirements for the delivery of restorative treatment are outlined in the General Dental Council's *The First Five Years: a framework for undergraduate dental education* (GDC 2002):

Paragraph 26.3 Students will need considerable experience in the operative procedures which dentists undertake in general practice, so that, on graduation, they are fit for independent practice, whilst at the same time being aware of their limitations and the need for specialist advice.

Paragraph 74 Restorative dentistry is concerned with the management of plaque-related diseases (dental caries and periodontal diseases) tooth wear and tooth loss. Management includes preventive, non-operative care as well as the restoration of teeth using the well-established techniques of restorative dentistry.

In restorative dentistry the students should have continuous responsibility for the care of a number of adults in order to assess their overall needs, the efficacy of preventive measures, their behaviour, management and long-term success or failure of restorative treatment...

All aspects of restorative dentistry may be required for medically compromised patients and those with special needs.

Paragraph 75 All restorative techniques can be invasive in nature, and some are irreversible. The GDC considers that dental students on graduation must be competent in procedures of restorative dentistry.... They should be fully aware when patients should be referred to specialists for advice and treatment.

Paragraph 77 The student should be aware of the presentation of dental and oral diseases in elderly people, and in the range of psychological and social factors involved in such situations. The student should be able to distinguish

Paragraph 77 – *continued*

between normal and abnormal consequences of ageing, and learn to avoid stereotyping elderly patients. Conditions including xerostomia, excessive tooth wear, root caries, recession of the gingival tissues and the special difficulty in providing removable prostheses, whilst not restricted to the elderly, are most prevalent in that group of patients. The student should be able to formulate management strategies for the dental care of elderly people, and to participate with members of the dental team in implementing them. Given the profound demographic changes affecting the population and the significant increase in the numbers of older adults with some natural teeth, the GDC would expect to see specific emphasis on this throughout the curriculum.

Restorative Dentistry and care for the elderly is also included in the Subject Benchmark for Dentistry (QAA 2002):

Assess patient risk for dental caries and non-bacterial tooth surface loss and be able to provide dietary counseling and nutritional education for the patient relevant to oral health and disease, based upon knowledge of disease patterns and aetiology.

Restore teeth to form, function and appearance with appropriate materials, using techniques that preserve health of the pulp and unnecessary loss of tooth tissues.

Manage and integrate the procedures necessary to provide biocompatible, functional and aesthetic dental prostheses (fixed and removable) in sympathy with patient requirements and needs.

Recognise the changes that occur with normal growth and ageing and apply their knowledge in the management of the oral environment.

Intended learning outcomes

Table 2.5.1 contains the intended learning outcomes incorporating those outlined in the *The First Five Years* (GDC 2002) the *American Dental Education Association Competencies for the New Dentist* (2003) and *Guidelines for Crown and Bridge* (British Society for Restorative Dentistry 1998).

Core skills in restorative dentistry

- ◆ History taking
- ◆ Clinical examination of teeth, periodontal tissues, oral mucosa and temporomandibular joints

Table 2.5.1 Intended learning outcomes for restorative dentistry

Be competent at	Have knowledge of	Be familiar with
Diagnosing active caries and planning appropriate non-operative care	Aetiology and histopathology of dental caries	
Using a rubber dam for the isolation of teeth	Aetiology and histopathology of xerostomia	Management of xerostomia
Designing cavities in relation to tooth anatomy, pathology and the characteristics of the restorative material	Management strategies for the carious process and protection of the dentino-pulpal complex	
The selection and handling of dental materials for restorative procedures based on a sound knowledge of their composition and physical properties		
Restore prepared cavities with the appropriate material	Methods to assess quality of restorations	
Diagnosing tooth wear and planning appropriate non-operative care	Aetiology of tooth wear	
Operative management of simple toothwear	Shortened dental arch concept	Management of advanced toothwear
Diagnose and manage traumatic injuries to teeth	Options for the replacement of the missing tooth or teeth	
Prescribing a maintenance programme for patients who have undergone restorative care		
Planning and providing oral care for the elderly	Demographic, medical, social and oral consequences of ageing	Domiciliary care
Patient referral for complex restorative care		
Prescribing maintenance care provided by Professions Complementary to Dentistry	Remit of activity of the Professions Complementary to Dentistry	

Table 2.5.1 Intended learning outcomes for restorative dentistry – *continued*

Be competent at	Have knowledge of	Be familiar with
Analysing failures to minimize future complications		
Planning for provision of indirect fixed restorations		
Tooth preparation, impression-making, temporization and provision of indirect fixed restorations		
Prescribing for indirect fixed restorations	Laboratory stages in the provision of indirect, fixed restorations	
Critically evaluate and provide feedback on laboratory work		
	Principles of osseo-integration and implant provision	The surgical and prosthetic techniques involved in implant provision
	Maintenance for patients with implants	

- Special investigations
- Taking long cone periapical and bitewing radiographs; interpreting plain film radiographs and diagnosing film faults
- Vitality testing
- Preparation of study casts
- Diagnosis
- Formulation of a treatment plan
- Obtain written, informed consent
- Communication of maintenance protocol.

History taking

The student should demonstrate ability to take a history. This should precede any form of treatment, and should elicit:

- The patient's name, date of birth and address
- Their reason for attendance

- The nature and duration of the presenting complaint

- Details of previous dental history, including frequency of attendance; motivation towards treatment; past dental treatment; any adverse events

- Details of previous medical history, particularly details of allergies, current medications, bleeding problems, diabetes and epilepsy, cardiac valve disorders, infective endocarditis, hepatitis

- Social history, including whether the patient can attend for prolonged courses of treatment.

All of this information should be written legibly into the patient's records, signed and dated.

Clinical examination

The student should demonstrate ability to carry out a clinical examination. The examination should be systematic and a sequential examination of the extra- and intra-oral tissues should be recorded.

During the extra-oral examination, the student should demonstrate ability to examine and record the:

- Facial muscles and note any painful trigger points

- TMJ for clicking/crepitus

- Any facial asymmetry

- Lip competence

- Lip line.

During the intra-oral examination, the student should demonstrate ability to:

- Recognize the presence of pathological lesions of the oral mucosa and know when to organize a referral for specialist advice

- Undertake a basic periodontal examination (BPE) and assign a BPE score for the patient

- Detect the presence of caries and defective restorations

- Detect the presence of pathological tooth wear and establish the aetiology based on the appearance of the teeth

- Detect the presence of deflective occlusal contacts.

Special investigations

Radiographs

The student should demonstrate ability to:

- Prescribe a radiographic examination when it is appropriate

- Prescribe radiographs appropriately

◆ Take intra-oral plain film radiographs

◆ Identify the different dental hard tissues (enamel, dentine and pulp chamber, alveolar bone) on a radiograph

◆ Identify radiographic evidence of dental hard tissue pathology

◆ Determine the morphology of the root canal system.

Vitality tests

◆ The student should demonstrate ability to

◆ Demonstrate a knowledge as to when a vitality test is applied

◆ Use an electronic pulp tester and understand the relevance of the information it provides

◆ Demonstrate a knowledge of the limitations of the response of the pulpal tissues to thermal vitality tests such as ethyl chloride.

Study casts:

The student should demonstrate ability to:

◆ Record satisfactory impressions for the construction of study casts

◆ Mount these casts on a semi-adjustable articulator using a facebow

◆ Critically assess the adequacy of the casts for diagnostic purposes

◆ Use study casts to communicate a treatment plan to the patient.

Diagnosis

The student should be demonstrate ability to reach a diagnosis on whether a restorative procedure is indicated based on the information collected during history taking and the examination. There should be a demonstrable recognition that the diagnosis is based on the:

◆ Patient's motivation for treatment

◆ Patient's medical history

◆ Condition of the gingival and periodontal tissues

◆ Condition of the remaining tooth structure

◆ Health of the pulp of the tooth/teeth involved

◆ Long-term prognosis for the remaining teeth.

Formulation of a treatment plan

The student should demonstrate ability to formulate a definitive treatment plan which is based on the:

- Prognosis for the teeth
- Patient's aspirations for treatment
- Individual circumstances such as ability to implement satisfactory plaque control measures and accept long periods in the dental chair
- Possible changes in circumstances, including further loss of teeth.

Consent

The student should demonstrate:

- Knowledge of the rationale for obtaining consent.
- Ability to obtain written informed consent prior to embarking on restorative care for a patient.

Communication of maintenance protocol

The student should demonstrate knowledge of the rationale of the need to maintain the health of the oral and dental tissues and the concept of whole patient care.
   The student should demonstrate ability to:

- Show a patient plaque removal techniques including flossing and the use of interdental toothbrushes
- Be familiar with the need to reinforce this information, particularly in the elderly patient
- Demonstrate a knowledge of the consequences of personal habits, such as smoking, for the health of oral tissues
- Demonstrate a knowledge of the sequencing of review appointments, the frequency of which should be based on individual risk of dental disease.

Specific skills in modalities of restorative dentistry

1. Caries management and protection of the pulp
2. Management of tooth wear
3. Management of dental trauma
4. Restorative care of the elderly patient
5. Preparation of teeth for indirect restorations including bridgework
6. Manipulation of impression materials
7. Construction of temporary restorations
8. Evaluation of laboratory work
9. Provision of indirect restorations for the patient
10. Use of dental implants.

Caries management and protection of the pulp

Aetiology

The student should demonstrate a knowledge of the:

◆ Major aetiological features of caries. This will include the specific anatomic features of enamel, dentine and cementum, the micro-organisms associated with caries, the role of diet, and the influence of time.

◆ Influence of factors including medical, behavioural, environmental, social, and intra-oral considerations on caries development.

Histopathology

The student should demonstrate knowledge of the:

◆ Stages of the disease process, the influence of the structure and composition of enamel, dentine, and cementum and the pulpal responses to the disease process

◆ Relationship between the histopathology of the disease process and its diagnosis and management strategies.

Diagnosis

The undergraduate should demonstrate knowledge of the:

◆ Features in a history that would lead to a diagnosis of caries including medical, behavioural, environmental and social factors, oral disease, and previous disease history

◆ Concept of caries activity, including determinants of caries activity especially lesion texture, colour, location, size and cavitation

◆ Aetiology and diagnosis of xerostomia

◆ Rationale for the use of special tests, especially radiographs

◆ Rationale for non-invasive diagnostic techniques including caries detecting dyes, fibre-optic transillumination (FOTI) and laser based diagnostic systems.

In order to diagnose caries the clinician should demonstrate ability to:

◆ Carry out an examination utilising the prerequisites for examination including adequate lighting, vision, removal of deposits and prostheses

◆ Prescribe, take and interpret appropriate intra-oral radiographs.

Treatment

The undergraduate should demonstrate understanding of the:

◆ Rationale for treatment strategies influenced by caries activity and stage of disease progression

◆ Principles of conventional caries removal, chemomechanical caries removal and atraumatic restorative treatment (ART)

- Principles of protection of the dentino-pulpal complex
- Properties of dental materials used in lining, basing and restoring cavities from which caries has been removed and apply this to the selection of appropriate materials for the restoration of a specific lesion. The range of materials should include calcium hydroxide, zinc phosphate, zinc oxide and eugenol, dentine bonding agents, glass ionomer cement, light-cured glass ionomer cement, amalgam and composite resin
- Relationship between the properties of amalgam, composite and glass ionomer cement and their clinical applications
- Relationship between the properties of restorative dental materials and cavity design
- Safety implications of the use of amalgam, composite resin and glass ionomer cement.

    Treatment strategies would encompass a demonstrable ability to:

- Apply the prevention of caries to its aetiological features
- Analyse a patient's dietary history and deliver appropriate dietary counselling
- Deliver oral hygiene instruction
- Prescribe and apply appropriate chemotherapeutic anti-caries agents to early carious lesions
- Develop a preventive regime for a patient suffering from xerostomia which would encompass the ability to prescribe appropriate saliva substitutes
- Identify hand and rotary instruments used in caries removal describing their characteristics and function
- Differentiate between sound and carious tooth tissue
- Carry out conventional caries removal
- Carry out ART
- Carry out appropriate protective lining and basing to protect the dentino-pulpal complex
- Apply matrices where appropriate
- Restore prepared cavities with amalgam, composite or glass ionomer cement
- Use safely amalgam, composite and glass ionomer cement, including personal protection and disposal of the materials
- Critically evaluate the quality of their operative procedures.

Tooth wear

Upon graduation, the student should:

1. Be familiar with the aesthetic and functional consequences of pathological and advanced physiological tooth wear

2. Have knowledge of the aetiology of pathological tooth wear

3. Furthermore an understanding of the influence of factors including medical, behavioural, environmental and social considerations should be manifest

4. Demonstrate ability to diagnose tooth wear

5. Be able to formulate a treatment plan for patients with advanced physiological or pathological tooth wear

6. Have knowledge of the need for maintenance in patients with tooth wear

7. Have knowledge of when it is appropriate to refer patients with advanced tooth wear for specialist advice and possible treatment.

Tooth wear in context

The undergraduate should demonstrate knowledge of:

◆ The difference between physiological and pathological tooth wear

◆ The aesthetic and functional consequences of tooth wear

◆ The concepts of:

  ▪ Attrition

  ▪ Abrasion

  ▪ Erosion

  ▪ Abfraction.

Aetiology

Demonstrate an understanding of the major aetiological features of tooth wear. This will include the role of diet, medical history, occupation, environment, oral hygiene practices, habits, occlusion and iatrogenic factors.

Diagnosis

The undergraduate should demonstrate an understanding of:

◆ Features in a history that would lead to a diagnosis of tooth wear including dietary, medical, behavioural, environmental, social and occlusal factors, and previous dental treatment.

◆ The rationale for the use of special tests, especially diet analysis and study models.

In order to diagnose tooth wear the clinician should demonstrate ability to:

◆ Carry out an examination including assessment of:

  ▪ Facial height

  ▪ Intra-oral soft tissue lesions

  ▪ Occlusal examination including premature contacts

  ▪ Teeth affected by tooth wear

  ▪ Surfaces of teeth affected by tooth wear

  ▪ Involvement of enamel, dentine or pulp

  ▪ Condition of existing restorations.

- Prescribe and take study models.
- Prescribe and take appropriate intra-oral radiographs.
- Prescribe and take photographs.
- Refer the patient for appropriate medical consultation.

Treatment planning

The undergraduate should demonstrate an understanding of:

- The rationale for treatment strategies influenced by tooth wear activity and stage of disease progression
- The principles of conventional lesion restoration, modification of the vertical dimension and selective over eruption
- The properties of dental materials used in restoring teeth and surfaces affected by tooth wear and apply this to the selection of appropriate materials for the restoration of a specific lesion. The range of materials should include dentine bonding agents, glass ionomer cement, light-cured glass ionomer cement, composite resin, gold alloy, porcelain and resin-bonded metals
- The relationship between the properties of, composite resin, glass ionomer cement, gold alloy, porcelain and resin-bonded metals and their clinical applications
- Relate the properties of restorative dental materials to tooth preparation.

  Treatment strategies would encompass a demonstrable ability to:

- Apply the prevention of tooth wear to its aetiological features
- Analyse a patient's dietary history and deliver appropriate dietary counselling
- Deliver oral hygiene instruction
- Prescribe and apply appropriate desensitizing agents to tooth wear lesions affected by sensitivity
- Select and apply appropriate adhesive materials for the restoration of tooth tissue lost due to tooth wear
- Carry out splint therapy to ameliorate the effect of excessive occlusal loading
- Carry out splint therapy to modify the patient's vertical dimension of occlusion
- Provide removable prostheses in cases of advanced tooth wear.

Maintenance

The undergraduate should demonstrate an understanding of:

- The rationale for recall to monitor patients who may be suffering from tooth wear
- The rationale for recall and maintenance of patients who have undergone treatment for tooth wear.

The undergraduate should demonstrate ability to:

♦ Formulate a recall programme for a patient who may be suffering from tooth wear

♦ Formulate a recall and maintenance programme for a patient who has undergone treatment for tooth wear.

Referral

The undergraduate should demonstrate ability to recognize and refer appropriately patients with tooth wear when:

♦ A medical or psychiatric consultation is required

♦ The complexity of restorative treatment contemplated would require specialist care.

Dental trauma

Upon graduation, the student should:

♦ Be familiar with the consequences of dental trauma

♦ Have knowledge of the aetiology of dental trauma

♦ Demonstrate ability to diagnose dental trauma

♦ Be able to formulate a treatment plan for patients with dental trauma

♦ Have knowledge of when it is appropriate to refer patients with severe dental trauma for specialist advice.

Consequences of dental trauma

The undergraduate should demonstrate knowledge of:

♦ The aesthetic consequences of dental trauma

♦ The functional consequences of dental trauma

♦ The dentino-pulpal consequences of dental trauma

Aetiology

Demonstrate an understanding of the major aetiological features of dental trauma. This will include the role of habits, occlusion and iatrogenic factors.

Diagnosis

The undergraduate should demonstrate an understanding of:

♦ Factors in a history that would lead to a diagnosis of dental trauma including dietary, medical, behavioural, environmental, social, occlusion, and previous dental treatment.

♦ The rationale for the use of special tests, especially radiographs.

In order to diagnose dental trauma the clinician should demonstrate ability to:

- Carry out an examination including:

  - Soft tissue trauma

  - Occlusal examination

  - Teeth affected by dental trauma

  - Surfaces of teeth affected by dental trauma

  - Involvement of enamel, dentine or pulp

  - Condition of existing restorations

- Prescribe and take appropriate intra-oral radiographs

- Carry out vitality testing

- Prescribe and take photographs

- Refer the patient for appropriate medical consultation.

Treatment planning

The undergraduate should demonstrate an understanding of:

- The principles of acute care and long-term care

- When it is more appropriate to extract a tooth/teeth affected by dental trauma

- Appropriate management and/or referral of soft tissue lesions as a consequence of dental trauma

- The properties of dental materials used in restoring teeth and surfaces affected by dental trauma and apply this to the selection of appropriate materials for the restoration of a specific lesion. The range of materials should include dentine bonding agents, glass ionomer cement, light-cured glass ionomer cement, composite resin, gold alloy, porcelain and resin-bonded metals

- The relationship between the properties of composite resin, glass ionomer cement, gold alloy, porcelain, and resin-bonded metals and their clinical applications

- Relate the properties of restorative dental materials to tooth preparation.

Treatment strategies

These would encompass a demonstrable ability to:

- Apply the prevention of dental trauma to its aetiological features

- Prescribe and apply appropriate desensitizing agents to lesions affected by trauma

- Select and apply appropriate adhesive materials for the restoration of tooth tissue lost due to trauma

- Carry out endodontic therapy when there is pulpal involvement as a result of dental trauma

- Carry out appropriate long-term treatment of the endodontically treated tooth.

Maintenance

The undergraduate should demonstrate an understanding of:

◆ The rationale for recall and maintenance of patients who have undergone treatment for dental trauma.

The undergraduate should demonstrate ability to:

◆ Formulate a recall programme for a patient who may be suffering from dental trauma

◆ Formulate a recall and maintenance programme for a patient who has undergone treatment for dental trauma.

Referral

The undergraduate should demonstrate ability to recognize and refer appropriately patients with dental trauma when:

◆ The complexity of restorative treatment contemplated would require specialist care.

Restorative care for the elderly patient

Upon graduation, the student should demonstrate:

◆ Knowledge of changing patterns of oral and dental disease in older adults.

◆ Knowledge of the challenges to oral health in older adults, including xerostomia, root caries, recession of the gingival tissues, prosthetic difficulties, tooth wear, and oral pathology.

◆ Familiarity with the distinction between ageing and poor health.

◆ Knowledge of consequences of ageing on oral and dental tissues and the impact of this on oral health and the response to treatment.

◆ Familiarity with the desirability of maintaining a functional, aesthetic, and healthy dentition for life for older adults.

◆ Ability to assess treatment need in older adults; be familiar with the principle of functionally oriented treatment planning for older adults, including the shortened dental arch concept

◆ Ability to communicate a treatment plan to an older adult.

◆ Knowledge of the rationale for maintenance in older adults, both with and without intra-oral prostheses.

Epidemiology of oral health of older adults

The undergraduate should demonstrate knowledge of:

◆ The demographic changes and their causes that have occurred in the elderly population

◆ The projected demographic changes in the elderly population and their impact on the delivery of health care

◆ The heterogeneity of the elderly population with particular emphasis on the distinction between ageing and poor health.

Oral health and the elderly

The undergraduate should demonstrate knowledge of:

- The changes in oral health and their causes that have occurred in the elderly population
- The projected changes in oral health in the elderly population and their impact on oral health care
- The aetiology, clinical consequences and diagnosis of xerostomia
- The aetiology and diagnosis of tooth wear, discrimination should be made between physiological and pathological tooth wear
- The aetiology and diagnosis, with particular emphasis on disease activity, of root caries
- The aetiology and diagnosis, with particular emphasis on disease activity, of gingival recession and periodontal disease
- The systemic, behavioural, oral, and iatrogenic factors which may contribute towards difficulties in wearing prosthetic appliances
- The aetiology and diagnosis of oral pathology, especially oral cancer.

Systemic ageing

The undergraduate should demonstrate knowledge of:

- What constitutes true ageing
- Factors which may influence the ageing process including:
  - Attitudinal
  - Medical
  - Psychiatric
  - Therapeutic
  - Nutritional
  - Social
  - Occupational
  - Environmental.

The oral effects of ageing

The undergraduate should demonstrate knowledge of:

- What constitutes true oral ageing together with the superimposed effects on the oral tissues of pathology and iatrogenic factors
- The effects of ageing on oral tissues including:
  - Bone
  - Oral mucosa

- Salivary glands
- Muscles of mastication
- Blood vessels
- Nerves
- Taste buds
- Periodontal ligament
- Enamel
- Dentine
- Cementum
- The dental pulp.

◆ The effects of ageing of the oral tissues on oral care including:

- Prevention
- Xerostomia
- Periodontal treatment
- Dental caries
- Tooth wear
- Endodontics
- Provision of fixed prostheses
- Provision of removable prostheses
- Implants.

Treatment goals for the elderly

The undergraduate should demonstrate knowledge of:

◆ The desirability of maintaining a functional, aesthetic and healthy dentition for life for older adults

◆ The importance of patient feedback and the avoidance of stereotyping the elderly as a homogenous group with a uniform set of expectations.

Treatment planning for the elderly patient

The undergraduate should demonstrate knowledge of:

◆ The principles of information gathering as a basis for formulating a treatment plan. This should include:

- History, with particular emphasis on patient demands and needs, medical history and social history
- Examination including extra-oral examination, intra-oral examination and examination of any existing prosthesis

- Special tests including radiographs, study models, vitality tests, salivary testing, dietary analysis and medical consultation.
- Functionally oriented treatment planning, including the shortened dental arch concept.
- The sequence of treatment planning:
  - Information gathering
  - Acute care
  - Control of pathology, including preventive care
  - Rehabilitation
  - Maintenance.
- The remit of treatment which can be carried out in a domiciliary environment.
- The medico-legal constraints under which domiciliary care can be delivered.
- The logistics of the delivery of domiciliary care.

The undergraduate should demonstrate the ability to:
- Carry out information gathering as a basis for developing a treatment strategy for elderly patients
- Formulate treatment strategies for elderly patients.

Communication with elderly patients
The undergraduate should demonstrate knowledge of:
- Sensory age changes which can affect communication
- Attitudinal factors on the part of clinician and patient which can act as barriers to effective communication.

The undergraduate should demonstrate the ability to communicate effectively with an elderly patient
In terms of:
- Information gathering
- Formulating a treatment plan together with the patient
- Provide feedback to the patient especially with regard to prevention and alternative treatment strategies
- Respond to feedback from the patient as treatment progresses.

Treatment of elderly patients
The undergraduate should demonstrate the ability to:
- Carry out treatment for elderly patients including:

- Preventive advice and care
- Management of xerostomia
- Periodontal therapy
- Management of root caries
- Management of simple tooth wear
- Endodontics when canals are locatable and negotiable
- Provision of fixed prostheses
- Provision of removable prostheses
- Refer patients where appropriate including:
  - Complex medical history
  - Complicated endodontics
  - Implants
  - Patient is housebound and requires domiciliary care.

Maintenance and the elderly patient

The undergraduate should demonstrate an understanding of:

- The importance of maintenance in the care of an elderly patient
- How maintenance programmes need to be tailored for specific patients based on factors including:
  - Medical state
  - Physical state
  - Medication
  - Dexterity
  - Past oral disease history
  - Level of treatment which has been provided
  - Presence of a removable prosthesis
  - Ability to attend for review
- The role of other members of the dental team, especially carers, dental hygienists and therapists in providing maintenance care.

The undergraduate should demonstrate the ability to:

- Formulate an appropriate maintenance programme for an elderly patient
- Deliver a programme of maintenance care for an elderly patient
- Prescribe a regime of maintenance care to be carried out in conjunction with a carer, dental hygienist or dental therapist.

Tooth preparation for indirect restorations including fixed prostheses (bridgework)

Upon graduation, the student should demonstrate the ability to:

◆ Undertake the necessary investigations prior to providing partial or full veneer crowns for a patient

◆ Execute preparations for partial and full veneer crowns

◆ To record and critically appraise impressions prior to sending them to a dental laboratory

◆ Manufacture and fit temporary restorations for patients following tooth preparation for partial and full veneer crowns

◆ Complete a prescription, including shade selection, and direct the dental technician in constructing partial and full veneer crowns

◆ Critically assess the quality of technical work returned from the dental laboratory, and to decide if it is appropriate to fit it in the patient's mouth

◆ Lute partial or full veneer crowns to teeth

◆ Communicate a maintenance protocol for crown work to the patient

◆ Recognize failure of indirect restorations, identify their causes and replace or repair the restorations with concomitant preventive strategies.

Upon graduation, the student should demonstrate knowledge of the:

◆ Indications for providing full and partial veneer crowns.

◆ Design principles for bridgework including fixed-fixed, fixed-moveable, cantilever and hybrid designs.

◆ Different principles of tooth preparation, temporization and cementation of conventional and resin-bonded bridgework.

◆ Principles of tooth preparation for indirect restorations.

◆ Rationale for the use of diagnostic and provisional restorations.

Caries management prior to tooth preparation for indirect restorations

The student should recognize that removal of tooth tissue during crown preparations can compromise the vitality of the pulpal tissues. They should be able to decide when previous restorations should be removed prior to crown preparation, and be able to choose suitable plastic restorative materials when a core is required. During the course of tooth preparation for full and partial veneer crowns, the student should:

◆ Recognize carious tissue and remove this entirely

◆ Demonstrate an understanding of the properties required for a core material, including the effect of this material on the pulpal tissues.

Preparation of the tooth to allow room for a partial or full veneer crown

The student must recognize that removal of tooth tissue during crown preparation is an invasive and irreversible procedure. This procedure must be undertaken with care and should be as minimally invasive as possible with a view to maintaining pulp vitality in the long term. The student should:

+ Be familiar with the depth of preparation required for gold, porcelain and porcelain fused to metal crowns

+ Recognize the degree of taper required during tooth preparation to provide adequate resistance and retention form

+ Recognize the amount of occlusal/incisal reduction required to give adequate occlusal/incisal clearance

+ Demonstrate knowledge of clinical situations when the degree of tooth reduction required would lead to compromised pulpal integrity and that endodontic or orthodontic treatment options should be considered.

Veneers

Upon graduation, the student should also:

+ Have knowledge of the relative merits of composite and porcelain laminate veneers.

+ Have knowledge of the indications for porcelain laminate veneers.

+ Be competent at preparing teeth for porcelain laminate veneers.

+ Be competent at recording impressions for porcelain laminate veneers.

+ Be competent at prescribing technical features of porcelain laminate veneers for the dental technician.

+ Be competent at assessing the quality of porcelain laminate veneers returned from the dental laboratory.

+ Be familiar with the techniques available for bonding porcelain laminate veneers to teeth.

+ Have knowledge of the need for maintenance of porcelain laminate veneers.

Fixed prostheses

In addition to the procedures outlined above for partial and full veneer crowns, the student should be able to undertake tooth replacement with simple fixed prostheses. Upon graduation, the student should:

+ Be competent at assessing patients with missing teeth and be familiar with the options available for replacing missing teeth.

+ Be competent at discussing with the patient indications for the various treatment options for replacing missing teeth using fixed prostheses.

- Be competent at undertaking preparations for conventional and resin bonded fixed prostheses.
- Be competent at recording and critically appraising impressions prior to sending them to a dental laboratory.
- Be competent at manufacturing and fitting temporary restorations for patients following tooth preparation for fixed prostheses.
- Be competent at completing a prescription, including shade selection, and directing the dental technician in constructing conventional and resin bonded fixed prostheses.
- Be competent at critically assessing the quality of technical work returned from the dental laboratory, and deciding if it is appropriate to fit it in the patient's mouth.
- Be familiar with the possibilities for cementing and bonding fixed prostheses to teeth.
- Have knowledge of the need for maintenance of fixed prostheses.
- Have knowledge of when it is appropriate to refer patients with missing teeth for specialist advice.

Manipulation of impression materials, occlusal registration and prescription
See Chapter 1.15.

Construction of temporary restorations
The student must appreciate that function, comfort, appearance, occlusal stability, and gingival health must be maintained during the interim period between tooth preparation for indirect restorations and return of the laboratory work. Consequently, the student must recognize that good quality temporary restorations are essential. The student should be able to critically evaluate:

- Whether the temporary crown/bridge is free from critical voids or fractures
- The marginal fit of the temporary crown/bridge
- The gingival emergence profile and embrasure form
- The occlusion of the temporary restorations with the opposing natural dentition and judge correctly that contact and guidance are evident where needed.

Upon graduation the student should:
- Demonstrate knowledge of the rationale for temporary restoration fabrication
- Demonstrate knowledge of the different techniques for temporary restoration fabrication
- Demonstrate knowledge of the materials available for temporary restoration fabrication and the appropriate luting agents
- Be competent at the fabrication of temporary restorations

◆ Demonstrate ability to critically evaluate the desirable criteria for a satisfactory temporary restoration

◆ Be competent at cementing a temporary restoration

◆ Be competent at removing a temporary restoration minimizing tissue loss or trauma to the hard or soft tissues.

Evaluation of laboratory work

When assessing the quality of laboratory work, the student should draw on their knowledge of dental materials, laboratory and clinical procedures. The student should demonstrate an appreciation of the need to have a well fitting, aesthetic restoration which is in harmony with the patient's occlusion. The student should:

◆ Have knowledge of the procedures involved in manufacturing indirect restorations, including:

  ■ Cast post and cores

  ■ Precious, semi-precious and non-precious metal alloy restorations

  ■ Porcelain and porcelain fused to metal restorations

  ■ Composite resin restorations

  ■ Resin-bonded restorations.

◆ Be able to recognize deficiencies, including:

  ■ Porosities in metal restorations

  ■ Perforation in metal restorations

  ■ Poor finishing of porcelain, including contamination with foreign bodies, crazing and failure to develop appropriate aesthetics

  ■ Damage/poor quality preparation of die materials

  ■ Be able to evaluate a laboratory prescription form

    • Assess if this has been used by the dental technician

    • Provide structured feedback to the dental technician.

Provision of laboratory work for the patient

When placing indirect restorations in the patient's mouth, the student should:

◆ Be familiar with the concepts of cementation and bonding restorations to tooth tissue

◆ Demonstrate ability to identify and rectify faults in an unsatisfactory indirect restoration

◆ Demonstrate knowledge of when it is appropriate to cement or bond a restoration to teeth

◆ Be able to assess the marginal fit of the restoration

- Be able to assess the contour of the restoration
- Be able to assess whether the restoration is in occlusal harmony with the opposing teeth
- Be able to assess the proximal contacts of the restoration and decide if these are acceptable
- Have knowledge of pontic designs for fixed prostheses and the impact of these on oral hygiene
- Have knowledge of finishing procedures such as minor occlusal adjustment and reglazing of porcelain restorations
- Demonstrate ability to assess the cosmetic qualities of a restoration
- Be able to communicate maintenance requirements to the patient
- Demonstrate ability to review indirect restorations post cementation/bonding.

Use of dental implants

The recent development of endosseous dental implants has implications for the management of tooth loss in partially dentate and edentulous patients. The use of dental implants is beyond the competence of undergraduate dental students. Nevertheless, the student should:

- Be familiar with the process of osseointegration and how implants are used to retain intra-oral prostheses
- Demonstrate an understanding of the principles of patient assessment for implants
- Be familiar with the surgical techniques involved in implant provision
- Be familiar with the fixed and removable prosthetic techniques involved in implant provision
- Be able to communicate to patients what the process involves
- Recognize when it is appropriate to refer patients for specialist advice
- Be competent to prescribe and execute a maintenance programme for a completed implant patient.

Checklist 41 **Assessment of operative management of caries**

	Yes	No
Adequate access		
No excessive tissue loss		
Caries remaining at amelo–dentinal junction		
Softened dentine remaining over pulp		
Complete caries removal		
Pulp exposure		
Selection of liner		
Application of liner		
Selection of base		
Placement of base		

Checklist 42 **Restoration evaluation**

Feature	Yes	No
Tooth-restoration junction not detectable with explorer		
Cusp planes, grooves, and marginal ridges continuous with existing tooth form		
Occlusal contact and anatomy restored		
Surface of restoration uniformly smooth		
Axial contour continuous with existing tooth form		
Proximal embrasures and proximal contact restored		
Perfect shade match		

Checklist 43 Assessment of tooth preparation for full or partial veneer crowns including impression-making

Feature	Yes	No
Sufficient occlusal clearance for the proposed material		
Free from undercut		
Sufficiently retentive		
Reduction of the buccal aspect in two planes sufficient to conform with the adjacent teeth		
Proximal contact adequately cleared at the finishing line		
Adjacent tooth been damaged during preparation		
Finish line smooth, with no lipping		
Finish line been positioned appropriately		
Surface of the preparation smooth with no sharp edges		
Obvious contamination of impression evident		
Margin of preparation detectable		
Air blows present		
Creases/folds present		
Entire dental arch recorded		
Is the laboratory prescription completed appropriately?		

Checklist 44 Assessment of laboratory work for indirect restorations

Feature	Yes	No
Quality of porcelain finish acceptable		
Metal free from porosities		
Damaged die detected		
Die overtrimmed		
Die undertrimmed		
Prescription followed by technician		

References and further reading

Allen P. F. (2002) *Teeth for Life for Older Adults*. London, Quintessence.

American Dental Education Association (2003) Competencies for the new dentist. *Journal of Dental Education* 67, 793–5.

Basker R., Cerny D., Burke F. *et al.* (2001) Restorative dentistry. In D. B. Shanley (ed.) *Dental Education in Europe. Towards convergence*, pp. 68–75. Dental Press Kft, Budapest, Hungary.

British Society for Restorative Dentistry (1998) *Guidelines for Crown and Bridge*. Available at: http://ww.bsrd.org/objects/downloads/cb_guide.doc

British Society for the Study of Prosthetic Dentistry: *Guidelines in Prosthetic and Implant Dentistry*. London, Quintessence.

Burke F. J. T., Grummitt J. M., Shearer A. C. and Wilson N. H. F. (1997) *A Strategy For Planning Restorative Dental Care*. British Society for Restorative Dentistry. Available at: http://www.bsrd.org/objects.downloads/rc_strategy.doc

Burke F. M. and Samarawickrama D. Y. D. (1995) Progressive changes in the pulpo-dentinal complex and their clinical consequences. *Gerodontology* 12, 57–66.

GDC (2002) *The First Five Years: a framework for undergraduate dental education*, 2nd edn. London, The General Dental Council.

http://www.dpb.nhs.uk/download/digest/digest_2003.pdf

http://www.qaa.ac.uk/crntwork/benchmark/phase2/Dentistry.pdf

National Institute of Clinical Excellence (2004) *Dental Recall. Recall interval between routine dental examinations*. Available at http://www.nice.org.uk/page,aspx?o=228919

Nuttall N. *et al.* (2001) *A Guide to the Adult Dental Health Survey 1998*. London, BDJ Books.

QAA (2002) *Dentistry: academic standards*. Subject benchmark statements. Gloucester, Quality Assurance Agency for Higher Education.

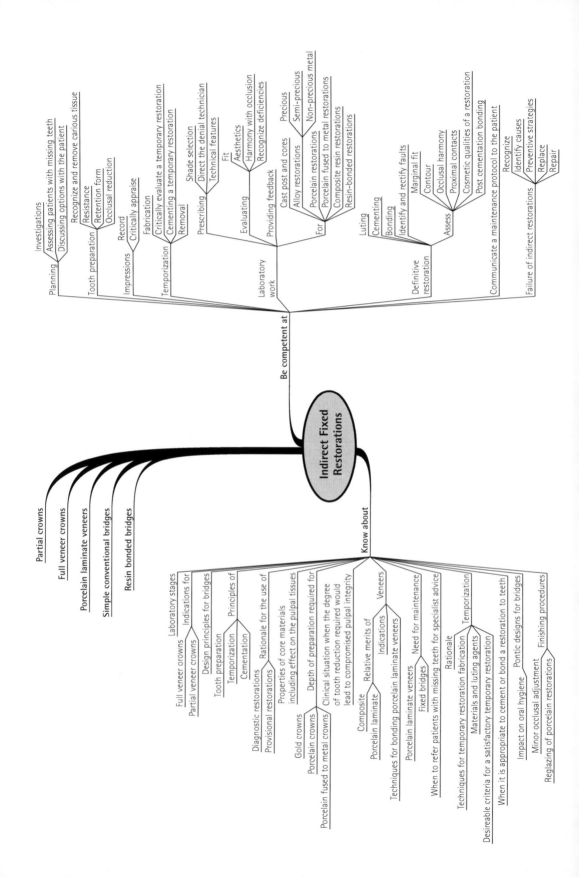

Indirect Fixed Restorations

Be competent at

- Partial crowns
- Full veneer crowns
- Porcelain laminate veneers
- Simple conventional bridges
- Resin bonded bridges

- Planning
  - Investigations
  - Assessing patients with missing teeth
  - Discussing options with the patient
- Tooth preparation
  - Recognize and remove carious tissue
  - Resistance
  - Retention form
  - Occlusal reduction
- Impressions
  - Record
  - Critically appraise
- Temporization
  - Fabrication
  - Critically evaluate a temporary restoration
  - Cementing a temporary restoration
  - Removal
- Laboratory work
  - Prescribing
    - Shade selection
    - Direct the denial technician
    - Technical features
  - Evaluating
    - Fit
    - Aesthetics
    - Harmony with occlusion
    - Recognize deficiencies
  - Providing feedback
  - For
    - Cast post and cores
    - Alloy restorations
      - Precious
      - Semi-precious
      - Non-precious metal
    - Porcelain restorations
    - Porcelain fused to metal restorations
    - Composite resin restorations
    - Resin-bonded restorations
- Definitive restoration
  - Luting
  - Cementing
  - Bonding
  - Identify and rectify faults
  - Assess
    - Marginal fit
    - Contour
    - Occlusal harmony
    - Proximal contacts
    - Cosmetic qualities of a restoration
    - Post cementation bonding
- Communicate a maintenance protocol to the patient
- Failure of indirect restorations
  - Recognize
  - Identify causes
  - Preventive strategies
  - Replace
  - Repair

Know about

- Laboratory stages
- Full veneer crowns
  - Indications for
- Partial veneer crowns
  - Design principles for bridges
- Tooth preparation
  - Principles of
  - Temporization
  - Cementation
  - Rationale for the use of
- Diagnostic restorations
- Provisional restorations
  - Properties of core materials including effect on the pulpal tissues
- Gold crowns
  - Depth of preparation required for
- Porcelain crowns
  - Clinical situation when the degree of tooth reduction required would lead to compromised pulpal integrity
- Porcelain fused to metal crowns
  - Veneers
    - Composite
    - Porcelain laminate
    - Relative merits of
    - Indications
- Techniques for bonding porcelain laminate veneers
  - Porcelain laminate veneers
  - Fixed bridges
    - Need for maintenance
- When to refer patients with missing teeth for specialist advice
  - Rationale
  - Temporization
- Techniques for temporary restoration fabrication
- Materials and luting agents
- Desireable criteria for a satisfactory temporary restoration
- When it is appropriate to cement or bond a restoration to teeth
  - Pontic designs for bridges
  - Impact on oral hygiene
  - Minor occlusal adjustment
  - Finishing procedures
  - Reglazing of porcelain restorations

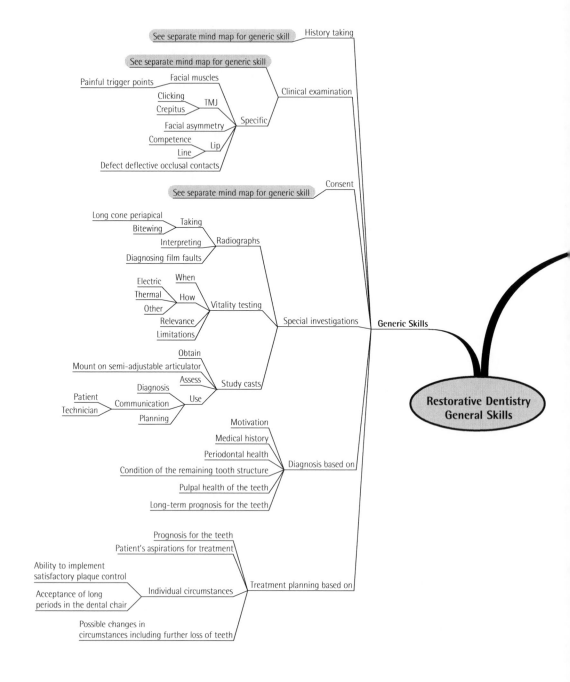

History taking
See separate mind map for generic skill

Clinical examination

See separate mind map for generic skill

Facial muscles — Painful trigger points

Specific

TMJ — Clicking
Crepitus

Facial asymmetry

Lip — Competence
Line

Defect deflective occlusal contacts

Consent
See separate mind map for generic skill

Special investigations

Radiographs

Taking — Long cone periapical
Bitewing

Interpreting

Diagnosing film faults

Vitality testing

When — Electric
Thermal

How — Other

Relevance

Limitations

Study casts

Obtain

Mount on semi-adjustable articulator

Assess

Use

Communication — Diagnosis
Patient
Technician

Planning

Diagnosis based on

Motivation

Medical history

Periodontal health

Condition of the remaining tooth structure

Pulpal health of the teeth

Long-term prognosis for the teeth

Treatment planning based on

Prognosis for the teeth

Patient's aspirations for treatment

Individual circumstances

Ability to implement
satisfactory plaque control

Acceptance of long
periods in the dental chair

Possible changes in
circumstances including further loss of teeth

Generic Skills

**Restorative Dentistry
General Skills**

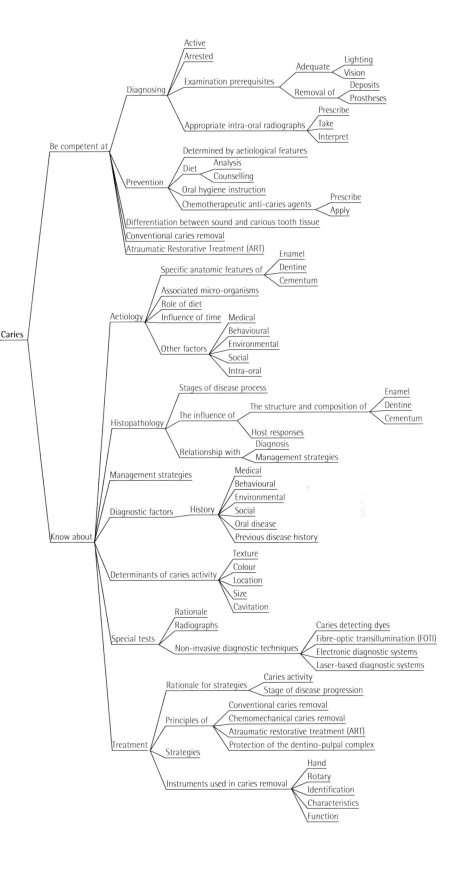

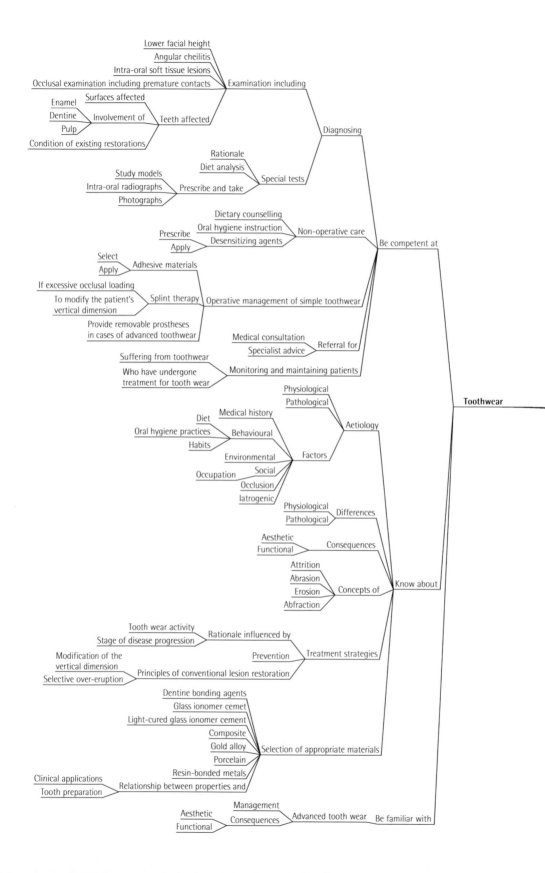

Lower facial height
Angular cheilitis
Intra-oral soft tissue lesions
Occlusal examination including premature contacts
Examination including

Enamel
Surfaces affected
Dentine — Involvement of — Teeth affected
Pulp
Condition of existing restorations

Diagnosing

Rationale
Diet analysis
Special tests
Study models
Intra-oral radiographs — Prescribe and take
Photographs

Dietary counselling
Oral hygiene instruction — Non-operative care
Prescribe — Desensitizing agents
Apply

Select
Apply — Adhesive materials
If excessive occlusal loading
To modify the patient's — Splint therapy — Operative management of simple toothwear
vertical dimension
Provide removable prostheses
in cases of advanced toothwear

Medical consultation
Specialist advice — Referral for
Suffering from toothwear
Who have undergone — Monitoring and maintaining patients
treatment for tooth wear

Be competent at

Physiological
Pathological
Medical history — Aetiology
Diet
Oral hygiene practices — Behavioural
Habits
Environmental — Factors
Occupation — Social
Occlusion
Iatrogenic

Physiological
Pathological — Differences
Aesthetic — Consequences
Functional

Attrition
Abrasion
Erosion — Concepts of
Abfraction

Know about

Toothwear

Tooth wear activity
Stage of disease progression — Rationale influenced by
Prevention — Treatment strategies
Modification of the
vertical dimension
Selective over-eruption — Principles of conventional lesion restoration

Dentine bonding agents
Glass ionomer cemet
Light-cured glass ionomer cement
Composite
Gold alloy — Selection of appropriate materials
Porcelain
Resin-bonded metals
Clinical applications
Tooth preparation — Relationship between properties and

Management
Aesthetic — Consequences — Advanced tooth wear — Be familiar with
Functional

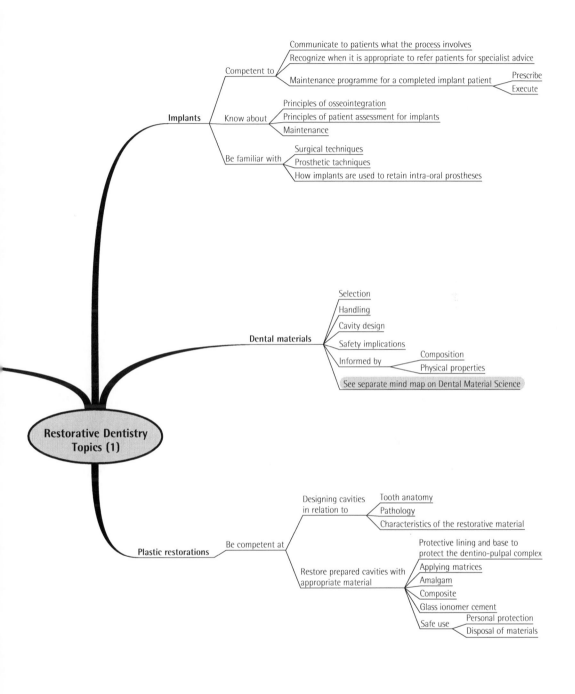

Restorative Dentistry
Topics (1)

Implants
- Competent to
  - Communicate to patients what the process involves
  - Recognize when it is appropriate to refer patients for specialist advice
  - Maintenance programme for a completed implant patient
    - Prescribe
    - Execute
- Know about
  - Principles of osseointegration
  - Principles of patient assessment for implants
  - Maintenance
- Be familiar with
  - Surgical techniques
  - Prosthetic tachniques
  - How implants are used to retain intra-oral prostheses

Dental materials
- Selection
- Handling
- Cavity design
- Safety implications
- Informed by
  - Composition
  - Physical properties
- See separate mind map on Dental Material Science

Plastic restorations
- Be competent at
  - Designing cavities in relation to
    - Tooth anatomy
    - Pathology
    - Characteristics of the restorative material
  - Restore prepared cavities with appropriate material
    - Protective lining and base to protect the dentino-pulpal complex
    - Applying matrices
    - Amalgam
    - Composite
    - Glass ionomer cement
    - Safe use
      - Personal protection
      - Disposal of materials

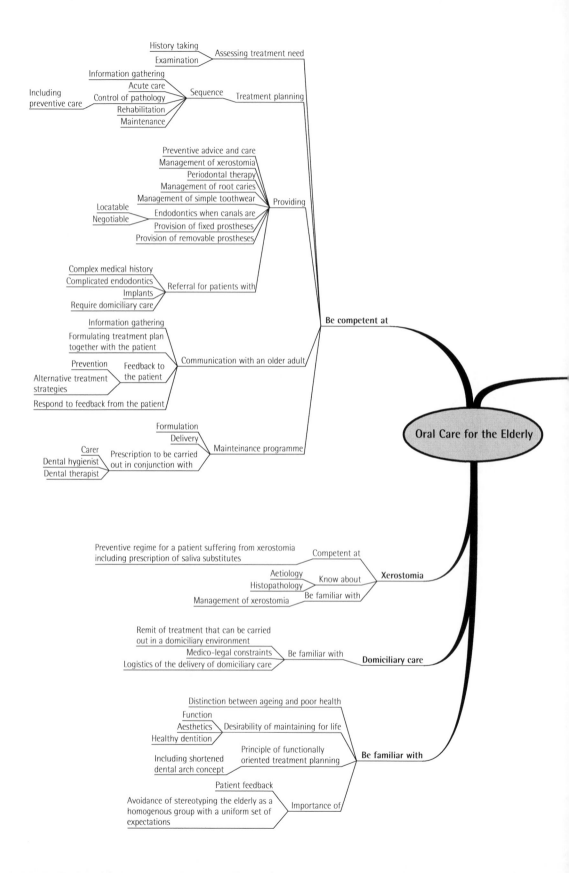

History taking
Examination
Assessing treatment need

Information gathering
Acute care
Control of pathology
Rehabilitation
Maintenance

Including preventive care

Sequence
Treatment planning

Preventive advice and care
Management of xerostomia
Periodontal therapy
Management of root caries
Management of simple toothwear
Endodontics when canals are
Provision of fixed prostheses
Provision of removable prostheses

Locatable
Negotiable

Providing

Complex medical history
Complicated endodontics
Implants
Require domiciliary care

Referral for patients with

Information gathering
Formulating treatment plan together with the patient
Prevention
Alternative treatment strategies
Respond to feedback from the patient

Feedback to the patient

Communication with an older adult

Formulation
Delivery

Carer
Dental hygienist
Dental therapist

Prescription to be carried out in conjunction with

Mainteinance programme

Be competent at

Oral Care for the Elderly

Preventive regime for a patient suffering from xerostomia including prescription of saliva substitutes

Competent at

Aetiology
Histopathology

Know about

Xerostomia

Management of xerostomia

Be familiar with

Remit of treatment that can be carried out in a domiciliary environment
Medico-legal constraints
Logistics of the delivery of domiciliary care

Be familiar with

Domiciliary care

Distinction between ageing and poor health

Function
Aesthetics
Healthy dentition

Desirability of maintaining for life

Including shortened dental arch concept

Principle of functionally oriented treatment planning

Patient feedback

Avoidance of stereotyping the elderly as a homogenous group with a uniform set of expectations

Importance of

Be familiar with

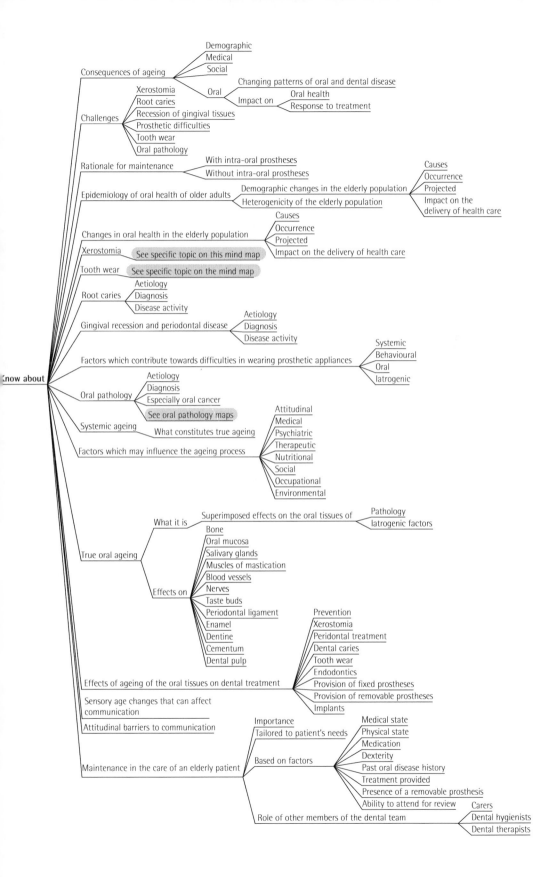

Know about

Consequences of ageing
- Demographic
- Medical
- Social
- Oral
  - Changing patterns of oral and dental disease
  - Impact on
    - Oral health
    - Response to treatment

Challenges
- Xerostomia
- Root caries
- Recession of gingival tissues
- Prosthetic difficulties
- Tooth wear
- Oral pathology

Rationale for maintenance
- With intra-oral prostheses
- Without intra-oral prostheses

Epidemiology of oral health of older adults
- Demographic changes in the elderly population
  - Causes
  - Occurrence
  - Projected
  - Impact on the delivery of health care
- Heterogenicity of the elderly population

Changes in oral health in the elderly population
- Causes
- Occurrence
- Projected
- Impact on the delivery of health care

Xerostomia   See specific topic on this mind map

Tooth wear   See specific topic on the mind map

Root caries
- Aetiology
- Diagnosis
- Disease activity

Gingival recession and periodontal disease
- Aetiology
- Diagnosis
- Disease activity

Factors which contribute towards difficulties in wearing prosthetic appliances
- Systemic
- Behavioural
- Oral
- Iatrogenic

Oral pathology
- Aetiology
- Diagnosis
- Especially oral cancer
- See oral pathology maps

Systemic ageing
- What constitutes true ageing

Factors which may influence the ageing process
- Attitudinal
- Medical
- Psychiatric
- Therapeutic
- Nutritional
- Social
- Occupational
- Environmental

True oral ageing
- What it is
  - Superimposed effects on the oral tissues of
    - Pathology
    - Iatrogenic factors
- Effects on
  - Bone
  - Oral mucosa
  - Salivary glands
  - Muscles of mastication
  - Blood vessels
  - Nerves
  - Taste buds
  - Periodontal ligament
  - Enamel
  - Dentine
  - Cementum
  - Dental pulp

Effects of ageing of the oral tissues on dental treatment
- Prevention
- Xerostomia
- Peridontal treatment
- Dental caries
- Tooth wear
- Endodontics
- Provision of fixed prostheses
- Provision of removable prostheses
- Implants

Sensory age changes that can affect communication

Attitudinal barriers to communication

Maintenance in the care of an elderly patient
- Importance
- Tailored to patient's needs
- Based on factors
  - Medical state
  - Physical state
  - Medication
  - Dexterity
  - Past oral disease history
  - Treatment provided
  - Presence of a removable prosthesis
  - Ability to attend for review
- Role of other members of the dental team
  - Carers
  - Dental hygienists
  - Dental therapists

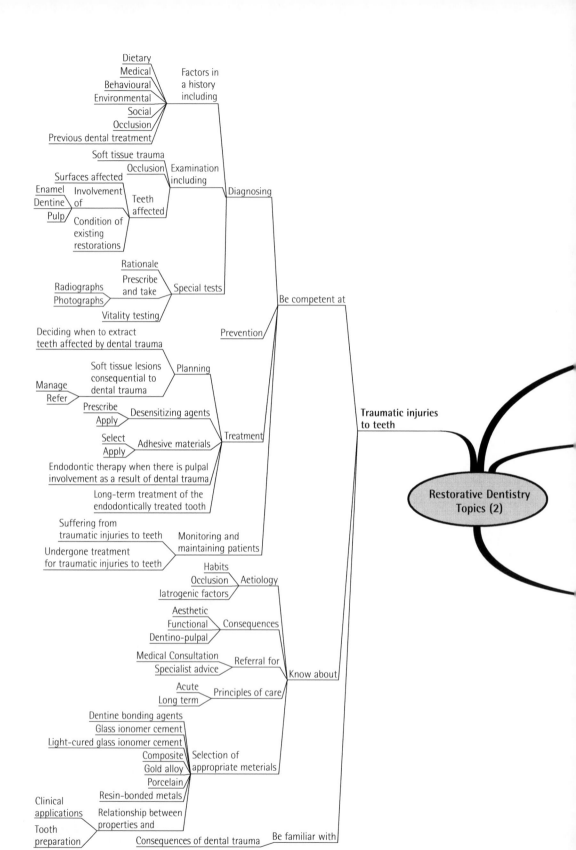

Dietary
Medical
Behavioural
Environmental
Social
Occlusion
Previous dental treatment

Factors in
a history
including

Soft tissue trauma
Occlusion
Surfaces affected
Enamel
Dentine
Pulp

Involvement
of

Examination
including

Teeth
affected

Condition of
existing
restorations

Diagnosing

Rationale
Prescribe
and take

Radiographs
Photographs

Special tests

Vitality testing

Be competent at

Prevention

Deciding when to extract
teeth affected by dental trauma

Soft tissue lesions
consequential to
dental trauma

Planning

Manage
Refer

Prescribe
Apply

Desensitizing agents

Select
Apply

Adhesive materials

Treatment

Endodontic therapy when there is pulpal
involvement as a result of dental trauma

Long-term treatment of the
endodontically treated tooth

Suffering from
traumatic injuries to teeth

Undergone treatment
for traumatic injuries to teeth

Monitoring and
maintaining patients

Habits
Occlusion
Iatrogenic factors

Aesthetic

Functional
Dentino-pulpal

Aetiology

Consequences

Medical Consultation
Specialist advice

Acute
Long term

Referral for

Principles of care

Traumatic injuries
to teeth

Know about

Dentine bonding agents
Glass ionomer cement
Light-cured glass ionomer cement
Composite
Gold alloy
Porcelain
Resin-bonded metals

Selection of
appropriate meterials

Clinical
applications
Tooth
preparation

Relationship between
properties and

Consequences of dental trauma

Be familiar with

Restorative Dentistry
Topics (2)

Be competent at
- Using rubber dam for the isolation of teeth
- Referral for complex restorative care
- Analysing failures to minimize future complications
- Critical evaluation of quality of operative procedures

Have knowledge of
- Management strategies for protection of the dentino-pulpal complex
- Methods to assess quality of restorations
- Shortened dental arch concept
- Options for replacement of missing teeth
- Remit of activity of Professions Complementary to Dentistry

Prescribing maintenance for patients
- Self delivered
- DCP delivered
- Dentist delivered
  - Be competent at
    - Communication of the protocol
    - Advising and instructing on plaque removal techniques including
      - Flossing
      - Use of interdental toothbrushes
  - Knowledge of the
    - Consequences of personal habits such as smoking for the health of oral tissues
    - Sequencing of review appointments' frequency based on individual risk of dental disease
  - Be familiar with the need to reinforce this information, particularly in the elderly patient

2.6 Endodontics

Bill Saunders

Key points

- The graduating dentist should demonstrate competency in the diagnosis of diseases of the dental pulp and periradicular tissues and treatment of these diseases in both deciduous and permanent teeth.

- This should include aspects of dental traumatology, and interrelationships of endodontics with other clinical dental disciplines to ensure comprehensive patient care.

- A core of knowledge including basic science and practical skills must be learned and assessed to ensure patient safety.

Introduction

Endodontology is defined as the study of the form, function and health, injuries to and diseases of the dental pulp and periradicular tissues, their prevention and treatment (*International Endodontic Journal*, European Society of Endodontology 1998). Endodontics is the practice of this science. The aetiology of the most common diseases of the dental pulp and periradicular tissues is microbial (Kakehashi *et al.* 1966) and the objective of endodontic treatment is to eliminate microbial irritation of the pulpal and periradicular tissues. Dental caries and its subsequent removal and replacement with restorations and traumatic injuries to the teeth are the most common sources of microbial contamination of the dental pulp and periradicular tissues. Endodontic treatment must be part of holistic care to ensure that oral and general health of the patient is maintained.

> Undergraduate education in endodontics expects competence to be achieved in practical procedures, involving management of the dental pulp and root canal treatment in both single- and multi-rooted teeth.
>
> **GDC (2004, paragraph 75)**

The Quality Assurance Agency benchmarking committee for dentistry has recommended that the newly qualified dentist should be able to manage diseases and conditions involving the pulpal and periradicular tissues in both primary and permanent teeth (QAA 2002, paragraph 3.14).

The European Society of Endodontology have produced undergraduate curriculum guidelines for endodontology. These include a series of competencies which includes theoretical and practical knowledge. Elements of didactic teaching, preclinical operative techniques classes and clinical treatment of patients will contribute to this curriculum. Clinical endodontics should ideally be supervized by specialists or at least by staff with a special knowledge and interest in endodontics. Both formative and summative assessment procedures should be part of the curriculum in endodontology.

Table 2.6.1 Intended learning outcomes in endodontics

Be competent at	Have knowledge of	Be familiar with
Communicating with patients in order to elicit appropriate details	The importance of record keeping	Epidemiology and biostatistics related to endodontology
Undertaking a clinical examination of soft and hard tissues	Which endodontic procedures may pose a risk, and particularly those in relation to a specific medical history	Literature to ensure 'best practice' is undertaken
Chart teeth and recognize the presence of dental caries, intact and failing intra- and extra-coronal restorations	The occlusal relations of the mandibular to the maxillary teeth, to include static and dynamic relationships	The principles and practice of dental traumatology
Undertaking special tests appropriate for endodontic therapy	Principles and practice of intra-oral radiography	
Planning treatment in a logical sequence to include treating the immediate problem and then linking with other treatment goals	Methods of determining pulp sensitivity	
Differentiating between a surgical and non-surgical approach	The principles of surgical endodontics	
Non-surgical endodontics for deciduous teeth	Biology, anatomy and physiology of the oral and perioral tissues	
Non-surgical endodontics for immature permanent teeth	Biomaterials science in relation to endodontics	
	Pharmacological agents used in the management of pulpal and periradicular tissues	

Checklist for skills in endodontics

1. History taking
2. Clinical examination – extra-oral and intra-oral
   - Extra-oral:
     - temporomandibular joints
     - submandibular and cervical lymph nodes
     - soft tissue evaluation including swelling
   - Intra-oral:
     - soft tissues; sinus tracts, swelling
     - teeth including carious lesions, existing and failing restorations
     - occlusion; static and dynamic (lateral and protrusive)
     - periodontal tissues
3. Special investigations
   - Sensitivity tests:
     - cold, heat and electrical, test cavity
   - Radiological:
     - periapical and parallax
4. Diagnosis and recording the 'diagnostic statement'
5. Treatment plan and objectives
6. Nonsurgical endodontic treatment including treatment by indirect and direct pulp capping and non-surgical root canal treatment and re-treatment
   - Principals of surgical root canal treatment
7. Letter of referral for secondary endodontic care

All the tasks will be described in the two stage format:

1. The standards expected for that particular task;
2. A checklist to enable the supervision of the task and enable the assessment of level of competency that the student has achieved.

History taking in endodontics

Standards

The student should:

1. Appreciate that history taking is part of a sequence as follows:
2. History taking $\Rightarrow$ examination $\Rightarrow$ diagnosis $\Rightarrow$ treatment
3. Be competent at communicating with patients in order to elicit appropriate details as follows:

- ◆ Patient's name, date of birth, age and address
- ◆ Reason for attendance: Many of the patients who require endodontic treatment present with pain and it is important to establish the cause of pain and make a suitable differential diagnosis of orofacial pain of odontogenic and non-odontogenic origin.
- ◆ Assess the patient's motivation for endodontic treatment and identify the expectations of the patient. This should include a risk assessment of all endodontic treatment options. The previous dental treatment history will help to establish the level of commitment by the patient.
- ◆ Describe in appropriate detail and language (without jargon) what endodontic treatment might entail.
- ◆ Medical history: demonstrate a knowledge of aspects of the history which are particularly relevant to endodontics such as the following:
  - ▪ Conditions requiring antimicrobial prophylaxis
  - ▪ Conditions that may preclude long appointments especially in the supine position eg chronic obstructive airway disease
  - ▪ Allergies. Patients with multiple allergies are liable to experience an increased incidence of flare-up during root canal treatment (Torabinejad *et al.* 1988)
  - ▪ Bleeding tendencies
  - ▪ Diabetes
  - ▪ Epilepsy
- ◆ Social history: to include occupation, ability to attend for treatment and smoking and alcohol consumption
- ◆ Record dated, accurate, concise and legible entries in the patient's case notes.

Underpinning knowledge

The student should have knowledge of:

- ◆ the importance of good record keeping
- ◆ which endodontic procedures may pose a risk, and particularly those in relation to a specific medical history.

History taking in endodontics

The checklist should include:

- ◆ Introduction and explanation of procedure to patient
- ◆ Recording of basic identification and demographic details
- ◆ Establishing reasons for attendance

- Taking history of patient's presenting complaint, using appropriate questions and answers
- Systematic and appropriate medical history details
- A dental history with specific mention of:
  - previous endodontic and restorative dental treatment experience
  - anaesthetic experience
- Making enquiries about social history and ability to attend
- Recording the above concisely and legibly in patient's notes.

Clinical examination

The undergraduate should be able to perform an examination of the patient with an endodontic-related problem, evaluate the status of the dental pulp and periradicular tissues of teeth and provide good quality endodontic treatment in the context of the overall welfare of the patient.

Extra-oral examination

The student should be competent at undertaking a clinical examination to include:
- prior explanation of the procedure
- examination of the face to establish any asymmetry and presence of facial swelling
- clinical examination of the temporomandibular joints by palpation to determine whether there is pain, clicking and deviation on opening and closing, or limitation of movement
- examination of the muscles of mastication and to understand the significance of muscle tenderness
- examination of the submandibular and cervical lymph nodes by palpation.

Intra-oral examination

The student should:
- have knowledge of the occlusal relations of the mandibular to the maxillary teeth, to include static and dynamic relationships.
- be competent to undertake an examination of the soft tissues of the oropharynx, including cheeks, soft and hard palate, posterior wall of pharynx, tonsils, tongue, floor of mouth, alveolar mucosa and lips
- be competent in undertaking a detailed examination of the periodontal status of the patient
- chart the teeth and recognize the presence of dental caries, intact and failing intra- and extra-coronal restorations

♦ be competent at palpating and percussing teeth to determine mobility, fremitus and tenderness

♦ carry out all the above taking cognisance of cross-infection control procedures

♦ communicate effectively with the patient during the course of the examination.

Special investigations

The student should demonstrate:

♦ a detailed knowledge of the principles and practice of intra-oral radiography including the use of film-holders. It is essential that radiographs are of suitable diagnostic quality and that the findings are recorded carefully in the patient's case notes

♦ how the use of parallax may help in the location of root canals in teeth

♦ a knowledge of the methods of determining pulp sensitivity using heat, cold and electrical stimulation and the use of a test cavity

♦ knowledge of the principles of pulpal blood flow and how this may be measured using laser doppler flowmetry

♦ a detailed knowledge of how a sinus tract may be explored

♦ how to use selective anaesthesia to help determine painful teeth

♦ how to use transillumination to determine cracked teeth and carious lesions

♦ knowledge of the use of microbiological sampling techniques, including needle aspiration biopsy, to investigate infections within the root canal and soft tissue swellings.

Diagnostic statement

The student should:

Be able to formulate a diagnostic statement based upon all the information gathered during the history taking and examination. This statement will be specifically concerned with the endodontic pathology of one or a number of teeth but it is important that the diagnosis is not made in isolation but is based upon the complete examination of the patient and includes any other findings of note.

A diagnosis of both the pulpal and periradicular status of the tooth/teeth should be made.

Pulp

It is difficult to know the histopathological status of the pulp and thus diagnosis is made on clinical criteria. The student should be aware of the following differential diagnoses:

♦ Acute reversible pulpitis

♦ Acute irreversible pulpitis

♦ Chronic asymptomatic pulpitis

♦ Necrosis.

Periradicular tissues

♦ Acute (symptomatic) periradicular periodontitis

♦ Chronic (asymptomatic) periradicular periodontitis

♦ Chronic suppurative periradicular periodontitis (chronic abscess)

♦ Acute apical abscess.

Other diagnoses

The student should have detailed knowledge of how to diagnose the following:

♦ Cracked teeth

♦ Internal and external root resorption

♦ Fractured roots, including both horizontal and vertical root fractures.

Treatment plan

The planning of treatment should be made after discussion with the patient. The student should be competent at:

♦ planning treatment in a logical sequence to include treating the immediate problem and then linking the endodontic treatment with other treatment goals

♦ identifying patient expectations regarding endodontic treatment and present realistic treatment outcomes

♦ assessing patient acceptance of treatment modalities in endodontics

♦ undertaking treatment for different patient groups including the elderly

♦ liaising with colleagues for multidisciplinary planning and management of treatment

♦ understanding of the relationship of endodontics with other dental and medical disciplines and the possibilities for adjunctive treatment:

- diagnosis and management of periodontal disease and the interaction between endodontic and periodontal disease

- diagnosis and management of tooth surface loss

- diagnosis and management related to fixed and removable prosthodontics and implants

- understanding the role of orthodontics and paediatric dentistry in the management of endodontically related problems

♦ differentiating between a surgical or non-surgical approach to endodontic treatment.

Undergraduate students will be expected to have the requisite technical skills to undertake non-surgical root canal treatment but only to have knowledge of the principles and practice of surgical endodontics.

The examination can only be undertaken, the diagnosis made, and the treatment plan executed if the student has a sound knowledge of the principles of basic science in relation to endodontics.

The student should have knowledge of:

◆ the biology, anatomy and physiology of the oral and perioral tissues to include:

  ▪ the development of the tooth and local anomalies of tooth development including those affecting the morphology of the root canal system

  ▪ the physiological and anatomical changes that take place in the pulpo-dentinal complex of teeth as a result of dental caries, trauma, tooth surface loss and age

  ▪ the relationship of the teeth with local structures in respect to those involved in disease of endodontic origin

  ▪ the microbiology and immunology of pulpal and periradicular disease

  ▪ biomaterials science in relation to endodontics

  ▪ the pharmacotherapeutic agents used in the management of pulpal and periradicular disease

  ▪ the principles and practice of prevention of diseases of the pulp and periradicular tissues.

The student should be familiar with:

◆ the epidemiology and biostatistics related to endodontics

◆ the endodontic literature to ensure 'best practice' is undertaken.

Treatment

Endodontic treatment includes indirect and direct pulp capping, non-surgical root canal treatment and re-treatment, surgical root canal treatment (including root-end resection and root-end filling, root resection and guided tissue regenerative techniques). The treatment of dental trauma is also part of endodontic care for patients, as these injuries very often damage the dental pulp.

The student should have knowledge of:

◆ The principles and practice of local anaesthesia for the treatment of pulpal and periradicular disease and:

  ▪ practical competence in the use of infiltration and regional anaesthesia in endodontic treatment

  ▪ intrapulpal, intraligamental and intraosseous techniques for anaesthesia

◆ The principles of and competence in the use of rubber dam in endodontically related procedures and to have extensive experience of the application of rubber dam in a variety of cases

- The principles of and be competent in the practice of the management of endodontic emergencies, including toothache, flare-ups and acute abscesses
- The principles of and be competent at the practice of vital pulp therapy and preventive endodontics. These must include:
  - indirect pulp capping and stepwise excavation of dental caries
  - direct pulp capping and the agents used to pulp cap
  - pulpotomy
- The principles of and be competent at the practice of non-surgical root canal treatment for vital and non-vital *de novo* cases. Students must demonstrate satisfactory non-surgical root canal treatment of single and multi-rooted teeth. This must include:
  - providing adequate anaesthesia
  - preparing the tooth and the field of operation and rubber dam placement
  - access cavity preparation
  - shaping and cleaning the root canal system
  - determining working length
  - irrigation of the root canal system
  - placement of an inter-appointment dressing
  - obturation of the root canal system
  - provide appropriate instructions concerning post-operative discomfort, pain and swelling
  - an understanding the iatrogenic errors that may occur during non-surgical root canal treatment and how to avoid them
- The principles of, and be familiar with, the practice of non-surgical root canal re-treatment
  - have experience of non-surgical root canal re-treatment of single rooted and multi rooted teeth
  - observe and, if possible, perform dismantling of teeth restored with bridgework, crowns and post-retained restorations for the purpose of root canal treatment
  - observe and if possible perform removal of root canal filling materials
  - observe removal of fractured root canal instruments
  - observe internal repair of perforations
- The principles and practice of dental traumatology. These must include:
  - crown fractures
  - crown-root fractures

- root fractures, including vertical root fractures
- luxation injuries
- avulsion

◆ Able to advise various authorities on the prevention of dental traumatology especially during sporting pursuits

◆ The principles of and be competent at the practice of non-surgical endodontics for deciduous teeth and immature permanent teeth. These must include:

- devitalization
- pulp capping
- apexogenesis (root development)
- apexification (root-end closure)

◆ The principles of and be competent at the practice of the management of endodontic emergencies

◆ The principles of and be competent at procedures to restore the root filled tooth to function using intra-coronal and extra-coronal restorations

◆ The procedures to restore the aesthetics of the root filled tooth using non-vital bleaching techniques and restorative procedures

◆ Cross-infection control measures in endodontics

- have the ability to chemically disinfect cabinetry and dental unit surfaces
- have the ability to clean and autoclave dental handpieces and hand instruments
- have the ability to adopt appropriate barrier techniques for the practice of endodontics.

Checklist 45 **Root canal preparation**

	Yes	No
General		
Introduction and explanation of procedure to patient		
Initial diagnosis – demonstrate made a correct diagnosis		
Interpretation of pre-operative radiograph		
Delivery of local anaesthetic		
Rubber dam placement		
• causes minimal injury to the soft tissues		
• prevent any possible swallowing		
• no leakage around the tooth		

Checklist 45 **Root canal preparation** – *continued*

	Yes	No
Access cavity		
• position and shape		
• whole of the roof of the chamber has been removed		
• straight-line access to the apex of each root canal can be achieved		
• canal openings at the periphery of the access cavity		
Coronal preparation		
Choice of irrigant		
Working length		
• estimated working length		
• patency with a fine file and lubrication		
Working length radiograph		
• whole tooth on film, together with at least 3 mm of tissue surrounding the apex		
• no distortion and processed		
• tip of the instrument within 2 mm of the apical constriction		
• avoid perforation of the radiographic apex		
Apical preparation		

Checklist 46 **Root canal obturation**

	Yes	No
Placement of rubber dam		
Removal of temporary dressing		
Irrigation of root canal		
• Irrigate with a chelating agent e.g. EDTA or citric acid to remove the $Ca(OH)_2$ from the canal		
• final rinse with NaOCl		
Fitting of gutta percha point		
• Fit a cone that matches the ISO size of the master apical file		
• friction fit at the working length		
• modify accordingly		

Checklist 46 **Root canal obturation** – *continued*

	Yes	No
Depth of penetration of spreader		
Final irrigation and drying of canal		
Choice of sealer		
Quality of lateral condensation		
Cleanliness of access cavity		
Intermediary dressing – choice of material and placement		
• Quality of temporary restoration		
Postoperative radiograph		

Checklist 47 **Indirect pulp capping/stepwise excavation**

	Yes	No
General understanding of procedure		
Introduction and explanation of procedure to patient.		
You should be able to explain and show knowledge of what you intend to do		
Delivery of local anaesthetic		
Rubber dam placement. Ensure that the rubber dam is placed such that it causes minimal injury to the soft tissues. The dam should be positioned to prevent any contamination of the cavity. It should not leak around the tooth		
Removal of soft caries. The caries is removed at the periphery of the lesion		
Application of calcium hydroxide sublining. The setting calcium hydroxide should be placed over the deepest part of the cavity ensuring that it does not extend to the periphery of the cavity		
Dressing the cavity. A reinforced zinc oxide eugenol dressing should be placed. The occlusion should be checked. If a class II cavity has been cut it is important to ensure that a contact area is produced		
Arrangements for recall. It is essential that the patient is recalled to allow the dressing to be removed, the remaining caries removed and a permanent restoration placed		

Checklist 48 **Direct pulp capping**

	Yes	No
Introduction		
Explanation of procedure to patient		
Delivery of local anaesthetic		
Rubber dam placement		
Removal of soft caries		
• at the periphery of the lesion		
Care of the exposure site		
• irrigated with chlorhexidine or a weak solution of NaOCl		
• Bleeding should be allowed to occur to release tissue pressure		
• The bleeding stopped with sterile cotton wool pledget dampened in sterile saline		
Calcium hydroxide is be placed over the exposure – intimate contact with the pulpal tissue		
Restoration of the tooth		
Arrangements for recall		

References and further reading

GDC (2002) *The First Five Years: a framework for undergraduate dental education*, 2nd edn. London, The General Dental Council.

Education Committee of the European Society of Endodontology (2001) Undergraduate Curriculum Guidelines for Endodontology (2001) *International Endodontic Journal* 34, 574–80.

European Society of Endodontology (1998) Guidelines for speciality training in endodontology. *International Endodontic Journal* 31, 67–72.

Kakehashi S., Stanley H. R. and Fitzgerald R. J. (1966) The effects of surgical exposures of dental pulps in germfree and conventional laboratory rats. *J South Calif Dent Assoc* 34, 449–51.

QAA (2002) *Dentistry: academic standards*. Subject benchmark statements. Gloucester, Quality Assurance Agency for Higher Education.

Torabinejad M., Kettering J. D., McGraw J. C., Cummings R. R., Dwyer T. G. and Tobias T. S. (1988) Factors associated with endodontic interappointment emergencies with necrotic pulps. *J Endod* 14, 261–6.

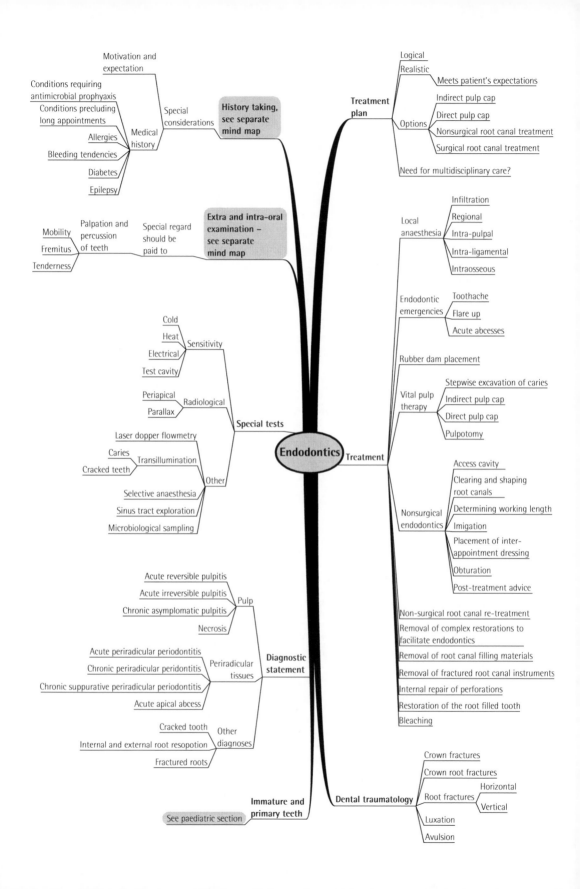

Endodontics

History taking, see separate mind map

Medical history — Special considerations
- Motivation and expectation
- Conditions requiring antimicrobial prophyaxis
- Conditions precluding long appointments
- Allergies
- Bleeding tendencies
- Diabetes
- Epilepsy

Extra and intra-oral examination – see separate mind map

Special regard should be paid to — Palpation and percussion of teeth
- Mobility
- Fremitus
- Tenderness

Special tests
- Sensitivity
  - Cold
  - Heat
  - Electrical
  - Test cavity
- Radiological
  - Periapical
  - Parallax
- Other
  - Laser dopper flowmetry
  - Transillumination
    - Caries
    - Cracked teeth
  - Selective anaesthesia
  - Sinus tract exploration
  - Microbiological sampling

Diagnostic statement
- Pulp
  - Acute reversible pulpitis
  - Acute irreversible pulpitis
  - Chronic asymplomatic pulpitis
  - Necrosis
- Periradicular tissues
  - Acute periradicular periodontitis
  - Chronic periradicular periodontitis
  - Chronic suppurative periradicular periodontitis
  - Acute apical abcess
- Other diagnoses
  - Cracked tooth
  - Internal and external root resopotion
  - Fractured roots

Immature and primary teeth — See paediatric section

Treatment plan
- Logical
- Realistic
  - Meets patient's expectations
- Options
  - Indirect pulp cap
  - Direct pulp cap
  - Nonsurgical root canal treatment
  - Surgical root canal treatment
- Need for multidisciplinary care?

Treatment
- Local anaesthesia
  - Infiltration
  - Regional
  - Intra-pulpal
  - Intra-ligamental
  - Intraosseous
- Endodontic emergencies
  - Toothache
  - Flare up
  - Acute abcesses
- Rubber dam placement
- Vital pulp therapy
  - Stepwise excavation of caries
  - Indirect pulp cap
  - Direct pulp cap
  - Pulpotomy
- Nonsurgical endodontics
  - Access cavity
  - Clearing and shaping root canals
  - Determining working length
  - Imigation
  - Placement of inter-appointment dressing
  - Obturation
  - Post-treatment advice
- Non-surgical root canal re-treatment
- Removal of complex restorations to facilitate endodontics
- Removal of root canal filling materials
- Removal of fractured root canal instruments
- Internal repair of perforations
- Restoration of the root filled tooth
- Bleaching

Dental traumatology
- Crown fractures
- Crown root fractures
- Root fractures
  - Horizontal
  - Vertical
- Luxation
- Avulsion

2.7 Prosthodontics

Damien Walmsley and John Drummond

Key points

- The undergraduate prosthodontics course must reflect the range of skills and knowledge outlined in this chapter and must be constructed in such a way that the student has the opportunity to acquire the requisite knowledge and skills.

- Effective communication with dental technicians is an essential skill in the construction of fixed and removable prostheses.

- Dental technology teaching should be aimed towards ensuring that students have sufficient understanding of the clinical preparations for the laboratory, and the subsequent laboratory processes, so that they can appropriately evaluate their own clinical work and the work provided to and received from dental technicians.

- Students should be aware that there are a number of areas relevant to prosthodontics where they gain little or no undergraduate experience, including advanced restorative procedures, overdentures, obturators, interdisciplinary work, and implant surgery.

Introduction

In 1968 over one third of the total adult population of the UK had no natural teeth, and only a small number of people of pensionable age had any teeth at all. The *1998 Adult Dental Health Survey* (ADHS 1998) shows that a major change has occurred in the past thirty years – currently only 13 per cent of adults have no teeth and, even more impressively, over half those of pensionable age have some of their natural teeth. The ADHS 1998 also shows that older people now are much more concerned with preserving their natural teeth than was the case before. Over the last decade a growing proportion of dentate 65–74 year olds would consider having a tooth crowned; in addition, a growing proportion of those aged over 55 expect to keep some of their natural teeth for life. Predictions from the ADHS 98 indicate that the proportion of UK adults with no natural teeth will fall to 8 per cent in 2008 and 5 per cent in 2018. The proportion of adults of pensionable age with some natural teeth will increase dramatically over the next two decades: for example by 2018, 56 per cent of people aged 85 and over will have some natural teeth, compared with a figure of 19 per cent in 1998.

These statistics by no means suggest that there will be little requirement for removable appliance therapy in the medium term future. Rather, we have moved from a situation where edentulous levels were of epidemic proportions to a less extreme situation. The demand for partial and complete dentures will, however, still be relatively high and patient's expectations, in terms of function and aesthetics, will without doubt be greater. Regional variations in edentulous levels suggest too that there will be significant areas of the UK where denture wearing will remain common, particularly in the older age groups. It is, therefore, essential that the graduate has a comprehensive knowledge and provision of removable prosthodontics, in order to offer a high level of care to their patients.

The graduate has to be able to screen patients who have edentulous spaces within the mouth. They must be able to diagnose, treat, monitor, and maintain patients with a removable prosthesis. Not all edentulous spaces require replacement and sensible treatment planning is a necessary skill. It is also essential that the graduate is aware of their limitations, and is able to recognize the more demanding prosthetic rehabilitation that is required. The ability to liase and refer to a specialist in fixed and removable prosthodontics is another important skill.

The undergraduate dental course needs to deliver the education and experience as outlined in the General Dental Council (GDC) document *The First Five Years* (GDC 2002). The requirements for the delivery of restorative care are given in paragraphs 74 and 75 of the report and in paragraph 76 for technical support. The intended learning outcomes for restorative dentistry are shown in Table 2.7.1.

Paragraph 74 Restorative dentistry is concerned with the management of the plaque-related diseases (dental caries and periodontal diseases), tooth wear and tooth loss. Management includes preventive, non-operative care as well as the restoration of teeth using the well-established techniques of conservative dentistry, including the replacement of teeth by means of prostheses, and the treatment and maintenance of the supporting structures of the teeth by procedures of periodontology. In restorative dentistry students should have continuous responsibility for the care of a number of adults in order to assess their overall needs, the efficacy of preventive measures, their behaviour, management and long-term success or failure of restorative treatment. Students should learn to manage adults requiring emergency care, carry out diagnostic procedures in such circumstnaces, formulate treatment plans and relate them to comprehensive dental care. All aspects of restorative dentistry may be required for medically compromised patients and those with other special needs. In its advanced forms restorative dentistry can involve extensive occlusal rehabilitation, sometimes requiring the use of dental implants. Students should appreciate that these forms of treatment may be delivered by specialists as secondary or tertiary care. They should be aware of when to refer such cases, understand the principles involved in their management and observe such treatment being carried out.

Paragraph 75 All restorative techniques can be invasive in nature, and some are irreversible. The GDC considers that dental students on graduation must be competent in procedures of restorative dentistry including non-surgical treatment of single- and multi-rooted teeth, crowns and simple bridges, removable partial and complete dentures and periodontal therapy. They should be fully aware of when patients should be directed to specialists for advice and treatment.

Paragraph 76 To meet the needs of this part of the curriculum, students will learn how to communicate effectively with a dental technician, so that indirect restorations and fixed and removable prostheses can be constructed. Students should be aware of the importance of high standards in that work and have practical experience of the processes involved. It is important that experience is gained in constructing indirect restorations and fixed and removable prostheses. However, once that experience has been gained, students should be able to have the appliances and restorations required by their patients manufactured by dental technicians. The primary purpose of dental technology teaching should be to ensure that students have sufficient understanding of the clinical preparations and laboratory processes so that they can appropriately evaluate their own clinical work and the work provided to and received from dental technicians. Students should appreciate the relevance of their preparations to the quality of technical work that can be produced.

Paragraph 77 The student should be aware of the presentation of dental and oral diseases and disorders in elderly people, and the range of psychological and social factors involved in such situations. The student should be able to distinguish between normal and abnormal consequences of ageing, and learn to avoid stereotyping elderly patients.

Prosthodontics is also referred to in the Subject Benchmark Statements for Dentistry (QAA 2002):

Paragraph 3.15 Graduating dentists should be able to manage and integrate the procedures necessary to provide biocompatible, functional and aesthetic dental prostheses (fixed and removable) in sympathy with patient requirements or needs.

Intended learning outcomes

In light of these recommendations, the aim of this chapter is to outline the specific competencies that are necessary for an undergraduate course for removable prosthodontics and should include the following:

1. Have the theoretical knowledge required to practise prosthetic dentistry.

Table 2.7.1 Intended learning outcomes for prosthodontics

Be competent at	Have knowledge of	Be familiar with
Completing a range of procedures in restorative dentistry including partial and complete dentures	How missing teeth should be replaced, choosing between the alternatives of no replacements, bridges, dentures or implants	The role of prosthodontics in overall patient care
Designing effective complete and partial dentures	The design and laboratory procedures used in the production of partial and complete dentures and be able to make appropriate chair-side adjustment to these	Treatment planning and management of patients requiring more advanced forms of removable prosthesis including overdentures and implants
Recognizing their limitations in managing patients required removable prostheses, and making appropriate referrals based on assessment.	Biomedical sciences, of oral physiology and craniofacial, oral and dental anatomy in relation to prosthodontic treatment	The range of contemporary prosthodontic treatment techniques
Communicating effectively with patients, their families and associates and with other health care professionals involved in their care	Clinical prosthodontics to the extent that they can explain and discuss treatments with patients and their parents	
	How the provision of removable prosthesis is incorporated in restorative treatment planning	

2. To establish proficiency in clinical and technical procedures in relation to treatment of patients requiring:

   ◆ Complete dentures using both conventional and copy techniques.

   ◆ Partial dentures constructed in either cobalt/chromium or acrylic resin.

   ◆ To provide opportunity to develop knowledge and clinical skills in other areas such as:

      ▪ Immediate dentures

      ▪ Relines and rebases

      ▪ Additions and repairs

      ▪ Overdentures

- Onlay appliances
- Osseo-integrated implants

3. To provide the theoretical knowledge of prosthetic dentistry in its relationship to other dental disciplines including specifically restorative dentistry.

Whilst the outcomes above relate to the GDC's document and relate directly to removable prosthodontics, there are others that impact on removable prosthodontics, for example occlusion, history taking (Chapter 1.1), local anaesthesia (Chapter 1.9), cross-infection (Chapter 1.5), patient referral (Chapter 1.13) and management of the medically compromised patient (Chapter 2.2).

This chapter outlines the learning outcomes that are appropriate for dental undergraduates as well as taking a more detailed look at the skills dental students will need to develop during their undergraduate course in removable prosthodontics, in order to offer comprehensive care for their patients on graduation.

Removable prosthodontics learning outcomes

This section contains a list of the learning outcomes (Table 2.7.1) that are felt appropriate for the undergraduate in removable prosthodontics. Each of the outcomes should be tested during a student's training, achieving a particular outcome can be assessed by using a variety of methods including competency tests, written examinations, viva, objective structured clinical examination (OSCE) clinical assessment, continual assessment etc. The methods of assessment will be discussed later in this chapter.

Curriculum guidelines in undergraduate prosthodontics education

This section lists the key areas that will be covered during an undergraduate course in removable prosthodontics.

Background knowledge

It is essential that the graduate has good background knowledge in order to understand disease processes and how this has led to the loss of teeth. The speciality of prosthodontics must always be placed in the context of restorative treatment planning and consider the holistic care of individual patients.

Basic sciences

Anatomy

Be aware of the anatomy (and applied anatomy) of the dentate and edentulous mouth and how this relates to its function, diseases of the teeth and their supporting structures and their management.

Microbiology

Be aware of the microflora of the mouth and of dental plaque, both in health and disease, as well as the micro-organisms implicated in various diseases including denture-induced stomatitis.

Physiology
Have a basic understanding of the physiology and biochemistry of saliva and how it aids in the retention of removable prosthesis.

Tooth loss
Be aware of the events leading to and subsequent to tooth loss and how this may influence treatment with removable prosthesis.

Epidemiology
Have an understanding of the epidemiology of tooth loss and the provision of removable prostheses.

Systemic disease
Be aware of the links between denture wearing and systemic disease and how systemic diseases can influence the success of a removable prosthesis.

Pharmacology
Be aware of a patient's medical history and how the basic pharmacology of these agents may influence the success of a removable prosthesis.

Gerontology
Be aware of the basic science of cellular, organ, and species ageing particularly as it relates to the structure and function of the mouth and related structures.

Materials
Be familiar with the different materials used in prosthetic dentistry including:
- Impression materials
- Registration materials
- Laboratory materials
- Articulators and the difference of articulation between the natural and artificial dentitions
- Implants.

Instrumentation
Be aware of the use of articulators and the theoretical knowledge behind their use.
- To have a knowledge of the different instrumentation used in the construction of removable prostheses.

Clinical skills
The development of clinical skills is essential to the practice of dentistry, and this applies equally to removable prosthodontics. The graduate needs to be able to diagnose and manage the edentulous space.

History taking

- ◆ To be able to take a comprehensive and relevant dental history

- ◆ To be able to ask questions that have particular relevance to the provision of removable prosthodontics e.g. history of tooth loss, previous denture-wearing history, care of teeth, oral hygiene regime, smoking history (including frequency, type, duration), drug therapy, diet with respect to erosion and caries experience and interpret the impact of such information.

- ◆ To take a thorough medical and social history and be aware of the relevance in relation to the provision of prosthodontics.

Examination

- ◆ Be able to examine the patient extra-orally and note any pathology associated with lymph nodes, muscles of mastication, tempromandibular joints etc. It is also important to be aware of the significance of any findings, and manage such findings (e.g. facial asymmetry) in an appropriate manner.

- ◆ Be able to carry out a thorough intra-oral examination including:

  - ▪ The oral soft tissues, and be able to identify any abnormal lesions or those associated with ageing that may be mistaken for disease e.g. sublingual varicosity

  - ▪ An assessment of oral hygiene in relation to plaque and calculus deposits

  - ▪ To undertake a basic periodontal examination (see periodontal competencies)

  - ▪ The identification of mobile teeth and classify them using a mobility index

  - ▪ To make an assessment of the hard dental tissues

  - ▪ To examine the edentulous areas

  - ▪ To examine the abutment teeth

  - ▪ An ability to recognize and record evidence of parafuctional activity

  - ▪ An assessment of the occlusion (both statically and dynamically), in regard to premature contacts, patterns of guidance, interferences and relate these to periodontal disease experience.

  - ▪ The ability to carry out a Basic Periodontal Examination (BPE) and be aware of the implications and limitations of the results.

Special tests

Radiographs

- ◆ To be able to determine what radiographs are appropriate for each individual case.

- ◆ To have knowledge of the limitations and advantages of each appropriate type of radiograph (long cone paralleling periapicals, vertical bitewings and orthopantomagram).

- To be able to interpret radiographs in relation to type and quantity of bone loss, apical pathology and perio-endo lesions.

- To be able to document in the patient records a concise and accurate report of the radiographic features.

- Aware of legislation IR(MA) 2000.

Vitality testing

To be able to determine the vitality of a tooth using thermal and electrical test methods and be aware of the sensitivity of such tests.

Diagnosis

It is, obviously, essential that a correct diagnosis is arrived at, so that the disease can be correctly managed and the appropriate removable prosthodontic device constructed.

Treatment planning

- When to refer a patient

- Writing a referral letter:
  - Be able to write, a suitable, referral letter to a specialist, giving the salient points required to allow for expedient patient management by the clinician receiving the referral.

- Be aware of the issues relating to the management of patients with complex medical histories.

- Be able to integrate periodontal therapy with other specialties (orthodontics, restorative dentistry, oral surgery, oral medicine etc.) to formulate a coherent treatment plan.

- Be aware that the undergraduate course although comprehensive needs to be reinforced at regular intervals by continued professional education.

Areas that are covered in the undergraduate curriculum but where clinical experience is limited, and further postgraduate education will be required include advanced prosthodontics techniques such as osseointegrated implants

Complete dentures

General considerations of competency

An undergraduate student will be able to complete a treatment plan for their patient. This will be dependant upon any presenting complaints together with the findings from a clinical examination. This treatment plan should include any preliminary requirements followed by the intended technique of denture construction including any special considerations. Understanding of the four different design considerations for complete dentures conventional, biometric, copy dentures and neutral zone technique.

Key skills

Diagnosis

* History and examination
* Diagnosis
* Treatment planning.

Communication

* Ability to present and discuss treatment options with the patient
* With other team members particularly the dental technician.

Knowledge

* Understanding of normal and pathological anatomy of the denture-bearing tissues
* Knowledge of the biological and mechanical properties of materials used in the laboratory and clinic.

Practical skills

* Handling of impression materials
* Handling of registration materials
* Selection appropriate anterior and posterior teeth
* Delivery of finished denture
* Advice and aftercare of patient
* Identification of problem.

Treatment: conventional complete denture construction

Preliminary impressions

Preliminary impressions are taken in stock trays using a suitable high viscosity material, which will be self-supporting. Such trays may need modification (usually reduction in form) to improve their suitability for the patient. Understanding of different materials that may be used at this stage is required.

Laboratory communication and prescription

Prior to recording master impressions it is essential at this and subsequent stages to indicate precisely what the technical requirements are for the case. The prescription on the laboratory card should be clear and comprehensive. If there is any possibility of confusion then it is valuable to discuss the case personally with the technician involved. The responsibility for the clinical and laboratory work will remain with the clinician.

Individual trays – requirements

* Construction of individual trays in acrylic or other materials, e.g. shellac.
* Understanding of whether such trays should be close-fitting or spaced dependent on material used.

◆ Laboratory features of tray – the peripheral border of all trays should finish 2 mm short of the depth of the sulcus when the spacer is in place. This is approximately the position of the muco-gingival line.

Master impressions

The impression should record detail of the denture bearing area together with the functional depth and width of the sulcus so that the finished denture maintains an effective border seal. In some cases the tray will require modification to its peripheral border. This should be carried out using autopolymerizing acrylic resin prior to the impression being recorded. It is important to preserve the width of the sulcus on the resultant cast.

Laboratory prescription

Casts should be poured in dental stone and a prescription provided regarding the construction of occlusal rims. The material to be used for the occlusal rim bases must be specified and the baseplate must be rigid to withstand subsequent clinical use. Understanding of the postdam function and position on the upper cast and indicate the position of a palatal relief if required.

Recording jaw relations

◆ Relevance of previous dentures:

  ▪ Understanding that previous dentures may provide information on the appropriate jaw relationship, occlusal plane, incisal level and the relationship of teeth to soft tissues. Any alterations in these factors which may be required should have been noted at the treatment planning stage.

◆ Understanding and competence in the use of the following materials for occlusal rims:

  ▪ Wax

  ▪ Shellac or polystyrene base

  ▪ Heat cured baseplates

◆ Ability to check stability, retention, and peripheral extension of upper and lower occlusal rims and modify if necessary.

◆ Able to measuring free way space (FWS). Measurements of the RVD should normally be made therefore with the lower rim in place.

◆ Able to adjust the upper rim so that:

  ▪ Incisal height and plane are correct

  ▪ Occlusal plane is correct (parallel to the ala-tragus and interpapillary lines).

  ▪ Labial and buccal contour is correct

  ▪ The centre line is marked.

◆ Adjust the lower rim to correct bucco-lingual contour posteriorly and correct labial contour anteriorly:

- The rim should sit in the neutral zone with an understanding of the concept of the neutral zone

- Trim the lower rim to establish even bilateral contact with the upper at the retruded contact position

- Some authorities might recommend that the muscular position is recorded if the patient has a controlled and reproducible closure pattern.

◆ Able to assist the patient in achieving the retruded position (if this is to be recorded) by asking them to curl the tongue back to contact the posterior border of the upper occlusal rim. In cases where this technique fails to easily produce the retruded position then there should be knowledge of other ways of obtaining the position e.g. placing the patient in a supine position.

◆ Assess rest vertical dimension and vertical dimension of occlusion both from facial appearance and from measurement using the Willis gauge or the two dots technique. Ensure that there is an adequate inter-occlusal clearance and understand the variation in FWS that may be needed depending on such factors as past denture history and age.

◆ At the correct vertical dimension of occlusion, use of an appropriate technique to seal rims together in the retruded (or muscular) contact position. For example:

- Locating mark on both upper and lower rims.

- Cut 'V'-shaped notches in upper rim at the buccal locating mark.

- Remove 2 mm (or less if using a light viscosity occlusion recording paste) of occlusal rim height from the mesial aspect of the locating mark to the distal end of the rim on the lower.

- Use of softened modelling wax (or a bite-recording paste) on the trimmed posterior surface of the lower rim to record the upper notch. After removing rims from the mouth, check that casts can be placed into the rims without any premature contacts distally. Rims can be separated and re-located accurately.

◆ Select teeth which are appropriate for the age, sex and racial characteristics of the patient. Reference may be made to previous dentures if the patient was happy with their appearance.

◆ Prepare the post dam on your master cast and outline any areas of the cast requiring relief (this will have been done at an earlier stage if heat-cured bases are used).

Laboratory prescription

Record the shade, mould, and material to be used for the artificial teeth on the laboratory card. Indicate the type of articulator (average movement or semi-adjustable or plane line if using cuspless posterior teeth) on which the dentures are to be set up and indicate any aspects of the occlusal rims which are to be copied in the trial dentures. Indicate the type of bases you require for the trial dentures. Use of split cast mounting technique.

- Neutral zone impression:

  - If the lower record rim is unstable then a neutral zone impression may be required. An understanding of why such an impression is required

  - Competent in handling viscogel and knowledge of its clinical handling.

Trial dentures

Understanding of occlusal balance and how to examine and check a completed set up on the articulator before trying in the mouth.

In the mouth carry out a complete assessment of the trial dentures including:

- Stability and retention.

- Peripheral extension and shape of polished surfaces including an assessment of the degree of undercut engagement by the flanges.

- Positioning of teeth in relation to the neutral zone.

- Occlusion – this should be assessed visually.

- Inter-occlusal clearance – check that a satisfactory inter-occlusal clearance is present.

- Appearance – check carefully the shade, mould and position of the anterior teeth and the contour of the labial flanges. Check that the appearance is natural (a completely even arrangement of teeth usually looks unnatural), and modify if necessary. Understand the need to engage the patient and sometimes others in this process. Remember that modification of the positions of the anterior teeth may result in occlusal interference. Therefore re-check occlusion if modifications are carried out.

- Able to undertake a new jaw registration if existing occlusal and vertical dimension of occlusion is incorrect.

Laboratory prescription

This should state definitely whether dentures can be finished or if a further trial is required. If the jaw relationship has been re-recorded the casts must be re-mounted on the articulator and a second trial stage carried out. If the dentures are to be processed use of the split cast technique will avoid occlusal errors due to processing. Instructions should be given for any special colouring (i.e. ethnic) or contouring of the acrylic matrix.

Denture insertion

Check the processed dentures for any sharp edges, acrylic 'pearls', or excessive undercuts on the fitting surface. Insert each denture separately and check on fit and comfort to patient.

Able to check the occlusion in the mouth either:

- Visually – by observing and asking the patient when he closes gently if the teeth are meeting with equal pressure on both sides of mouth.

- By using articulating paper to confirm your findings and to locate precisely any premature contacts.

- Identify artefacts, such as those produced by tilting of the dentures.

- Remember if any occlusal faults are diagnosed it is a clinical and not a laboratory error providing the split cast technique has been used.

Check record

- Clinical decision to adjust minor occlusal discrepancies at the chair-side and when to use the check record. A check record is advisable for the correction of occlusal errors which are too large to adjust easily at the chairside.

- Use of narrow wax wafers, sealed to the occlusal surfaces of the lower posterior teeth. Registration is obtained but teeth do not penetrate through the wax.

- Re-mounted on an average movement, or semi-adjustable, articulator.

- Able to convey instructions to the laboratory for set up and adjustment.

Advice to patient

To be able to draw up and discuss with the patient a printed leaflet giving instructions in respect of new dentures. To include:

- the importance of good denture hygiene

- type of immersion cleaner to be used (preferably a hypochlorite type)

- mechanical cleaning with a brush that allows access and adaptability to all surfaces of the denture

- Discussion of potential problems and preparation for a review appointment which will be arranged for a weeks time.

Review

Obtain a careful history of any complaints. Undertake a thorough examination – identification of mucosal damage even when the patient has reported that the dentures are comfortable. Always re-check the occlusion before adjusting the fitting surface. Carry out any necessary adjustments to the dentures.

Arrange further appointments as necessary. Arrange for and make sure the patient understands the need for periodic recall to assess the dentures and the general health of the mouth.

Copy dentures

Introduction

This section will cover those skills over and above previous skills required in conventional complete dentures.

Understanding when an examination, diagnosis and treatment plan will involve copy dentures. Knowledge of the potential advantages of a copy denture technique.

Distinguish between clinical needs where either only minor changes to polished surfaces, tooth positions and arch form required or major alteration to polished surfaces, tooth positions and arch form required:

First visit – mould production

◆ Able to correct under extension with a suitable autopolymerizing acrylic and then record occlusion

◆ Use of registration materials such as bite registration paste or modelling wax.

◆ Able to produce a replica mould (+ template if mould not sent to the laboratory, and stone replica if record of original denture required)

◆ Knowledge of using a recognized replica/mould technique involving

▪ Alginate in a soap box/custom metal box

▪ Silicone putty in stock trays.

Second visit – impressions and registration

◆ Modify templates with wax to prescribed new design (where this necessitates an additional visit)

◆ Wash impressions with a suitable impression material. (This may be left to the end of the trial denture stages)

◆ Record occlusion and select tooth shade as for conventional dentures

◆ Try-in, insertion and review as for conventional complete dentures

Removable partial dentures

A removable prosthesis restores and maintains oral function by the replacement of missing teeth in a partially edentulous mouth by the replacement of missing teeth and associated structures with a removable prosthesis. This replacement may also be undertaken with a fixed restoration such as a bridge or implant. An understanding of treatment options for restoration of the edentulous space is also required.

An undergraduate student will be able to complete a treatment plan for their patient with considerations of the placement of a removable partial denture in the restorative treatment plan. This will be dependant upon any presenting complaints together with the findings from a clinical examination. This treatment plan should include any preliminary requirements followed by the intended technique of denture construction including any special considerations.

Preliminary impressions

Able to select the correct stock tray and modify with impression compound or autopolymerizing acrylic as appropriate.

Competent in the use of a high viscosity alginate to compensate for the lack of fit of the stock tray.

Laboratory prescription

It is essential at this and subsequent stages to indicate *precisely* what is required for the next appointment. The prescription on the laboratory card must be clear and comprehensive. If there is any possibility of confusion it is essential to discuss the case personally with the technician involved. All casts at this stage should be poured in dental stone and the type and material of individual trays indicated.

Removable partial denture design

The design of a partial denture should be determined *before* master impressions are recorded. In this respect where there are opposing natural teeth in contact, casts must be mounted on an articulator and surveyed to produce the desired design. In many cases where there are sufficient teeth, casts can be placed in occlusion by hand prior to mounting. In other situations it will be necessary to construct occlusal rims to register the jaw relationship of the patient.

Be knowledgeable of the Kennedy and support classifications for partially dentate arches. Understanding of the rational and technique of surveying of dental casts prior to the drawing up a partial denture design.

◆ Competent to survey and analyse casts especially in identifying, marking, measuring and eliminating undercuts.

◆ Survey initially to vertical path of insertion.

◆ In very few cases a second survey will be necessary to a modified path of insertion.

◆ Produce design for removable partial denture.

◆ Understand the system of partial denture design to consider

- Saddles – placement and design

- Support – tooth, mucosa and tooth/mucosa. Rests and their placement

- Retention – types of retention, clasps materials used and their placement

- Reciprocation – types of reciprocation, materials used, bracing components of a denture

- Connection – types of connection for both upper and lower dentures

- Indirect retention – indications and placement.

◆ Consideration of acrylic partial dentures and in particular the Every design for upper removable partial dentures.

◆ A decision should be made on the need for possible tooth preparation or modification. This may indicate that the following may be necessary:

◆ Rest seat preparation to provide sufficient space and a horizontal surface for any support component.

◆ Modification of tooth contour, by grinding or the addition of light-cured composite resin, to improve the action of clasp arms or the occlusal relationship.

The proposed design drawn up on the laboratory card and also transferred to the study cast which should be retained for reference until the trial stage has been completed. The design prescription must be clear and comprehensive. If surgical, conservative or periodontal treatment is indicated this must be completed before recording master impressions. Understanding that the type of denture required may influence the overall treatment plan, e.g. rest seats incorporated into Class II restorations, full veneer crowns contoured to provide undercut areas for retention, or tooth extraction as a result of over-eruption.

Master impressions

Normally the next visit will be for master impressions if the preliminary casts have already been mounted and a design determined. In cases where the preliminary casts could not be mounted, however, the second visit will be devoted to recording the jaw relationship of the patient prior to mounting casts on the articulator and developing a design.

Recording jaw relationships

For the purpose of jaw relationships and their registration partially dentate patients can be divided
into two categories:

1. Patients without an occlusal stop to indicate the correct intercuspal position or vertical dimension of occlusion.

2. Patients with occlusal contact in the intercuspal position.

First category

In the first category the OVD is determined by establishing the RVD and modifying the occlusal rims until the OVD is some 2–4 mm short of the RVD, this distance indicating the amount of intero-cclusal clearance. The horizontal jaw relationship recorded should be the retruded contact position.

◆ In the mouth the fit and extension of the rim should be checked and modified if necessary to produce acceptable stability.

◆ The upper occlusal rim should be adjusted so that the occlusal plane is correct in relation to the remaining upper natural teeth. If there is an anterior saddle the rim must indicate the correct incisal level and degree of lip support.

◆ The retruded contact position should be recorded using wax or an occlusal registration material such as bite registration paste.

◆ The casts should be placed in occlusion using the occlusal rims and checked to determine that the tooth relationship on the casts is the same as in the mouth.

Second category

◆ The rims should be trimmed until the natural occlusal contact is observed.

◆ The occlusal contact should be checked with the natural teeth when the patient occludes with the upper rim in place.

◆ The lower rim should be adjusted until there is an even occlusion at the OVD determined by the intercuspal position.

- The intercuspal position recorded with the rims in place using wax or registration paste.

- The casts are placed in occlusion using the occlusal rims and checked to ensure that there is no premature contact between the heels of a cast and the opposing rim or cast.

Laboratory prescription

- Shade, material and mould of artificial teeth should be specified.

- If the next stage is the try-in of a metal framework, the design should be drawn on the laboratory card and full instructions given.

- If the metal denture is restoring lower free-end saddles consider the need for the altered cast technique. If the technique is to be employed request the addition of acrylic trays to the framework in the saddle areas.

- If the anterior teeth require metal backings, a wax trial denture should be requested for the next stage so that the appearance and position of the teeth can be approved before the metal framework is constructed.

Master impressions

- Wax stops should be placed on the fitting surface of the individual trays before modifying the peripheral extension if necessary.

- Any over-extension of the tray should be corrected using a blue stone.

- Any under-extension should be corrected with the addition of self curing acrylic resin. When mandibular free-end saddle areas are present, border moulding of the tray in the retro-mylohyoid areas should be undertaken routinely.

- A low viscosity alginate is used to record the impression. In some cases silicone based or rubber based materials may be used.

- If the impression is satisfactory a cast should be poured in either dental stone (for acrylic dentures) or improved dental stone (for cobalt chromium dentures) as soon as possible.

- Altered cast technique – knowledge of and indication of the technique

Laboratory prescription
The laboratory prescription should indicate the material to be used for cast pouring. Bearing in mind that the occlusion has already been determined naturally or by occlusal rims prior to establishing a design, the subsequent stage should be either trial dentures or the production of a metal casting. In the former situation a shade and mould of teeth must be selected.

The metal framework

- The framework must conform to the original design.

- The framework must fit the master cast. If the fit is unsatisfactory on the cast it will also be unsatisfactory in the mouth.

- All components which are designed to be clear of the gingival margin area should be checked to ensure that the clearance is adequate.

- In the mouth, these aspects should be checked again, remembering that the likelihood of some instability in free-end saddle cases may be due to spacing beneath the mesh retention.

- The occlusion is examined to ensure that there are no premature contacts caused by support units. This should be done by visual examination, from comments by the patient and with the use of articulating paper or disclosing wax. Any premature contact should normally be removed at this stage.

Laboratory prescription

If the metal framework is satisfactory, request the setting of the teeth on the framework, after choosing an appropriate shade and mould of tooth.

The trial denture

A careful routine followed to prevent any mistakes continuing through to the finished dentures. The dentures should first be examined on the mounted casts in respect of:

- Adaptation of dentures on the casts

- Occlusion

- Position of artificial teeth with regard to adjacent natural ones

- The arrangement of anterior teeth

- Extension and contouring of wax flanges.

  In the mouth the trial dentures should be examined in respect of:

- Adaptation of the dentures.

- Occlusion including the vertical dimension of occlusion.

- Contouring of wax flanges with regard to peripheral extension, shaping of polished surfaces, coverage of gingival margins.

- Appearance. Modify positions of teeth and incisal edges of anterior teeth to achieve a pleasing result.

- Ask for patient's comments on appearance. Show the patient the dentures in the mirror and ensure that they are satisfied.

  If the occlusion is incorrect, modifications must be carried out before continuing with the next stages.

  If the occlusion has been re-recorded this will indicate a change in the jaw relationship. Accordingly the casts must be remounted to this relationship and the teeth set for a second trial.

Laboratory prescription

Carefully list and describe any modifications you wish the technician to carry out before finishing the dentures. To ensure that interference with insertion of the finished denture will not occur as a result of inadequately blocked out tooth undercuts the following instructions and procedure must be followed:

- Undercuts are blocked out in wax on the master cast, in respect of vertical path of insertion.

- The master cast should be duplicated.

- The denture should be processed on the duplicate cast.

- The processed denture should be fitted back on master cast.

Denture insertion

Examine the dentures and check there are no sharp edges or acrylic 'pearls' on the fitting surface of the saddle areas. Insert denture into the mouth. Relieve any undercut areas on the cast due to possible inadequate blocking out of the undercuts. Use of pressure relief cream to identify pressure areas

In the mouth, check for adaptation of components, retention and stability and occlusion

Occlusal contact is checked by asking for the patient's comments, by visual inspection, and by the use of articulating paper. Occlusal adjustment should be continued until both the patient's comments and visual inspection confirm that even contact has been achieved in the chosen jaw position. Attention should be given to occlusal contacts in lateral and protrusive positions. In many cases the dentures will be adjusted so that they conform to the occlusal guidance provided by the remaining natural teeth.

Advice to the patient

The patient must be taught the correct way to Insertion and removal of denture the denture.

A printed sheet of instructions is provided for the patient which covers cleaning/eating/wearing at night together with pain and need for regular recall – including recall with the hygienist.

- It is important to discuss these points verbally with the patient first of all. The purpose of the sheet is simply to act as an aide-memoir.

- Finally you should ensure that the patient knows who to contact in the event of problems arising with the denture.

Review appointment

Able to take a history of any presenting complaint. Able to examine the denture-bearing tissues and the occlusion and diagnose the cause of the complaint before making any adjustments.

Immediate dentures

An immediate denture may be defined as a denture that is made prior to the extraction of the natural teeth and which is inserted into the mouth immediately after the extraction of those teeth. The knowledge of a transitional approach to tooth loss should be appreciated.

+ Understand the advantages and disadvantages to clinician and patient.

+ Communication with the patient concerning the future treatment including the consequences of tooth loss and requirements for relining and rebasing with the provision of new dentures.

Whilst these competencies are directed at provision of a new complete immediate denture, an understanding of immediate addition of teeth to existing partial dentures is also required.

Preliminary impressions

For jaws where immediate dentures are to be provided, preliminary impressions are recorded in alginate. For master impressions spaced acrylic or shellac individual trays are requested.

Master impressions

These will normally be recorded in low viscosity alginate material.

Recording the occlusion

If tooth contact is insufficient to demonstrate the occlusal relationship, occlusal rims will be required. These will be constructed as wax occlusal rims with a shellac base plate. A decision is taken at this stage as to whether the denture is to have a flange or whether the replacement teeth are to be socketed. In general a flanged denture should be provided unless there are any specific contraindications. The depth of socketing is influenced by the bone level round the teeth involved, this is determined by using a periodontal probe and any available radiographs. Some authorities recommend minimal cast preparation.

+ Record the shade and mould of anterior teeth.

+ Teeth for extraction should be recorded on the master cast at the earliest opportunity. Posterior teeth may be best extracted in advance unless they provide information regarding the occlusion.

+ Specify undercuts which must be blocked out for an immediate partial denture

Try-in of posterior teeth

The removal of those teeth to be extracted from the cast and the placement of the teeth in wax is the responsibility of the clinician before giving the denture to the technician for processing.

Any particular aesthetic requirement requested by the patient for the arrangement of the anterior teeth is noted. It is useful to have a duplicate cast with a diagnostic wax up to show the patient the amount of tooth repositioning that may be required.

Insertion of immediate dentures

Ability to remove teeth using as atraumatic technique as possible and be able to follow appropriate procedures in the case of difficulties encountered during the extractions. Otherwise, as for complete dentures but avoid trauma to the anaesthetized tissues. Remove acrylic pearls and spicules, undercuts (helps insertion of denture). Obvious occlusal discrepancies and over-extension must be corrected.

Understand that definitive adjustment of occlusion is not possible because of swelling following tooth extraction.

Instructions to patient

Dentures should not be removed for 24 hours and post-extraction instructions are given as normal surgical procedures. Offer appropriate advice to the patient regarding problems, e.g. prolonged haemorrhage or after pain.

Review

At 24 hours

- ◆ Dentures removed from mouth and cleaned with brush, soap and water
- ◆ Mouth is examined for areas of soreness. Adjust border for:
  - ▪ over-extension
  - ▪ excessive pressure from denture base
  - ▪ obvious occlusal discrepancies.
- ◆ Oral and denture hygiene is given together with patient handout.

At one week

- ◆ All factors at 24 hour review checked again with evaluation and adjustment of occlusion.
- ◆ Regular review appointments (as appropriate, depending on number of teeth replaced on immediate denture) e.g.:
  - ▪ one month,
  - ▪ three months,
  - ▪ six months,
  - ▪ annually thereafter.

Relines and rebases

When the fit of a denture has deteriorated to an unacceptable degree and there are no other faults which require correction (such as the occlusion), relining or rebasing may be the treatment of choice. In the case of a rebase the patient must be willing to leave the denture to enable the laboratory work to be carried out.

A reline is usually considered to be the replacement or restoration of the fitting surface of a denture and is often done at the chairside using autopolymerizing resin. Generally it will increase the bulk of the denture. A rebase is replacement of the base of the denture (and other parts) by new material. It is a laboratory procedure produced in heat cured resin.

An outline of the clinical procedure for a rebase is as follows:

1. Remove all undercuts from the impression surface to allow the denture to be removed from the cast in the laboratory.

2. Adjust the periphery of the denture by trimming or border moulding as necessary to correct over or under extension.

3. Impression with silicone paste or zinc oxide impression paste of a low viscosity type and relocate accurately in the mouth. Border moulding is then carried out, patient to close the teeth gently together in intercuspal position so as to avoid altering the occlusal relationships.

Laboratory instructions

In the case of a rebase the following instructions are requested:

- Pour cast in stone preserving land area

- Remove all old acrylic, especially in palate

- Rewax (including new palatal coverage)

- Process in heat cured resin

- When fitting a re-based denture a check must be made on the occlusal relationships.

Advanced prosthetic skills

Overdentures

- Knowledge of overdentures including their advantages and disadvantages: why teeth are retained and how they may assist in the retention and stability of an overdenture.

- The care and maintenance of the retained tooth and/or root including the use of copings and precision attachments (such as bars, studs and magnets).

Implants

- Understanding of osseo-integration including biological principles underlying their use in prosthetic dentistry.

This is a constantly changing area and their popularity is increasing. The undergraduate should appreciate that this area of dentistry requires extensive postgraduate training and that specialization is required. The consequences of poor treatment planning should be understood.

Competency tests

The previous sections have attempted to build a comprehensive picture of the knowledge and skills a dental undergraduate should have gained during their course in removable prosthodontics, however it is not practical to test everyone to ensure that every student has gained each of these skills. Moreover, some of the skills outlined are more important than others, it is therefore important that we have a list of skills that every student must achieve in order successfully complete their course of study, i.e. the concept of Key competencies.

Assessing competency

If a student is said to be 'competent' in a certain skill, then he or she will need to achieve a certain level of skill and this will need to be assessed using a competency test. The outcome of this test can be either pass, (and they are competent in the particular skill), or fail (not be competent in the particular skill). So if in a course, a number of key skills (see previous section) have been identified that a student must achieve during the course of study, then these will need to be individually assessed to ensure competency.

Checklist 49 **Recording jaw relations**

	Yes	No	N/A
Introduction and explanation of procedure to patient			
Check stability, retention, and peripheral extension of upperand lower occlusal rims and modify if necessary			
Adjust the upper rim so that incisal height and plane are correct			
Occlusal plane is correct (parallel to the ala-tragus and interpapillary lines)			
Labial and buccal contour is correct			
The centre line is marked			
Adjust the lower rim to correct bucco-lingual contour posteriorly and correct labial contour anteriorly			
Trim the lower rim to establish contact with the upper at the retruded contact position			
Assist the patient in achieving the retruded position			
Measurement of the free way space			
Use appropriate technique to seal rims together in the retruded (or muscular) contact position			

Checklist 49 **Recording jaw relations** – *continued*

	Yes	No	N/A
Remove rims from the mouth and check that casts can be placed into the rims without any premature contacts distally			
Appropriate selection of teeth			
Prepare post dam on master cast and outline any areas of the cast requiring relief			
Instructions to laboratory			
Caring communication (empathy with patient)			

Checklist 50 **Trial dentures**

	Yes	No	N/A
Introduction and explanation of procedure to patient			
Carry out a complete assessment of the trial dentures including stability and retention			
Peripheral extension and shape of polished surfaces including an assessment of the degree of undercut engagement by the flanges			
Positioning of teeth in relation to neutral zone			
Occlusion – this should be assessed visually			
Inter-occlusal clearance – check that a satisfactory inter-occlusal clearance is present (free way space)			
Appearance – check carefully the shade, mould and position of the anterior teeth and the contour of the labial flanges			
Engage the patient and supporting staff or family in this process			
Re-check occlusion if modifications are carried out			
Undertake a new jaw registration if existing occlusal and vertical dimension of occlusion is incorrect			
Instructions to laboratory (should state definitely whether dentures can be finished)			
Caring communication (empathy with patient)			

Checklist 51 **Denture insertion**

	Yes	No	N/A
Introduction and explanation of procedure to patient			
Check the processed dentures for any sharp edges, acrylic 'pearls', or excessive undercuts on the fitting surface			
Insert each denture separately and check on fit and comfort to patient			
Check the occlusion in the mouth			
Adjust minor occlusal discrepancies at the chair-side			
Take check record for correction of occlusal discrepancy			
Provide advice to the patient regarding wear, care and potential problems			
Arrange for a review appointment			
Caring communication (empathy with patient)			

References and further reading

ADHS (1998) *Adult Dental Health Survey: oral health in the United Kingdom 1998*. London, The Stationery Office.

GDC (2002) *The First Five Years: a framework for undergraduate dental education*, 2nd edn. London: The General Dental Council.

QAA (2002) *Dentistry: academic standards*. Subject benchmark statements. Gloucester, Quality Assurance Agency for Higher Education

Scott B. J. J., Evans D. J. P., Drummond J. R., Mossey P. A. and Stirrups D. R. (2001) An investigation into the use of a structured clinical operative test for the assessment of a clinical skill. *European Journal of Dental Education* 5, 31–7.

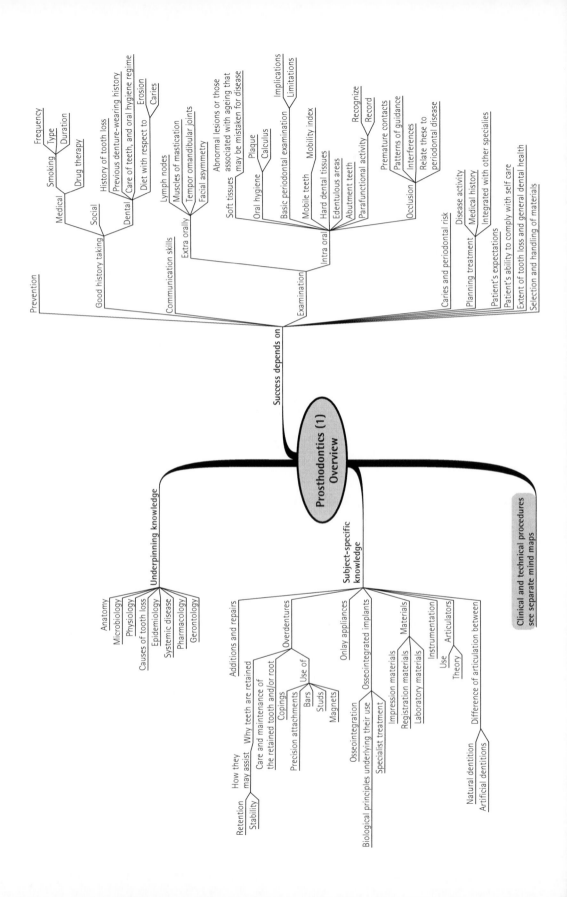

Prosthodontics (1) Overview

Success depends on

Prevention

Good history taking
- Medical
  - Smoking
    - Frequency
    - Type
    - Duration
  - Drug therapy
- Social
- Dental
  - History of tooth loss
  - Previous denture-wearing history
  - Care of teeth, and oral hygiene regime
  - Diet with respect to
    - Erosion
    - Caries

Communication skills

Examination
- Extra orally
  - Lymph nodes
  - Muscles of mastication
  - Temporomandibular joints
  - Facial asymmetry
- Intra oral
  - Soft tissues
    - Abnormal lesions or those associated with ageing that may be mistaken for disease
  - Oral hygiene
    - Plaque
    - Calculus
  - Basic periodontal examination
    - Implications
    - Limitations
  - Mobile teeth
    - Mobility index
  - Hard dental tissues
  - Edentulous areas
  - Abutment teeth
  - Parafunctional activity
    - Recognize
    - Record
  - Occlusion
    - Premature contacts
    - Patterns of guidance
    - Interferences
    - Relate these to periodontal disease
- Caries and periodontal risk
  - Disease activity
- Planning treatment
  - Medical history
  - Integrated with other specialies
- Patient's expectations
- Patient's ability to comply with self care
- Extent of tooth loss and general dental health
- Selection and handling of materials

Underpinning knowledge
- Anatomy
- Microbiology
- Physiology
- Causes of tooth loss
- Epidemiology
- Systemic disease
- Pharmacology
- Gerontology

Subject-specific knowledge

- Additions and repairs
- Overdentures
  - Why teeth are retained
    - How they may assist
    - Retention
    - Stability
  - Care and maintenance of the retained tooth and/or root
  - Use of
    - Copings
    - Precision attachments
    - Bars
    - Studs
    - Magnets
- Onlay appliances
- Osseointegrated implants
  - Osseointegration
  - Biological principles underlying their use
  - Specialist treatment
- Materials
  - Impression materials
  - Registration materials
  - Laboratory materials
- Instrumentation
  - Articulators
    - Use
    - Theory
    - Difference of articulation between
      - Natural dentition
      - Artificial dentitions

Clinical and technical procedures see separate mind maps

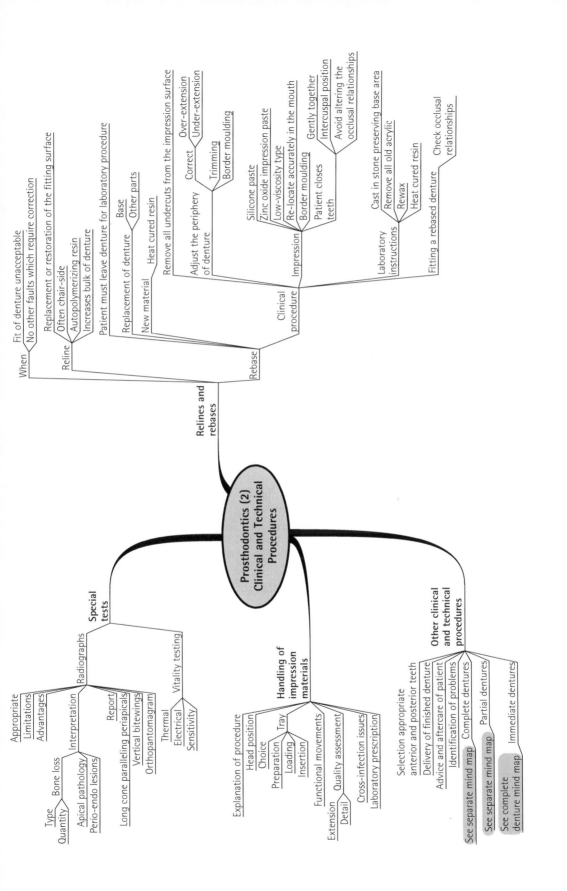

Prosthodontics (2) Clinical and Technical Procedures

Relines and rebases

Reline

When
- Fit of denture unacceptable
- No other faults which require correction
- Replacement or restoration of the fitting surface

- Often chair-side
- Autopolymerizing resin
- Increases bulk of denture
- Patient must leave denture for laboratory procedure

Rebase

Replacement of denture
- Base
- Other parts

New material
- Heat cured resin

Clinical procedure

Remove all undercuts from the impression surface

Adjust the periphery of denture
- Trimming
  - Correct
    - Over-extension
    - Under-extension
  - Border moulding

Impression
- Silicone paste
- Zinc oxide impression paste
- Low-viscosity type
- Re-locate accurately in the mouth
- Border moulding
- Patient closes teeth
  - Gently together
  - Intercuspal position
  - Avoid altering the occlusal relationships

Laboratory instructions
- Cast in stone preserving base area
- Remove all old acrylic
- Rewax
- Heat cured resin

Fitting a rebased denture
- Check occlusal relationships

Special tests

Radiographs
- Appropriate
- Limitations
- Advantages
- Interpretation
  - Type
    - Bone loss
    - Quantity
  - Apical pathology
  - Perio-endo lesions
  - Report
- Long cone paralleling periapicals
- Vertical bitewings
- Orthopantomagram

Vitality testing
- Thermal
- Electrical
- Sensitivity

Handling of impression materials

- Explanation of procedure
- Head position
- Tray
  - Choice
  - Preparation
  - Loading
  - Insertion
- Functional movements
  - Extension
  - Detail
- Quality assessment
- Cross-infection issues
- Laboratory prescription

Other clinical and technical procedures

- Selection appropriate anterior and posterior teeth
- Delivery of finished denture
- Advice and aftercare of patient
- Identification of problems
- Complete dentures — See separate mind map
- Partial dentures — See separate mind map
- Immediate dentures — See complete denture mind map

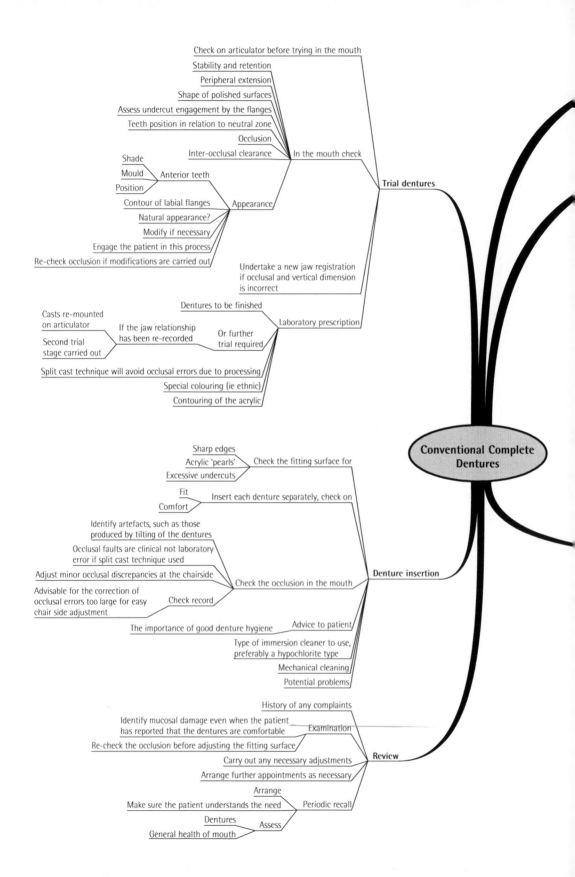

Conventional Complete Dentures

Trial dentures

In the mouth check
- Check on articulator before trying in the mouth
- Stability and retention
- Peripheral extension
- Shape of polished surfaces
- Assess undercut engagement by the flanges
- Teeth position in relation to neutral zone
- Occlusion
- Inter-occlusal clearance

Appearance
- Anterior teeth
  - Shade
  - Mould
  - Position
- Contour of labial flanges
- Natural appearance?
- Modify if necessary
- Engage the patient in this process
- Re-check occlusion if modifications are carried out

Undertake a new jaw registration if occlusal and vertical dimension is incorrect

Laboratory prescription
- Dentures to be finished
- Or further trial required
  - If the jaw relationship has been re-recorded
    - Casts re-mounted on articulator
    - Second trial stage carried out
- Split cast technique will avoid occlusal errors due to processing
- Special colouring (ie ethnic)
- Contouring of the acrylic

Denture insertion

Check the fitting surface for
- Sharp edges
- Acrylic 'pearls'
- Excessive undercuts

Insert each denture separately, check on
- Fit
- Comfort

Check the occlusion in the mouth
- Identify artefacts, such as those produced by tilting of the dentures
- Occlusal faults are clinical not laboratory error if split cast technique used
- Adjust minor occlusal discrepancies at the chairside
- Check record
  - Advisable for the correction of occlusal errors too large for easy chair side adjustment

Advice to patient
- The importance of good denture hygiene
- Type of immersion cleaner to use, preferably a hypochlorite type
- Mechanical cleaning
- Potential problems

Review

Examination
- History of any complaints
- Identify mucosal damage even when the patient has reported that the dentures are comfortable

- Re-check the occlusion before adjusting the fitting surface
- Carry out any necessary adjustments
- Arrange further appointments as necessary

Periodic recall
- Arrange
  - Make sure the patient understands the need
- Assess
  - Dentures
  - General health of mouth

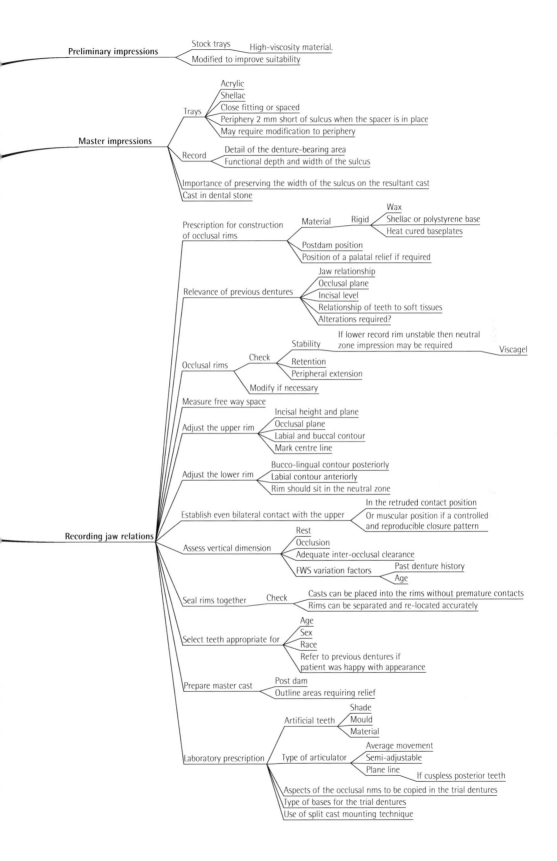

Preliminary impressions
- Stock trays — High-viscosity material.
- Modified to improve suitability

Master impressions
- Trays
  - Acrylic
  - Shellac
  - Close fitting or spaced
  - Periphery 2 mm short of sulcus when the spacer is in place
  - May require modification to periphery
- Record
  - Detail of the denture-bearing area
  - Functional depth and width of the sulcus
- Importance of preserving the width of the sulcus on the resultant cast
- Cast in dental stone

Recording jaw relations
- Prescription for construction of occlusal rims
  - Material — Rigid
    - Wax
    - Shellac or polystyrene base
    - Heat cured baseplates
  - Postdam position
  - Position of a palatal relief if required
- Relevance of previous dentures
  - Jaw relationship
  - Occlusal plane
  - Incisal level
  - Relationship of teeth to soft tissues
  - Alterations required?
- Occlusal rims
  - Check
    - Stability — If lower record rim unstable then neutral zone impression may be required — Viscagel
    - Retention
    - Peripheral extension
  - Modify if necessary
- Measure free way space
- Adjust the upper rim
  - Incisal height and plane
  - Occlusal plane
  - Labial and buccal contour
  - Mark centre line
- Adjust the lower rim
  - Bucco-lingual contour posteriorly
  - Labial contour anteriorly
  - Rim should sit in the neutral zone
- Establish even bilateral contact with the upper
  - In the retruded contact position
  - Or muscular position if a controlled and reproducible closure pattern
- Assess vertical dimension
  - Rest
  - Occlusion
  - Adequate inter-occlusal clearance
  - FWS variation factors
    - Past denture history
    - Age
- Seal rims together — Check
  - Casts can be placed into the rims without premature contacts
  - Rims can be separated and re-located accurately
- Select teeth appropriate for
  - Age
  - Sex
  - Race
  - Refer to previous dentures if patient was happy with appearance
- Prepare master cast
  - Post dam
  - Outline areas requiring relief
- Laboratory prescription
  - Artificial teeth
    - Shade
    - Mould
    - Material
  - Type of articulator
    - Average movement
    - Semi-adjustable
    - Plane line — If cuspless posterior teeth
  - Aspects of the occlusal nms to be copied in the trial dentures
  - Type of bases for the trial dentures
  - Use of split cast mounting technique

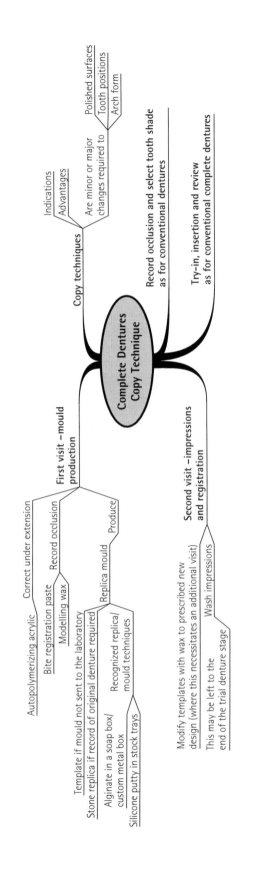

Complete Dentures Copy Technique

Copy techniques
- Indications
- Advantages
  - Are minor or major changes required to
    - Polished surfaces
    - Tooth positions
    - Arch form

Record occlusion and select tooth shade as for conventional dentures

Try-in, insertion and review as for conventional complete dentures

First visit – mould production
- Correct under extension
- Record occlusion
  - Autopolymerizing acrylic
  - Bite registration paste
  - Modelling wax
- Replica mould
  - Produce
  - Recognized replica/mould techniques
    - Template if mould not sent to the laboratory
    - Stone replica if record of original denture required
    - Alginate in a soap box/custom metal box
    - Silicone putty in stock trays

Second visit – impressions and registration
- Wash impressions
- Modify templates with wax to prescribed new design (where this necessitates an additional visit)
- This may be left to the end of the trial denture stage

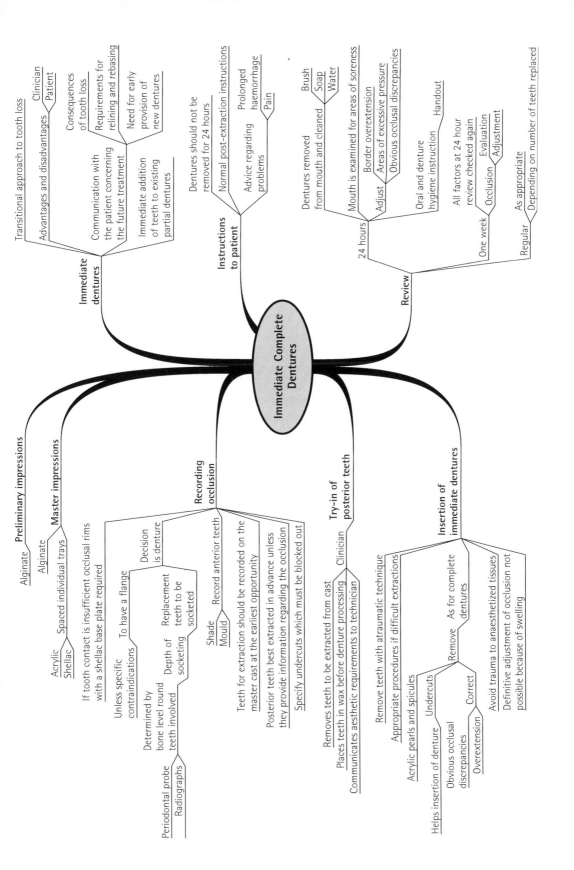

Immediate Complete Dentures

Immediate dentures
- Transitional approach to tooth loss
- Advantages and disadvantages
  - Clinician
  - Patient
- Consequences of tooth loss
- Requirements for relining and rebasing
- Need for early provision of new dentures
- Communication with the patient concerning the future treatment
- Immediate addition of teeth to existing partial dentures

Instructions to patient
- Dentures should not be removed for 24 hours
- Normal post-extraction instructions
- Advice regarding problems
  - Prolonged haemorrhage
  - Pain

Review
- 24 hours
  - Dentures removed from mouth and cleaned
    - Brush
    - Soap
    - Water
  - Mouth is examined for areas of soreness
    - Border overextension
    - Areas of excessive pressure
    - Obvious occlusal discrepancies
    - Adjust
  - Oral and denture hygiene instruction
    - Handout
- One week
  - All factors at 24 hour review checked again
    - Occlusion
      - Evaluation
      - Adjustment
- Regular
  - As appropriate
  - Depending on number of teeth replaced

Preliminary impressions
- Alginate

Master impressions
- Alginate
  - Acrylic
  - Shellac
- Spaced individual trays
- If tooth contact is insufficient occlusal rims with a shellac base plate required
- Decision is denture
  - To have a flange
    - Unless specific contraindications
  - Replacement teeth to be socketed
    - Depth of socketing
      - Determined by bone level round teeth involved
        - Periodontal probe
        - Radiographs

Recording occlusion
- Shade
- Mould
- Record anterior teeth
- Teeth for extraction should be recorded on the master cast at the earliest opportunity
- Posterior teeth best extracted in advance unless they provide information regarding the occlusion
- Specify undercuts which must be blocked out

Try-in of posterior teeth
- Clinician
  - Removes teeth to be extracted from cast
  - Places teeth in wax before denture processing
  - Communicates aesthetic requirements to technician

Insertion of immediate dentures
- Remove teeth with atraumatic technique
- Appropriate procedures if difficult extractions
- Remove
  - Acrylic pearls and spicules
  - Undercuts
    - Helps insertion of denture
- As for complete dentures
  - Obvious occlusal discrepancies
  - Overextension
    - Correct
- Avoid trauma to anaesthetized tissues
- Definitive adjustment of occlusion not possible because of swelling

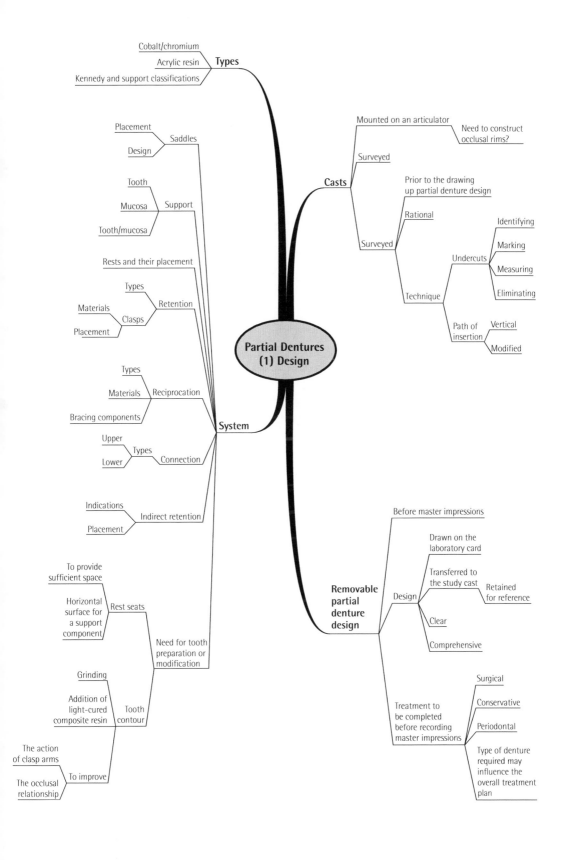

Partial Dentures (1) Design

Types
- Cobalt/chromium
- Acrylic resin
- Kennedy and support classifications

Casts
- Surveyed
  - Mounted on an articulator
    - Need to construct occlusal rims?
- Surveyed
  - Rational
    - Prior to the drawing up partial denture design
  - Technique
    - Undercuts
      - Identifying
      - Marking
      - Measuring
      - Eliminating
    - Path of insertion
      - Vertical
      - Modified

System
- Saddles
  - Placement
  - Design
- Support
  - Tooth
  - Mucosa
  - Tooth/mucosa
- Retention
  - Rests and their placement
  - Clasps
    - Types
    - Materials
    - Placement
- Reciprocation
  - Types
  - Materials
  - Bracing components
- Connection
  - Types
    - Upper
    - Lower
- Indirect retention
  - Indications
  - Placement
- Need for tooth preparation or modification
  - Rest seats
    - To provide sufficient space
    - Horizontal surface for a support component
  - Tooth contour
    - Grinding
    - Addition of light-cured composite resin
  - To improve
    - The action of clasp arms
    - The occlusal relationship

Removable partial denture design
- Design
  - Before master impressions
  - Drawn on the laboratory card
  - Transferred to the study cast
    - Retained for reference
  - Clear
  - Comprehensive
- Treatment to be completed before recording master impressions
  - Surgical
  - Conservative
  - Periodontal
  - Type of denture required may influence the overall treatment plan

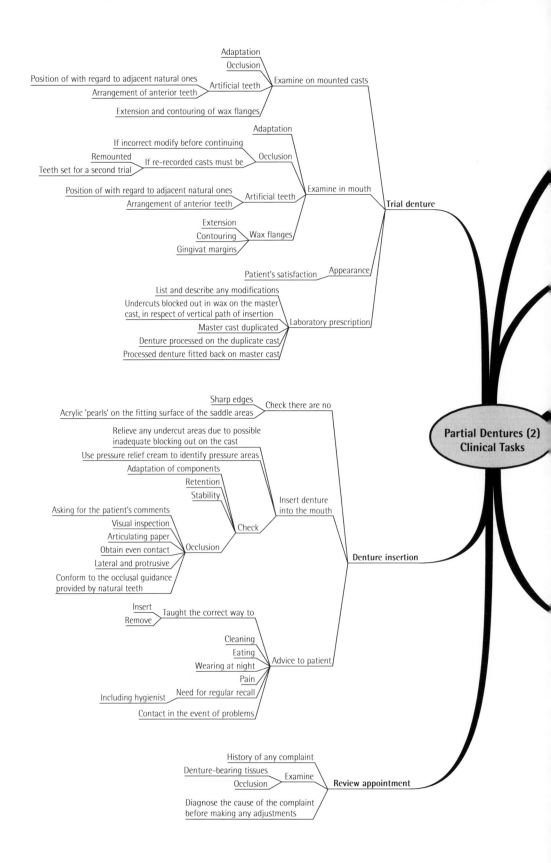

Adaptation
Occlusion
Position of with regard to adjacent natural ones
Arrangement of anterior teeth
Artificial teeth
Extension and contouring of wax flanges
Examine on mounted casts

If incorrect modify before continuing
Remounted
Teeth set for a second trial
If re-recorded casts must be
Adaptation
Occlusion
Position of with regard to adjacent natural ones
Arrangement of anterior teeth
Artificial teeth
Examine in mouth
Extension
Contouring
Gingival margins
Wax flanges

Patient's satisfaction
Appearance

List and describe any modifications
Undercuts blocked out in wax on the master
cast, in respect of vertical path of insertion
Master cast duplicated
Denture processed on the duplicate cast
Processed denture fitted back on master cast
Laboratory prescription

Trial denture

Sharp edges
Acrylic 'pearls' on the fitting surface of the saddle areas
Check there are no
Relieve any undercut areas due to possible
inadequate blocking out on the cast
Use pressure relief cream to identify pressure areas
Adaptation of components
Retention
Stability
Insert denture
into the mouth

Asking for the patient's comments
Visual inspection
Articulating paper
Obtain even contact
Lateral and protrusive
Conform to the occlusal guidance
provided by natural teeth
Occlusion
Check

Insert
Remove
Taught the correct way to

Cleaning
Eating
Wearing at night
Pain
Including hygienist
Need for regular recall
Contact in the event of problems
Advice to patient

Denture insertion

History of any complaint
Denture-bearing tissues
Occlusion
Examine
Diagnose the cause of the complaint
before making any adjustments
Review appointment

**Partial Dentures (2)
Clinical Tasks**

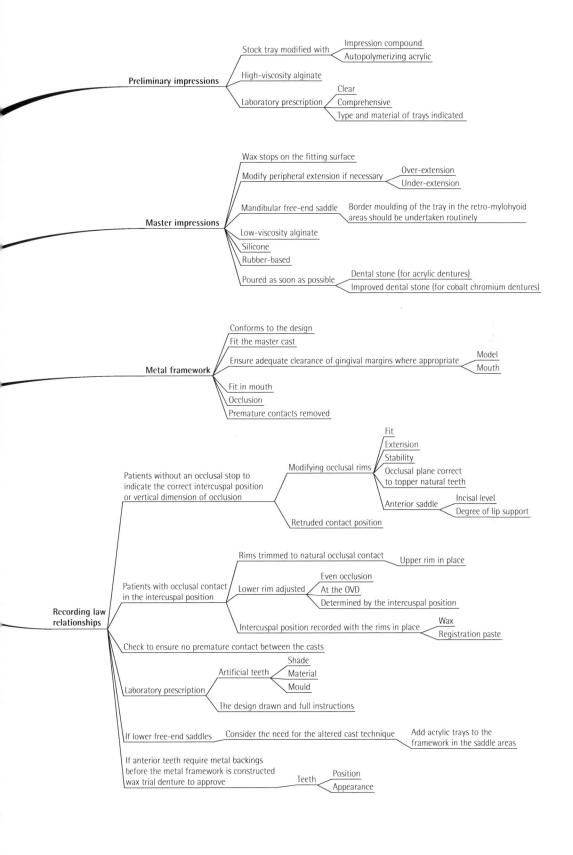

Preliminary impressions
- Stock tray modified with
  - Impression compound
  - Autopolymerizing acrylic
- High-viscosity alginate
- Laboratory prescription
  - Clear
  - Comprehensive
  - Type and material of trays indicated

Master impressions
- Wax stops on the fitting surface
- Modify peripheral extension if necessary
  - Over-extension
  - Under-extension
- Mandibular free-end saddle — Border moulding of the tray in the retro-mylohyoid areas should be undertaken routinely
- Low-viscosity alginate
- Silicone
- Rubber-based
- Poured as soon as possible
  - Dental stone (for acrylic dentures)
  - Improved dental stone (for cobalt chromium dentures)

Metal framework
- Conforms to the design
- Fit the master cast
- Ensure adequate clearance of gingival margins where appropriate
  - Model
  - Mouth
- Fit in mouth
- Occlusion
- Premature contacts removed

Recording law relationships
- Patients without an occlusal stop to indicate the correct intercuspal position or vertical dimension of occlusion
  - Modifying occlusal rims
    - Fit
    - Extension
    - Stability
    - Occlusal plane correct to topper natural teeth
    - Anterior saddle
      - Incisal level
      - Degree of lip support
  - Retruded contact position
- Patients with occlusal contact in the intercuspal position
  - Rims trimmed to natural occlusal contact — Upper rim in place
  - Lower rim adjusted
    - Even occlusion
    - At the OVD
    - Determined by the intercuspal position
  - Intercuspal position recorded with the rims in place
    - Wax
    - Registration paste
- Check to ensure no premature contact between the casts
- Laboratory prescription
  - Artificial teeth
    - Shade
    - Material
    - Mould
  - The design drawn and full instructions
- If lower free-end saddles — Consider the need for the altered cast technique — Add acrylic trays to the framework in the saddle areas
- If anterior teeth require metal backings before the metal framework is constructed wax trial denture to approve
  - Teeth
    - Position
    - Appearance

Surgical dentistry
Jonathan Pedlar

Key points

- Competence in diagnosis and practical management of surgical conditions of the jaws is essential in the graduating dentist.

- The removal of erupted and unerupted teeth and other minor surgical procedures require the ability to apply basic and medical sciences along with a high level of practical technical skill, as well as an understanding of the interaction of that surgery with medical illness and anxiety.

- Surgery forms a part of many aspects of dentistry. Students should be familiar with procedures such as those performed as part of facial deformity surgery, periodontal treatment, implant placement, cancer management, and rehabilitation following extensive tooth loss, where interaction with other specialists is required.

- Though highly specialized, students should be familiar with management of patients with oral and maxillofacial trauma, temporomandibular joint (TMJ) problems and patients with clefting and dento-facial deformities.

Introduction

The contemporary view of undergraduate learning should seek to integrate oral surgery, oral and maxillofacial surgery, oral medicine, oral pathology and oral radiology. A broad interdisciplinary approach and vertical integration would also improve the relevance of the pre-clinical and para-clinical subjects. Both *The First Five Years* (GDC 2002) and the QAA benchmark statement for dentistry (QAA 2002) include oral surgery in their description of the characteristics of an undergraduate programme in dentistry:

Paragraph 91 Practical experience in oral surgery should include those procedures commonly undertaken in general dental practice. On graduation, all dental students should be able to undertake extraction of teeth and removal of roots where necessary, utilising surgical techniques involving raising of a muco-periosteal flap, bone removal, tooth sectioning, the use of elevators and intraoral suturing. They should be able to assess a surgical extraction. They should be aware of their surgical limitations and understand when to refer for secondary or tertiary care.

Paragraph 92 In addition, the student should have an understanding of the range of surgical procedures which may be used to manage diseases and disorders of the mouth and jaws. They should also be aware of the principles of trauma management and have observed a selection of cases being treated. Dental students can gain valuable experience in oral and maxillofacial surgery, oral medicine and aspects of medicine and surgery by attendance at selected units in teaching and district general hospitals. However, when undertaking dental procedures at such units they must be supervised by staff who are appropriately qualified and registered with the GDC. (GDC 2002)

In the benchmarking statements, paragraph 3.17 deals with oral medicine, pathology and surgery as an integrated package:

Manage patients with facial pain, disease and disorders of the oral cavity and associated structures, including a recognition of when it is appropriate to refer for specialist help and advice;

Manage basic dento-alveolar surgical procedures, including intra- and post-operative complications and recognise when it is appropriate to refer for specialist help and advice;

Understand the importance of and procedures for submitting specimens for laboratory diagnosis and demonstrate the ability to interpret diagnostic reports.

Intended learning outcomes

These are defined using GDC definitions of 'competent at', 'have knowledge of' and 'be familiar with', but have been extended from the list of learning outcomes listed in *The First Five Years* and some aspects of oral medicine and restorative dentistry have been incorporated. This is in line with what is currently taught in most UK dental schools. The list is compliant with the European Union directive (available at www.dented.org/parse.php3?file=info/sect3.html) and is consistent with a list of competencies drawn from American dental schools (in this case, Baylor College).

Table 2.8.1 Intended learning outcomes for surgical dentistry

Be competent at	Have knowledge of	Be familiar with
Diagnosis and treatment planning for: • acutely painful conditions of dental origin • acute infection of dental origin	Diagnosis and treatment planning for: • maxillofacial trauma • facial deformity	Surgery for facial deformity and dento-facial anomalies, maxillofacial trauma, temporomandibular joint disorders, maxillofacial implants
Diagnosis of oral cancer and premalignant lesions and advising patients on prevention of malignant disease	Conditions of tissues adjacent to the mouth which may be caused by or may need to be distinguished from oral and dental conditions	Inpatient ward and operating theatre practices
The extraction of erupted teeth and the removal of roots and simpler unerupted teeth, including the design, raising and repair of a mucoperiosteal flap	Disorders of the masticatory muscles and temporomandibular joints	Construction of appliances for temporomandibular disorders
Minor surgery to oral soft tissue or alveolar bone	Common intra-bony pathological conditions such as cysts	
Applying principles of patient care, including control of pain, anxiety and cross-infection, to surgical procedures	Treatment planning for and outcomes of oral cancer	
	Appropriate special investigations and the interpretations of their results	
	Surgical endodontics	
	Incisional and excisional biopsy	

Competence at graduation

At graduation the dentist should be competent at:

Diagnosis and treatment planning

- ◆ For acutely painful conditions of dental origin, and
  - ▪ acute infection of dental origin.
- ◆ Identify from interview of the patient features of pain likely to indicate an origin from dental pulp, periodontal ligament, pericoronal tissues and the oral mucosa.
- ◆ Focus examination of the patient, seeking likely causes such as dental caries, large restorations, chronic periodontal disease, pericoronal infection, whilst not ignoring general aspects of examination.
- ◆ Select (propose) suitable special investigations to distinguish between various dental causes of pain, such as tenderness to pressure or percussion, radiography and vitality testing.
- ◆ Justify the choice of such special tests and explain the significance of the findings.
- ◆ Reach a diagnosis for a dental pain.
- ◆ Determine how best a painful dental condition may be treated and discuss the merits of various options with the patient in terms they can understand.
- ◆ Determine when it is not appropriate to restore the tooth and explain the implications of tooth loss to the patient.

These can be summarized as: Demonstrate ability to apply knowledge of common painful dental conditions to determining whether the patient may be better managed by tooth extraction, than by restorative management.

- ◆ Discriminate clearly acute infection which has spread beyond the alveolus from simpler painful dental conditions.
- ◆ Identify features likely to indicate a localized collection of pus, whether intra- or extra-oral.
- ◆ Distinguish the clinical patterns of spreading infection, abscess formation, bone infection, chronic infections such as actinomycosis, infection of salivary glands, infection of skin.
- ◆ Distinguish infection from neoplastic disease
- ◆ Identify those patients at more than average risk from infection because of medical conditions or drug therapy.
- ◆ Determine the severity and degree of spread of infection, including an assessment of the risk of serious outcomes such as airway obstruction or spread to the orbit or cavernous sinus.

- Determine which infection can safely be managed in a dental practice setting and when referral to a hospital specialist is indicated.
- Prescribe antibiotics for simpler dental infections and advise patients on other aspects of care.
- Determine when drainage of an abscess is indicated and incise an intra-oral abscess.
- Determine whether an infection is responding satisfactorily to treatment provided.

Diagnosis of oral cancer and premalignant lesions and advise patients on prevention of malignant disease

- Recognize mucosal lesions and conditions which have a potential for malignant change:
  - Red patches
  - White patches
  - Lichen planus
  - Submucous fibrosis
- and assess the likelihood of such change.
- Recognize oral cancers presenting at different stages in the various sites in the mouth, by history, appearance and on palpation.
- Apply the principles of staging of oral cancer to the assessment of a patient with cancer.
- Determine the urgency of referral of a patient with a suspicious lesion in the mouth.
- Advise patients about factors known to increase the risk of oral cancer.

Extraction of erupted teeth

- Determine which teeth should be extracted, rather than being managed conservatively.
- Achieve appropriate control of pain and anxiety for extraction.
- Select forceps or elevator suited to the extraction of a given tooth and hold them in an efficient and safe position in the hand.
- Position themselves and the patient for extraction and apply effective support with the hand during an extraction.
- Remove teeth efficiently, safely and with minimal distress to the patient.
- Give post-operative advice after tooth extraction.
- Distinguish, on the basis of clinical and radiographic features, those teeth likely to be difficult to remove with forceps, from the more straightforward cases, anticipating and if possible avoiding problems of tooth or root fracture.
- Anticipate difficulties with and complications of extraction, avoiding them where possible, recognizing, investigating and treating those which occur.

The extraction of simpler unerupted teeth and roots not amenable to removal with forceps or elevators alone

- Design and raise a mucoperiosteal flap to provide good access to the surgical site with minimal risk of damage to adjacent structures and amenable to simple repair with sutures, and resulting in minimal long-term damage to periodontal structures.
- Remove bone and divide a tooth with burs, making safe and effective access points for elevators or forceps.
- Clean and close the wound so formed with sutures.
- Provide post-operative care in the form of advice, medication and follow-up.
- Advise patients about the benefits and likely adverse effects or complications of minor surgery, including removal of lower third molars and agree a treatment plan.
- Anticipate difficulties with and complications of dento-alveolar surgery, other than simple extraction, avoiding them where possible, recognising, investigating and treating those which occur and recognising those which require referral for specialist opinion.

Minor surgery to oral soft tissue or alveolar bone

- Determine those minor soft tissue and bone abnormalities amenable to surgery in the dental practice setting.
- Perform simpler soft tissue surgery within the mouth, such as:
  - Excisional biopsy of fibro-epithelial polyps or viral warts
  - Maxillary labial fraenectomy in the edentulous patient
- Apply existing skills in soft tissue surgery to simple new settings, such as reduction in height of the maxillary tuberosity.
- Reduce, with burs, bony undercuts in edentulous areas via a mucoperiosteal flap.

Applying principles of patient care, including control of pain, anxiety and cross-infection to surgical procedures

Consent

See Chapter 1.3.

- Advise a patient about their condition, possible treatments, intended benefits, possible adverse outcomes, and engage with the patient to determine their consent to proposed treatment.

Control of pain and anxiety

See chapters 1.9 and 1.10.

- Application of local anaesthesia to achieve complete pain relief during extraction.
- Selection of patients who would benefit from additional support in the form of oral, inhalational or intravenous sedation and evaluating the interaction of each of these

techniques with the surgical process.

- Selection of patients who would benefit from general anaesthesia, including evaluating the risks associated with general anaesthesia in a particular patient:
  - Obesity
  - Cardiovascular disease
  - Respiratory disease
  - Neurological and neuromuscular disease
  - Other systemic disease
  - Smoking
  - Alcohol and substance abuse.
- Evaluate the social influences of these methods of pain and anxiety control for a patient.

Infection control
See Chapter 1.5.

- Evaluate and control specific risks associated with blood exposure
- Evaluate and control specific risks associated with sharp instruments in minor surgery
- Evaluate and control specific risks associated with open tissue wounds.

Prescription of analgesics
- Select and prescribe a suitable analgesic for post-operative pain relief and advise a patient on its administration.

Prescription of antibiotics
- Determine when it is appropriate to prescribe an antibacterial agent for prevention or control of infection associated with minor surgery in the mouth.

At graduation
The dentist should have knowledge of:

Diagnosis and treatment planning
For:

- maxillofacial trauma
- facial deformity
- conditions of tissues adjacent to the mouth which may be caused by or may need to be distinguished from oral and dental conditions
- disorders of the masticatory muscles and temporomandibular joints
- common intra-bony pathological conditions such as cysts.

Maxillofacial trauma

◆ Recognize clinical features of injuries of the soft tissues of the face and oral mucosa, jaws, and other facial bones, including swelling, localized tenderness, bone deformity, occlusal change and sensory nerve dysfunction.

◆ Recommend suitable radiographic investigation and interpret radiographic appearances of the commoner facial bone injuries.

◆ Describe the emergency care of patients with acute maxillofacial injuries.

◆ Describe the commoner types of treatment for maxillofacial injuries.

◆ Recognize the commoner complications associated with maxillofacial trauma and its treatment (e.g. occlusal discrepancy or persistent dysaesthesia).

Facial deformity

◆ Recognize abnormalities of facial form.

◆ Evaluate what types of treatment may be possible.

◆ Determine what investigations may be needed and evaluate from radiographic and modelling investigation the broad type of deformity present.

Conditions affecting tissues adjacent to the mouth

1. Salivary glands

   ◆ Recognize a history typical of obstructive or neoplastic disease of the parotid or submandibular gland

   ◆ Recognize enlargement, change in texture, tenderness of, or discharge from a salivary gland.

   ◆ Propose plain or contrast radiographic views for investigation of such a condition and interpret the results.

   ◆ Differentiate on clinical grounds between infection, obstruction, benign and malignant neoplasms of the salivary glands.

   ◆ Determine which such patients require referral and with what urgency.

   ◆ Describe the processes by which salivary stones may be managed.

2. Maxillary antrum

   ◆ Describe the relationship of the maxillary antrum to the oral structures.

   ◆ Recognize the clinical features of acute maxillary sinusitis and propose a treatment.

   ◆ Understand the common investigations and surgical procedures performed for antral disease and know when their use is indicated.

   ◆ Recognize situations where dental extraction/minor oral surgery may be complicated by the creation of an oro-antral communication or the displacement of a foreign body, tooth or root into the antrum.

- ◆ Know how to minimize the risk of these complications occurring, treat a newly formed oro-antral communication or foreign body in the antrum, anticipate and minimize the risk of a fracture of the maxillary tuberosity occurring during an extraction.

- ◆ Recognize the characteristic features of malignant disease of the maxillary antrum.

3. Lymph nodes (see Chapter 1.8)

- ◆ Distinguish swellings of lymph nodes from other disorders and evaluate the importance of further investigation in a given situation.

4. Masticatory muscles and temporomandibular joints (muscular disorders have few surgical implications but need to be distinguished from conditions which do):

- ◆ Recognize clinical features and imaging results for displacement with or without reduction of the intra-articular disk and advise a patient concerning the disorders.

- ◆ Describe the relationship between muscular and disk-related masticatory disorders.

- ◆ Describe the possible treatments for disk displacement disorders

- ◆ Recognize principal clinical and radiographic features of degenerative joint disease and systemic arthropathies

- ◆ Recognize ankylosis of the TMJ and describe possible treatments

- ◆ Recognize dislocation of the TMJ understand the principle of reduction.

5. Common intra-bony pathological conditions:

- ◆ Recognize clinical and radiographic features of odontogenic cysts

- ◆ Describe treatments and follow-up requirements for odontogenic cysts

- ◆ Recognize the commoner clinical and radiographic features of odontomes and determine the merits of their removal

- ◆ Recognize the principal clinical and radiographic features of odontogenic tumours and determine the urgency of referral of a patient suspected of having one

- ◆ Recognize the clinical and radiographic features suggestive of primary and secondary intra-osseous malignant disease.

Treatment planning for and outcomes of oral cancer

- ◆ Describe surgery for resection of cancer, the principles of surgical repair and indicate the main situations in which surgery would be chosen as a treatment modality.

- ◆ Describe radiotherapy, the way it is delivered for oral cancer and its principal effects.

- ◆ Anticipate the dental needs of patients with oral cancer and relate them to the likely treatments.

- ◆ Appreciate the potential outcomes of oral cancer and its treatment and apply that understanding sensitively in the management of cancer patients.

Appropriate special investigations and the interpretations of their results

◆ Recognize situations when it would be appropriate to order particular special investigations and assess the significance of the most important results of these:.

- Tests of pulp vitality
- Radiology: plain films, contrast films, imaging techniques such as MRI, CT, ultrasound, radionuclide imaging
- Haematology: full blood count, urea and electrolytes, bleeding and clotting screen, liver function tests, calcium, phosphorus and alkaline phosphatase
- Histopathology: biopsy of soft tissue or bone
- Microbiology: specimens for identification of organisms and antibiotic sensitivity.

Surgical endodontics

◆ Define the indications and contraindications to surgical endodontics.

◆ Design a suitable mucoperiosteal flap.

◆ Perform simple surgical endodontics with assistance.

◆ Select a suitable root-end sealant material.

◆ Justify an appropriate follow-up regime and determine whether surgery has been successful.

Incisional and excisional biopsy

◆ Determine when a biopsy is indicated, when and where it should be performed and select an appropriate technique.

◆ Perform a straightforward biopsy with appropriate guidance.

◆ Evaluate the applications of techniques such as smears, fine-needle aspiration and cutting needle biopsies.

At graduation

The dentist should be familiar with:

Surgery for facial deformity and dento-facial anomalies, maxillofacial trauma, temporomandibular joint disorders, maxillofacial implants

And be able to describe and apply an understanding of:

1. Facial deformity surgery:
    - Mandibular osteotomy techniques
    - Maxillary osteotomy techniques
    - The further implications of bimaxillary surgery
    - Segmental techniques
    - Distraction osteogenesis.

2. Cleft palate surgery:
   - Principles of primary cleft surgery
   - Secondary alveolar bone grafting.

3. Surgery for maxillofacial trauma:
   - Soft tissue injuries
   - Mandibular fractures (including the condyle)
   - Maxillary fractures
   - Orbital fractures
   - Nasal fractures.

4. Temporomandibular joint surgery:
   - For dislocation
   - Arthroscopy/arthrocentesis
   - Open surgery of the TMJ
   - TMJ replacement.

5. Surgery for maxillofacial implants:
   - Principles of selection of patients for implants
   - Techniques for implant placement
   - Special cases such as sinus lift procedures, zygomaticus implants, bone augmentation associated with implant placement, extra-oral implants.

Inpatient ward and operating theatre practices
Be able to describe and apply an understanding of:
- The formalities of inpatient hospital admission.
- The mechanisms guiding in-patient care, such as the role of the doctor or dentist on the ward, that of the nurse, ward rounds, control of drug administration, communication procedures, liaison with other specialties.
- The role of the accident and emergency department.
- The purpose and conduct of pre-admission assessment and determination of fitness of the patient to undergo the planned procedure.
- Patient identification practices.
- The role of the anaesthetist and the ODP.
- The 'scrub routine' and good practice at the operating table.
- Special care facilities such as ITU.
- Determining fitness for discharge.

Construction of appliances for temporomandibular disorders
Be familiar with a range of appliances that may be used in temporomandibular disorders such as the soft lower splint, the stabilization type appliance and the anterior repositioning appliance, and be able to justify the choice of an appliance in a given situation.

Checklist 52 (a) **Exodontia (uncomplicated)**

	Yes	No
Introduces themselves to patient and confirms the patient's identity		
Confirms diagnosis and that tooth requires extraction		
Correctly assesses likely difficulty of extraction		
Uses appropriate route, drug and dose of local anaesthetic		
Selects forceps appropriate to the tooth		
Holds forceps in hand in a way that maximizes control, applicable force and minimizes risk to the operator and patient		
Positions patient optimally		
Positions themselves optimally		
Applies appropriate control with supporting hand		
Applies forceps efficiently and safely		
Delivers tooth efficiently with method carrying minimal risk of tooth fracture or other injury to patient		
Confirms delivery of whole tooth, checks extraction site and compresses		
Confirms cessation of bleeding		
Gives postoperative instructions clearly in writing and orally		
Follows cross-infection procedure throughout		

Signing off will be declined for one 'No' in a shaded box or more than one 'No' in an unshaded box.

Checklist 52 (b) **Removal of retained roots**

	Yes	No
Confirms diagnosis and treatment plan		
Advises patient about nature of procedure		
Designs flap consistent with adequate access, minimal risk of avoidable damage and being repairable		
Raises flap with no tearing at margin, remaining subperiosteal at all times, to adequate extent		
Retracts flap with minimal risk of additional damage		
Safe finger rests during bone removal keeping shank of bur well clear of soft tissues		
Cuts bone without bur 'running' along bone surface		
Ensures adequate irrigation and cooling		
Clears adequate bone for access to roots, makes application point for elevator		
Divides roots if necessary, cutting in a safe direction and to a safe but adequate extent		
Elevator held safely in hand, with a secure finger rest and moved in a safe direction		
All roots removed or sound justification offered for leaving part of a root		
Bone edges smoothed, non-vital bone trimmed		
Wound cleaned		
Sutures well placed, appropriately tight		
Checks for haemostasis		
Postoperative instructions given		
Consideration of need for analgesia or antimicrobial therapy		

Signing off will be declined for one 'No' in a shaded box or more than one 'No' in an unshaded box.

References and further reading

European Union Advisory Committee on the Training of Dental Practitioners (2005) *Draft Competences for two specialist categories: Orthodontics and oral surgery.* Available at http://www.dented.org/parse.php3?file=info/sect3.html, accessed April 2005.

GDC (2002) *The First Five Years: a framework for undergraduate dental education*, 2nd edn. London, The General Dental Council.

Killey H. C., Seward G. R., Harris M. McGowan D. A. and Kay L. W. (1997) *An Outline of Oral Surgery.* London, Butterworth Heinemann.

Pedlar J. and Frame W. (2001) *Oral and Maxillofacial Surgery – an objective-based textbook.* Edinburgh, Churchill Livingstone.

QAA (2002) *Dentistry: academic standards.* Subject benchmark statements. Gloucester, Quality Assurance Agency for Higher Education.

Wray D., Stenhouse D. Lee D. and Clarke A. J. E. (2003) *Textbook of General and Oral Surgery.* Edinburgh, Churchill Livingstone.

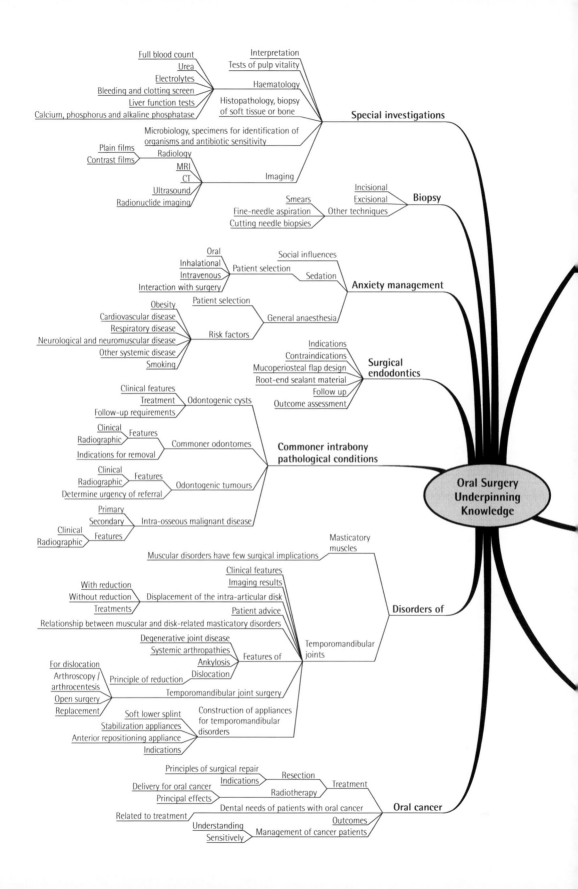

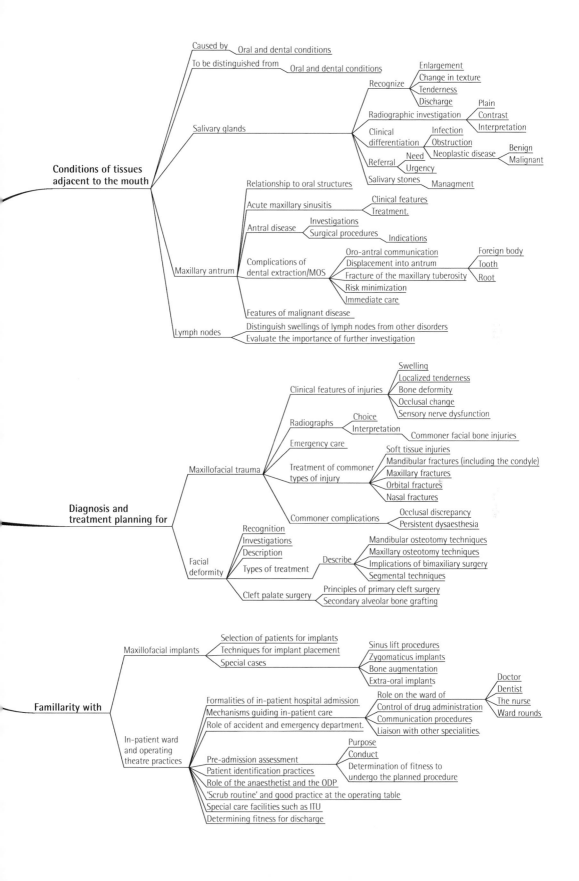

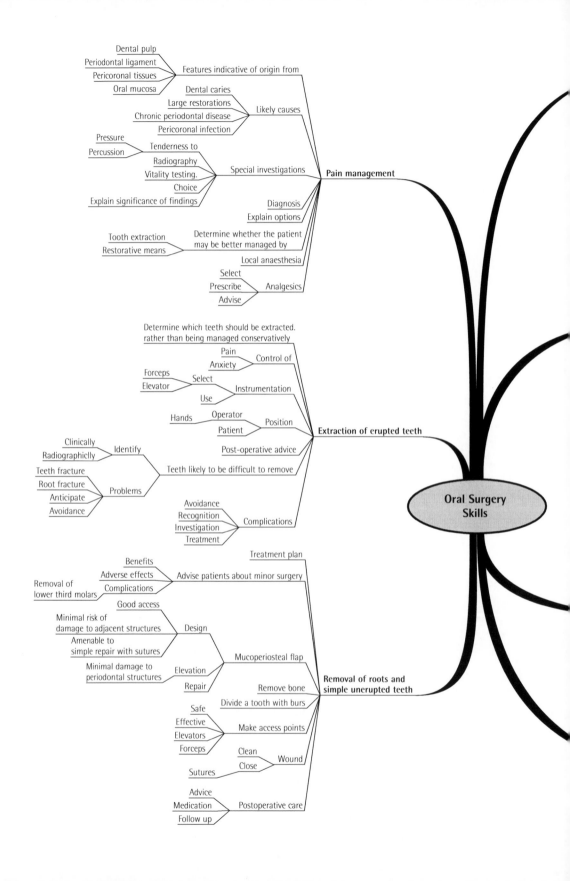

Oral Surgery Skills

Pain management

Features indicative of origin from
- Dental pulp
- Periodontal ligament
- Pericoronal tissues
- Oral mucosa

Likely causes
- Dental caries
- Large restorations
- Chronic periodontal disease
- Pericoronal infection

Special investigations
- Tenderness to
  - Pressure
  - Percussion
- Radiography
- Vitality testing.
  - Choice
- Explain significance of findings

- Diagnosis
- Explain options

Determine whether the patient may be better managed by
- Tooth extraction
- Restorative means

- Local anaesthesia

Analgesics
- Select
- Prescribe
- Advise

Extraction of erupted teeth

Determine which teeth should be extracted. rather than being managed conservatively

Control of
- Pain
- Anxiety

Instrumentation
- Select
  - Forceps
  - Elevator
- Use

Position
- Operator
  - Hands
- Patient

Post-operative advice

Teeth likely to be difficult to remove
- Identify
  - Clinically
  - Radiographiclly

Problems
- Teeth fracture
- Root fracture
- Anticipate
- Avoidance

Complications
- Avoidance
- Recognition
- Investigation
- Treatment

Removal of roots and simple unerupted teeth

Treatment plan

Advise patients about minor surgery
- Benefits
- Adverse effects
- Complications
- Removal of lower third molars

Mucoperiosteal flap
- Design
  - Good access
  - Minimal risk of damage to adjacent structures
  - Amenable to simple repair with sutures
  - Minimal damage to periodontal structures
- Elevation
- Repair

- Remove bone
- Divide a tooth with burs
- Make access points
  - Safe
  - Effective
  - Elevators
  - Forceps

Wound
- Clean
- Close
- Sutures

Postoperative care
- Advice
- Medication
- Follow up

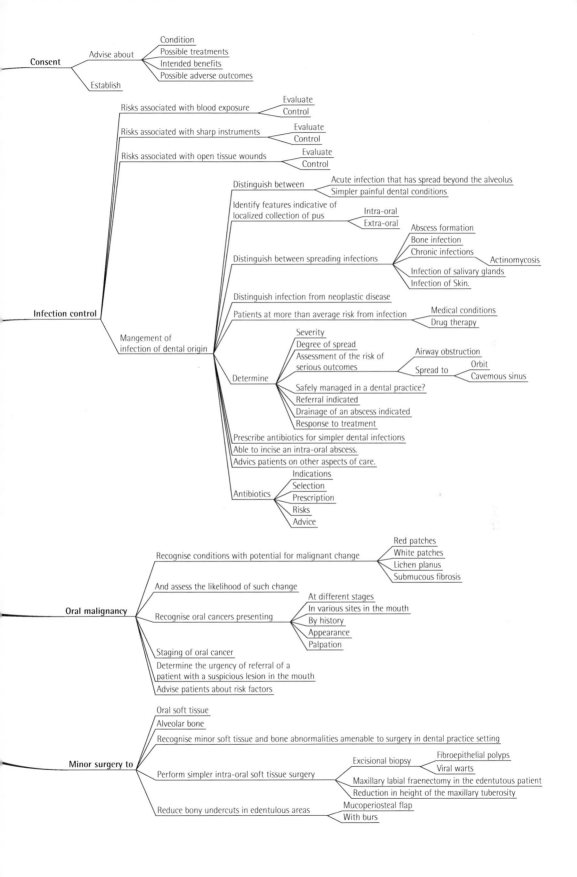

Consent
- Advise about
  - Condition
  - Possible treatments
  - Intended benefits
  - Possible adverse outcomes
- Establish

Infection control
- Risks associated with blood exposure
  - Evaluate
  - Control
- Risks associated with sharp instruments
  - Evaluate
  - Control
- Risks associated with open tissue wounds
  - Evaluate
  - Control
- Mangement of infection of dental origin
  - Distinguish between
    - Acute infection that has spread beyond the alveolus
    - Simpler painful dental conditions
  - Identify features indicative of localized collection of pus
    - Intra-oral
    - Extra-oral
  - Distinguish between spreading infections
    - Abscess formation
    - Bone infection
    - Chronic infections
      - Actinomycosis
    - Infection of salivary glands
    - Infection of Skin.
  - Distinguish infection from neoplastic disease
  - Patients at more than average risk from infection
    - Medical conditions
    - Drug therapy
  - Determine
    - Severity
    - Degree of spread
    - Assessment of the risk of serious outcomes
      - Airway obstruction
      - Spread to
        - Orbit
        - Cavernous sinus
    - Safely managed in a dental practice?
    - Referral indicated
    - Drainage of an abscess indicated
    - Response to treatment
  - Prescribe antibiotics for simpler dental infections
  - Able to incise an intra-oral abscess.
  - Advics patients on other aspects of care.
  - Antibiotics
    - Indications
    - Selection
    - Prescription
    - Risks
    - Advice

Oral malignancy
- Recognise conditions with potential for malignant change
  - Red patches
  - White patches
  - Lichen planus
  - Submucous fibrosis
- And assess the likelihood of such change
- Recognise oral cancers presenting
  - At different stages
  - In various sites in the mouth
  - By history
  - Appearance
  - Palpation
- Staging of oral cancer
- Determine the urgency of referral of a patient with a suspicious lesion in the mouth
- Advise patients about risk factors

Minor surgery to
- Oral soft tissue
- Alveolar bone
- Recognise minor soft tissue and bone abnormalities amenable to surgery in dental practice setting
- Perform simpler intra-oral soft tissue surgery
  - Excisional biopsy
    - Fibroepithelial polyps
    - Viral warts
  - Maxillary labial fraenectomy in the edentutous patient
  - Reduction in height of the maxillary tuberosity
- Reduce bony undercuts in edentulous areas
  - Mucoperiosteal flap
  - With burs

2.9 Oral medicine
Mike Lewis

Key points

+ The specialty of oral medicine, along with oral and maxillofacial surgery, oral radiology and oral pathology, bridges the gap between the medical and dental professions.

+ Appreciation and application of appropriate contemporary medical knowledge in an ever more complex era of medical science, diagnostics and therapeutics is a basic tenet of safe dental practice.

+ The contemporary undergraduate curriculum should integrate learning and teaching in the specialties of oral medicine, oral pathology, oral and maxillofacial surgery, oral microbiology, and oral radiology.

+ It is important for the student at graduation to be aware of the special medical investigations that are available in contemporary medical and dental practice, and to be able to interpret these or by consultation or referral to seek the appropriate expertise.

+ The undergraduate curriculum should emphasize the role of the dentist in preventive medicine, for example through smoking cessation advice, where the benefits are not confined to oral health.

Introduction

The European perspective on Dental Education is specified in a document known as the Dental Directives document 78/687/EEC. Since its appearance, a more focused and competency-based document has been produced by the Advisory Committee on the Training of Dental Practitioners (ACTDP), and this covers undergraduate competencies in Oral Medicine. However, all of these are also comprehensively covered by the *The First Five Years* (GDC 2002) and the QAA benchmark statement for dentistry (QAA 2002). From these documents, the description of the oral medicine input to the undergraduate programme in dentistry is recorded below.

Paragraph 93 It is important to ensure that the dental student is taught the clinical presentation, diagnosis and management of the common diseases of the oral mucosa, of other oral soft tissues, of the salivary glands, of the facial bones and joints, as well as the oral manifestations of systemic diseases. The various manifestations of facial pain of both dental and non-dental origin, its diagnosis and management must also be considered.

Paragraph 94 Teaching in oral surgery and oral medicine should include clinical instruction in the prevention, diagnosis and management of potentially malignant and malignant lesions and conditions of the oral mucosa.

(GDC 2002)

Paragraph 3.17 Graduating dentists should be able to:

- manage patients with facial pain, disease and disorders of the oral cavity and associated structures, including a recognition of when it is appropriate to refer for specialist help and advice.
- understand the importance of and procedures for submitting specimens for laboratory diagnosis and demonstrate the ability to interpret diagnostic reports.

(QAA 2002)

Intended learning outcomes

It is important to ensure that the dental student is taught the clinical presentation, diagnosis and management of the common diseases of the oral mucosa.

Table 2.9.1 Intended learning outcomes for oral medicine

Be competent at	Have knowledge of	Be familiar with
History taking (clinical, medical, social)	Special investigations (haematological, histopathological, biochemical and immunological) and their interpretation	Disease whose management would benefit from referral to other medical, surgical and dental specialists
Recording of clinical signs and symptoms	Chair-side investigations including urinalysis, blood glucose, salivary flow rate and Schirmer tests	The role of cryotherapy, laser and photodynamic therapy in the management of orofacial disease
Presenting a comprehensive patient history	The procedure of labial gland biopsy	

Table 2.9.1 Intended learning outcomes for oral medicine – *continued*

Be competent at	Have knowledge of	Be familiar with
Undertaking a general examination of the clothed patient, in particular the orofacial tissues	The role of clinical photography in patient management and the associated consent issues	
Perform a clinical examination, including when indicated:	Request appropriate radiographic examination relevant to the diagnostic needs of the patient and interpret and report the result	
• Cranial nerves (facial, trigeminal, hypoglossal)		
• Temporomandibular joint		
• Facial skeleton		
• Lymph nodes		
• Salivary glands		
• Lips and oral mucous membranes		
• Teeth and periodontium		
Recognizing variations in normal oral facial structures and the presence of disease	Request specialist imaging techniques appropriate to the diagnostic needs of the patient and be able to interpret the report	
Using terminology to describe mucosal disease	Oral malodour and chemosensory disorders	
Venepuncture for haematological investigations	Understand the role of hypersensitivity testing	
Microbiological investigations for mucosal disease	Detrimental oral habits including substance abuse and misuse	
Diagnosis and treatment of common mucosal diseases	Understand the clinical pharmacology of drugs used in the practice of oral medicine	
Diagnosis of facial pain of dental and non-dental origin	The need for drug monitoring and associated special investigations	

Table 2.9.1 Intended learning outcomes for oral medicine – *continued*

Be competent at	Have knowledge of	Be familiar with
Incisional and excisional biopsy	Understand the role of psychological intervention in patient management	
	Understand the principles involved in the management of oral malignancy and potentially malignant lesions	

At graduation

The dentist should be competent at:

History taking (clinical, medical, social), recording of clinical signs and symptoms and presenting a comprehensive patient history.
See Chapter 1.1 History and examination in dentistry.

Undertaking a general examination of the clothed patient, in particular the orofacial tissues.
See Chapter 1.8 Human disease and therapeutics.

Performing a clinical examination
Including when indicated:

◆ Cranial nerves (trigeminal, facial, hypoglossal)

◆ Temporomandibular joints

◆ Facial skeleton

◆ Lymph nodes (see Chapter 1.8)

◆ Salivary glands

◆ Lips and oral mucous membranes

◆ Teeth and periodontium.

Recognizing variations in normal oral facial structures and the presence of disease
See Chapters 1.1 and 2.3.

Using terminology to describe mucosal disease
See Chapters 1.1, 1.8 and 2.8.

Venepuncture for haematological investigations
- Recognize situations where haematological investigations are indicated.
- Be able to perform and interpret the results of the following investigations:
  - Full blood count
  - Serum ferritin
  - Vitamin B_{12}
  - Folic acid
  - Venous plasma glucose
  - Liver enzyme levels
  - Antibody titres (Hepatitis B, herpes simplex).

Microbiological investigations for mucosal disease
- Recognize situations where microbiological investigations are indicated.
- Be able to perform and interpret the results of microbiological investigations (see **Checklist 1**).
  - Fungal infection; smear, swab, imprint culture and oral rinse
  - Bacterial investigation: smear, swab, imprint culture and oral rinse
  - Viral investigation: swab.

Incisional and excisional biopsy of mucosal lesions
See Chapter 1.10.
- Determine when a biopsy is indicated.
- Be able to select site and the appropriate technique
- Be able to perform a simple biopsy.

Diagnosis and treatment of common mucosal diseases
Localized lesions
- Recognize the features of common localized lesions of the mucosa (fibro-epithelial polyp, squamous cell papilloma, haemangioma, pyogenic granuloma, pregnancy epulis, amalgam tattoo, geographic tongue, fissured tongue, exostosis).
- Advise and provide treatment for common localized lesions of the mucosa.

Traumatic ulceration
- Recognize the features of traumatic ulceration.
- Advise and provide treatment for traumatic ulceration.

Recurrent aphthous stomatitis (recurrent oral ulceration)

♦ Recognize the clinical presentation of the three subtypes of recurrent aphthous stomatitis (minor, major and herpetiform).

♦ Appreciation of proposed major aetiological factors of oral ulceration.

♦ Select special haematological investigations (FBC, ferritin, folate, vitamin B_{12}) and local factors implicated in recurrent aphthous stomatitis.

♦ Knowledge of the treatment of recurrent oral ulceration.

♦ Be able to provide topical treatment (chlorhexidine, benzydamine) and steroid preparations (hydrocortisone, triamcinolone) for recurrent aphthous stomatitis.

Candidosis

♦ Recognize the clinical presentation of forms of oral candidosis (pseudomembranous, acute erythematous, chronic erythematous, chronic hyperplastic).

♦ Appreciation of proposed major local and systemic aetiological factors of oral candidosis.

♦ Select special microbiological investigations (smear, swab, imprint, oral rinse) for oral candidosis.

♦ Select special haematological investigations (FBC, ferritin, folate, vitamin B_{12}, glucose) and local factors implicated in oral candidosis.

♦ Be able to provide appropriate treatment for oral candidosis, including use of topical antifungals (amphotericin, nystatin and miconazole) and systemic agent (fluconazole).

Angular cheilitis

♦ Recognize the clinical presentation of angular cheilitis.

♦ Appreciation of proposed major local and systemic aetiological factors of angular cheilitis.

♦ Select special microbiological investigations (smear, swab, imprint, oral rinse) for angular cheilitis.

♦ Select special haematological investigations (FBC, ferritin, folate, vitamin B_{12}, glucose) and local factors implicated in angular cheilitis.

♦ Be able to provide appropriate treatment for angular cheilitis, including use of topical antimicrobials (amphotericin, nystatin, miconazole, and fucidic acid) and systemic agent (fluconazole).

Primary and secondary herpes simplex infection

♦ Recognize the clinical presentation of primary (gingivostomatitis) and secondary (herpes labialis, oral ulceration) of herpes simplex infection.

♦ Appreciation of the aetiological of herpes simplex infection of the orofacial tissues.

- Select special investigations (virus isolation, tissue culture and serology) in diagnosis of herpes simplex infections.
- Be able to provide treatment, including use of nucleoside analogue drugs (aciclovir and penciclovir) in the management of herpetic infections.
- Teaching in oral surgery and oral medicine should include clinical instruction in the prevention, diagnosis and management of potentially malignant and malignant lesions and conditions of the oral mucosa.

Potentially malignant lesions

- Define leukoplakia and erythroplakia.
- Recognize the clinical presentation of pre-cancerous lesions (leukoplakia, erythroplakia) and pre-malignant conditions (submucous fibrosis, lichen planus) of the oral mucosa.
- Appreciation of proposed major aetiological factors (tobacco and alcohol) associated with potentially malignant lesions.
- Determine the need for special investigations (biopsy) and urgency of referral for specialist opinion.
- Advise patients on factors (tobacco, alcohol) known to increase likelihood of trans-formation (1–5 per cent).
- Be able to provide long-term follow-up of such lesions.

Oral cancer

- Appreciation of the increasing incidence of oral cancer in the UK (overall 3,000 cases per year), in particular in younger females.
- Recognize the clinical presentation of oral cancer (colour change, ulceration and swelling).
- Appreciation of proposed major aetiological factors (tobacco and alcohol) associated with oral cancer.
- Determine the need for special investigations (biopsy) and urgency of referral for specialist opinion.
- Awareness of the surgical and radiotherapy aspects of treatment of oral cancer and five-year survival (approximately 50 per cent).
- Be able to participate in long-term follow-up of oral cancer.

Lichen planus

- Recognize the clinical presentation of types of oral lichen planus (reticular, papular, plaque, atrophic, and erosive, including desquamative gingivitis).
- Determine presence of local factor (amalgam restorations).
- Select special investigation (biopsy).
- Be able to provide treatment, including use of steroid therapy (topical).
- Be able to refer patient for further specialist management.

Diagnosis and treatment of common salivary gland diseases

- Recognize the clinical presentation of forms of salivary gland disease (xerostomia, mucocele, salivary stone, bacterial sialadenitis, mumps, increased salivation, sialosis, and salivary neoplasia).
- Awareness of the features of Sjögren's syndrome.
- Select special investigations to diagnose cause of salivary gland disease.
- Be able to provide treatment, including use of artificial saliva and salivary stimulants.
- Importance of preventitive dentistry and long term follow-up.

Oral manifestations of systemic diseases

- Recognize the orofacial lesions may be presenting symptoms of HIV infection (pseudomembraneous candidosis, hairy leukoplakia, Kaposi's sarcoma, ulcerative gingivitis, necrotizing periodontitis).
- Recognize forms of vesiculo-bullous disorders that affect the oral mucosa (mucous membrane pemphigoid, pemphigus, angina bullosa haemorrhagica).
- Recognize that angular cheilitis, oral ulceration, candidosis, pigmentary changes, bleeding, or mucosa hyperplasia may be the presenting features of inflammatory bowel disease, haematinic deficiency, diabetes, connective tissue disease, leukaemia or pregnancy.
- Recognize the possible involvement of psychological disorders in orofacial disease.
- Appreciation of the appropriate liaison with medical practitioner and specialist services.

Oral manifestations of hypersensitivity and adverse reactions

- Recognize the orofacial presentation of allergic reactions within the orofacial tissues (orofacial granulomatosis, erythema multiforme and lichenoid reactions).
- Recognize the orofacial presentation of adverse reactions to drug therapy (xerostomia, hyperplasia, candidosis).
- The various manifestations of facial pain of both dental and non-dental origin, its diagnosis and management must also be considered.

Diagnosing facial pain of dental and non-dental origin

- Be able to assess the symptoms of orofacial pain (nature, duration, severity).
- Diagnosis of common forms of orofacial pain of non-dental (tooth) origin (trigeminal neuralgia, burning mouth syndrome, atypical facial pain, and temporomandibular joint dysfunction syndrome).

Trigeminal neuralgia

- Recognition of the clinical signs and symptoms of trigeminal neuralgia (sharp shooting, severe unilateral pain).

- Be able to diagnose trigeminal neuralgia.
- Be able to prescribe carbamazepine in management of trigeminal neuralgia.

Burning mouth syndrome

- Application of clinical (burning, cancerphobia, home circumstances) scales.
- Ability to diagnose burning mouth syndrome.
- Knowledge of the treatment of burning mouth syndrome.
- Provide reassurance.
- Contribute to joint management with general medical practitioner.

Atypical facial pain

- Recognition of the clinical signs and symptoms of atypical facial pain (unilateral or bilateral constant localized pain).
- Be able to diagnose atypical facial pain.
- Have a knowledge of the aetiology of atypical facial pain.
- Provide reassurance.
- Contribute to joint management with general medical practitioner.

Temporomandibular joint pain

- Recognition of the clinical signs and symptoms of temporomandibular joint pain (unilateral or bilateral localized pain with radiation to surrounding sites and muscle tenderness).
- Be able to diagnose temporomandibular joint pain.
- Have a knowledge of the aetiology of temporomandibular joint dysfunction (lack of posterior teeth, parafunctional habits and stress).
- Be able to provide acrylic splint therapy for temporomandibular joint pain.

At graduation the dentist should have knowledge of:

Special investigations (haematological, histopathological, biochemical and Immunological, psychological) and their interpretation

Histopathology

- Understanding of the range of histopathological investigations used in the diagnosis and management of orofacial disease.
- Knowledge of the methodology of histopathological sample collection.
- Ability to interpret results of histopathological investigations.
- Formalin-fixed paraffin-processed material and frozen section.
- Incisional or excisional biopsy.

Haematology

- Understanding of the range of haematological investigations used in the diagnosis and management of orofacial disease.
- Knowledge of the methodology of haematological sample collection.
- Ability to interpret results of haematological investigations.
- Antibody titres.

Immunological

- Use of direct (tissue) and indirect (serum) immunofluorescence in laboratory diagnosis.

Psychological

- Use of HAD scale in detection of anxiety and depression.

Chair-side investigations including urinalysis, salivary flow rate and Schirmer tests

- Understand the usefulness of urinalysis for detection of diabetes.
- Describe the procedures of salivary flow estimation.
- Describe the procedure of Schirmer test for estimation of lacrimal gland flow rate.

The procedure of labial gland biopsy

- Describe the procedure of labial gland biopsy.

The role of clinical photography in patient management and the associated consent issues

- Understand the usefulness of photography for the monitoring of mucosal abnormalities.

Request appropriate radiographic examination relevant to the diagnostic needs of the patient and interpret and report the result

- Describe the procedure of sialography for detection of salivary gland disease.

Request specialist imaging techniques appropriate to the diagnostic needs of the patient and be able to interpret the report

- Understand the role of salivary scintiscanning in salivary gland disease.

Oral malodour and chemosensory disorders
The role of hypersensitivity testing

- Describe the procedure of patch testing for demonstration of hypesensitivity (Benzoates (E210 – E219), cinnamon, acrylic and amalgam. Use of RAST.

Detrimental oral habits including substance abuse and misuse

◆ Recognize the effects of substance abuse (tobacco, alcohol, betel, cocaine) on the orofacial tissues.

The clinical pharmacology of drugs used in the practice of oral medicine

◆ Have an understanding of the drugs listed for prescribing in dental practice within the *British National Formulary.*

The need for drug monitoring and associated special investigations

◆ Have an understanding of the need to monitor FBC and liver enzyme levels when prescribing carbamazepine.

The role of psychological intervention in patient management

◆ Recognize the role of psychological aspects of orofacial disease.

The principles involved in the management of oral malignancy and potentially malignant lesions

◆ Be able to stage an carcinoma based on the results of full assessment of the patient.

◆ Describe the adverse effects of radiotherapy to the head and neck.

Understanding of the aetiology and management of orofacial disease

◆ Awareness of yeasts, *Candida albicans* and non-albicans candidal species (*C. glabrata, C. krusei*) within the oral flora and factors that predispose to candidosis.

◆ Understanding of herpes simplex virus. Varicella zoster virus, Epstein–Barr virus, human herpes virus 8, human papilloma viruses, coxsackie group viruses.

◆ Importance of short- and long-term management of dysplastic lesions.

◆ Awareness of the surgical and radiotherapy aspects of treatment of oral cancer.

◆ Use of steroid therapy (topical or systemic) and role of other agents (azathioprine, and anxiolytics) in treatment of lichen planus.

◆ Understanding of the investigation and treatment of primary Sjögren's syndrome (dry eyes and dry mouth) and secondary Sjögren's syndrome (connective tissue disease).

◆ Understanding of the special investigations and treatment (systemic and topical steroid therapy and immulomodulating drugs) in vesicullo-bullous disease.

◆ Understanding of the use of systemic drug therapy (tricyclics, SSRI, antipsychotic agents) in psychological disease.

At graduation the dentist should be familiar with:

Disease whose management would benefit from referral to other medical, surgical and dental specialists

For generic principles of patient referral see Chapter 1.13.

The role of cryotherapy, laser and photodynamic therapy in the management of orofacial disease

References and further reading

GDC (2002) *The First Five Years: a framework for undergraduate dental education*, 2nd edn. London, The General Dental Council.

Lamey P.-J. and Lewis M. A. O. (1997) *A Clinical Guide to Oral Medicine*. London, British Dental Association.

Lewis M. A. O. and Jordan R. C. K. (2004) *A Colour Handbook of Oral Medicine*. London, Manson Publishing.

QAA (2002) *Dentistry: academic standards*. Subject benchmark statements. Gloucester, Quality Assurance Agency for Higher Education.

Scully C. (2004) *Oral and Maxillofacial Medicine*. London, Elsevier Science Limited.

Wray D., Lowe G. D. O., Dagg J. H., Felix D. H. and Scully C. (1999) *Textbook of General and Oral Medicine*. Edinburgh, Churchill Livingstone.

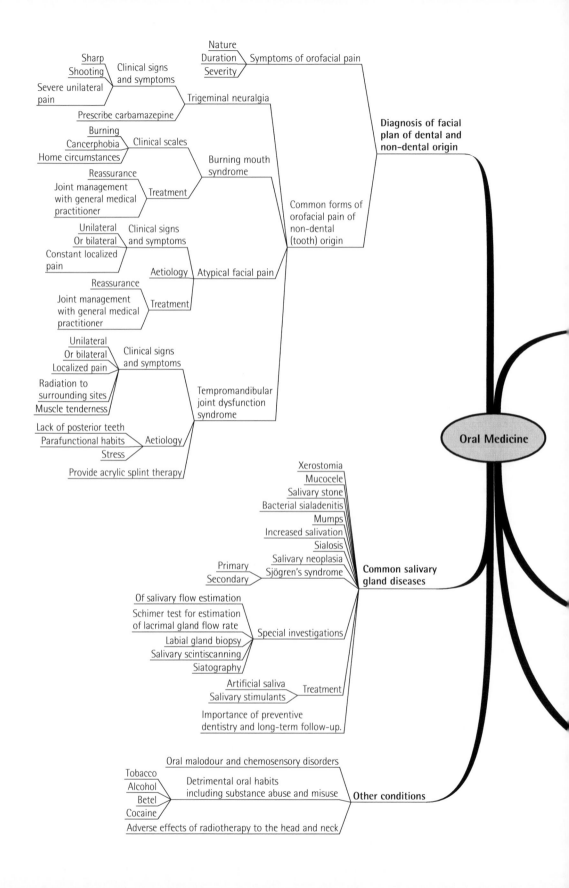

Oral Medicine

Diagnosis of facial plan of dental and non-dental origin

Symptoms of orofacial pain
- Nature
- Duration
- Severity

Common forms of orofacial pain of non-dental (tooth) origin

Trigeminal neuralgia
- Clinical signs and symptoms
  - Sharp
  - Shooting
  - Severe unilateral pain
- Prescribe carbamazepine

Burning mouth syndrome
- Clinical scales
  - Burning
  - Cancerphobia
  - Home circumstances
- Treatment
  - Reassurance
  - Joint management with general medical practitioner

Atypical facial pain
- Clinical signs and symptoms
  - Unilateral
  - Or bilateral
  - Constant localized pain
- Aetiology
- Treatment
  - Reassurance
  - Joint management with general medical practitioner

Tempromandibular joint dysfunction syndrome
- Clinical signs and symptoms
  - Unilateral
  - Or bilateral
  - Localized pain
  - Radiation to surrounding sites
  - Muscle tenderness
- Aetiology
  - Lack of posterior teeth
  - Parafunctional habits
  - Stress
- Provide acrylic splint therapy

Common salivary gland diseases
- Xerostomia
- Mucocele
- Salivary stone
- Bacterial sialadenitis
- Mumps
- Increased salivation
- Sialosis
- Salivary neoplasia
- Sjögren's syndrome
  - Primary
  - Secondary
- Special investigations
  - Of salivary flow estimation
  - Schimer test for estimation of lacrimal gland flow rate
  - Labial gland biopsy
  - Salivary scintiscanning
  - Siatography
- Treatment
  - Artificial saliva
  - Salivary stimulants
- Importance of preventive dentistry and long-term follow-up.

Other conditions
- Oral malodour and chemosensory disorders
- Detrimental oral habits including substance abuse and misuse
  - Tobacco
  - Alcohol
  - Betel
  - Cocaine
- Adverse effects of radiotherapy to the head and neck

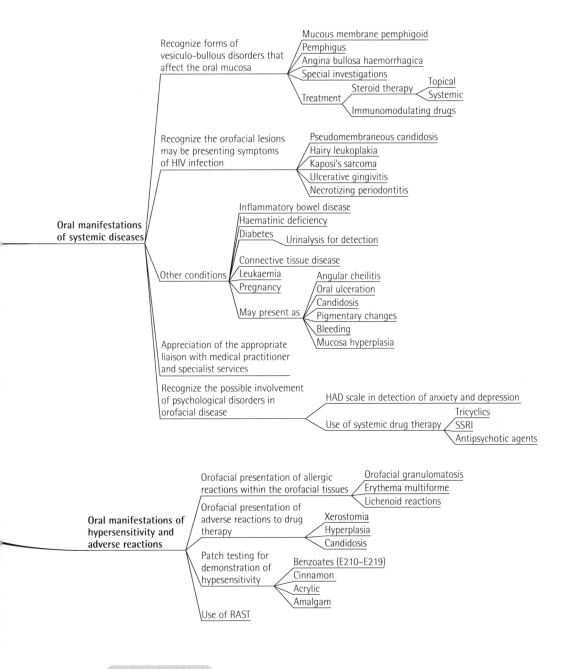

Oral manifestations of systemic diseases

Recognize forms of vesiculo-bullous disorders that affect the oral mucosa
- Mucous membrane pemphigoid
- Pemphigus
- Angina bullosa haemorrhagica
- Special investigations
- Treatment
  - Steroid therapy
    - Topical
    - Systemic
  - Immunomodulating drugs

Recognize the orofacial lesions may be presenting symptoms of HIV infection
- Pseudomembraneous candidosis
- Hairy leukoplakia
- Kaposi's sarcoma
- Ulcerative gingivitis
- Necrotizing periodontitis

Other conditions
- Inflammatory bowel disease
- Haematinic deficiency
- Diabetes
  - Urinalysis for detection
- Connective tissue disease
- Leukaemia
- Pregnancy
- May present as
  - Angular cheilitis
  - Oral ulceration
  - Candidosis
  - Pigmentary changes
  - Bleeding
  - Mucosa hyperplasia

Appreciation of the appropriate liaison with medical practitioner and specialist services

Recognize the possible involvement of psychological disorders in orofacial disease
- HAD scale in detection of anxiety and depression
- Use of systemic drug therapy
  - Tricyclics
  - SSRI
  - Antipsychotic agents

Oral manifestations of hypersensitivity and adverse reactions

Orofacial presentation of allergic reactions within the orofacial tissues
- Orofacial granulomatosis
- Erythema multiforme
- Lichenoid reactions

Orofacial presentation of adverse reactions to drug therapy
- Xerostomia
- Hyperplasia
- Candidosis

Patch testing for demonstration of hypesensitivity
- Benzoates (E210–E219)
- Cinnamon
- Acrylic
- Amalgam

Use of RAST

Mucosal diseases
see separate mind map

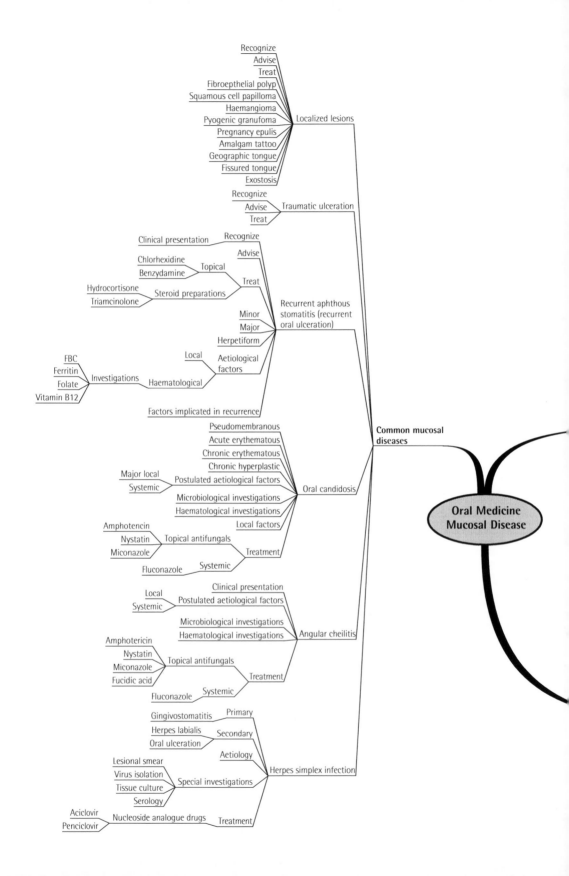

Recognize
Advise
Treat
Fibroepthelial polyp
Squamous cell papilloma
Haemangioma
Pyogenic granufoma
Pregnancy epulis
Amalgam tattoo
Geographic tongue
Fissured tongue
Exostosis

Localized lesions

Recognize
Advise
Treat

Traumatic ulceration

Clinical presentation
Recognize
Advise
Chlorhexidine
Benzydamine
Topical
Treat
Hydrocortisone
Triamcinolone
Steroid preparations
Minor
Major
Herpetiform

Recurrent aphthous
stomatitis (recurrent
oral ulceration)

FBC
Ferritin
Folate
Vitamin B12
Investigations
Local
Aetiological
factors
Haematological
Factors implicated in recurrence

Pseudomembranous
Acute erythematous
Chronic erythematous
Chronic hyperplastic
Major local
Systemic
Postulated aetiological factors
Microbiological investigations
Haematological investigations
Local factors

Oral candidosis

Amphotencin
Nystatin
Miconazole
Topical antifungals
Treatment
Fluconazole
Systemic

Local
Systemic
Clinical presentation
Postulated aetiological factors
Microbiological investigations
Haematological investigations

Angular cheilitis

Amphotericin
Nystatin
Miconazole
Fucidic acid
Topical antifungals
Treatment
Fluconazole
Systemic

Gingivostomatitis
Primary
Herpes labialis
Secondary
Oral ulceration
Aetiology
Lesional smear
Virus isolation
Tissue culture
Serology
Special investigations

Herpes simplex infection

Aciclovir
Penciclovir
Nucleoside analogue drugs
Treatment

Common mucosal
diseases

**Oral Medicine
Mucosal Disease**

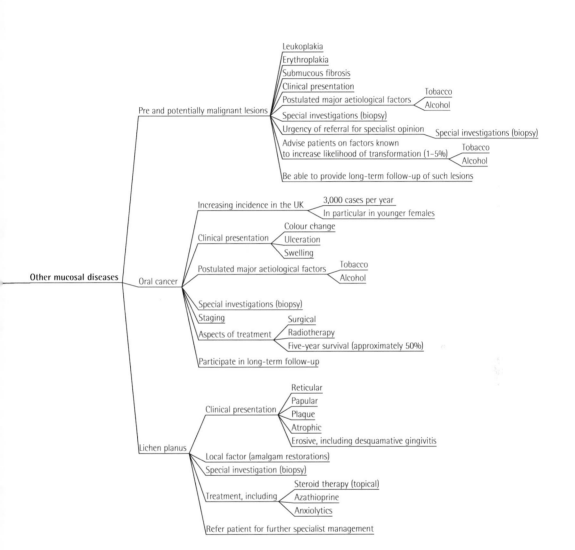

Other mucosal diseases

- Pre and potentially malignant lesions
  - Leukoplakia
  - Erythroplakia
  - Submucous fibrosis
  - Clinical presentation
  - Postulated major aetiological factors
    - Tobacco
    - Alcohol
  - Special investigations (biopsy)
  - Urgency of referral for specialist opinion — Special investigations (biopsy)
  - Advise patients on factors known to increase likelihood of transformation (1–5%)
    - Tobacco
    - Alcohol
  - Be able to provide long-term follow-up of such lesions

- Oral cancer
  - Increasing incidence in the UK
    - 3,000 cases per year
    - In particular in younger females
  - Clinical presentation
    - Colour change
    - Ulceration
    - Swelling
  - Postulated major aetiological factors
    - Tobacco
    - Alcohol
  - Special investigations (biopsy)
  - Staging
  - Aspects of treatment
    - Surgical
    - Radiotherapy
    - Five-year survival (approximately 50%)
  - Participate in long-term follow-up

- Lichen planus
  - Clinical presentation
    - Reticular
    - Papular
    - Plaque
    - Atrophic
    - Erosive, including desquamative gingivitis
  - Local factor (amalgam restorations)
  - Special investigation (biopsy)
  - Treatment, including
    - Steroid therapy (topical)
    - Azathioprine
    - Anxiolytics
  - Refer patient for further specialist management

Monitoring of mucosal abnormalities — Photographic

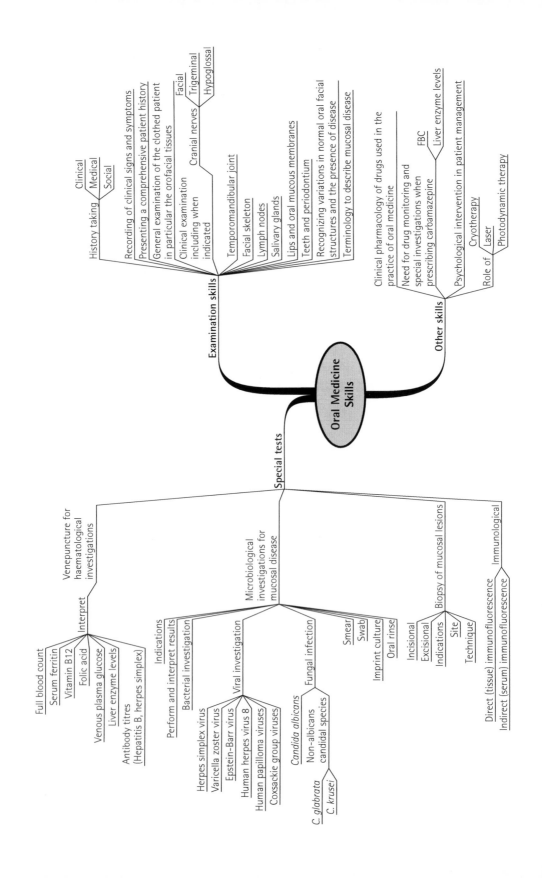

2.10 | Oral pathology
Edward Odell

Key points

+ The GDC, QAA, EU and national bodies all support the teaching of oral pathology with other clinical subjects in an integrated multidisciplinary course. Competences specific to oral pathology are therefore often difficult to identify.

+ Most of the learning objectives and competences defined for oral pathology are knowledge based rather than practical clinical competencies.

+ On qualification, students should know the classification, epidemiology, aetiology, genetics, molecular biology, microbiology, transmission, immunology, pathogenesis, macroscopic and microscopic structural changes, sequelae and complications of oral diseases and systemic diseases with oral or significant head and neck presentations, together with the links between these features and diagnosis, treatment and prognosis.

+ The competent student will be able to undertake the process of history taking, examination and differential diagnosis in a logical manner based on pathological knowledge, select and interpret relevant investigations, including performing an oral biopsy and submitting specimens appropriately.

+ The degree of competence required in diagnostic histopathology varies between UK dental schools.

Introduction

An understanding of oral disease underpins much of dentistry and it is therefore difficult to define the boundaries of the subject of oral pathology. Many competencies founded in pathological knowledge are to be found elsewhere in this book, particularly in sections on oral surgery, oral medicine, cariology and periodontology.

Competencies relating to oral pathology are given in the second edition of the General Dental Council's (GDC) *The First Five Years: a framework for undergraduate dental education* (GCD 2002) the Quality Assurance Agency's benchmark statement for dentistry (QAA 2000, 2002) and the European Union's Competences Required for the Practice of Dentistry in the European Union (European Union 1998). All three organizations actively promote the concept of interdisciplinary teaching and integrated courses. As a result competencies in oral pathology may be partly subsumed into problem-based learning, in courses including general pathology, medicine and surgery or in integrated courses in oral medicine, microbiology, pathology, surgery, radiology and therapeutics.

The GDC requirements for courses involving a significant oral pathology component are shown below:

Paragraph 92 (Main subject area oral surgery) The student should have an understanding of the range of surgical procedures which may be used to manage diseases and disorders of the mouth and jaws.

Paragraph 93 (Main subject area oral medicine) It is important to ensure that the dental student is taught the clinical presentation, diagnosis and management of the common diseases of the oral mucosa, of other oral soft tissues, of the salivary glands, of the facial bones and joints as well as the oral manifestations of systemic diseases. The various manifestations of facial pain of both dental and non-dental origin, its diagnosis and management must also be considered.

Paragraph 94 (Main subject area oral surgery and oral medicine) Teaching should include clinical instruction in the prevention, diagnosis and management of potentially malignant and malignant lesions and conditions of the oral mucosa.

Paragraph 95 (Main subject area oral pathology and oral microbiology) The course in oral pathology and oral microbiology should integrate with pathology and medical microbiology. Initially, the processes underlying the common oral diseases and methods of their diagnosis, prevention and management should be described. The teaching should continue through the clinical course and the full range of oral and dental diseases should be considered with particular attention being given to potentially malignant and malignant lesions and conditions of the oral mucosa.

The QAA Benchmark Statement on Dentistry (QAA 2000) also integrates oral pathology with other subjects and relevant benchmarking statements are within generic headings including history, examination and diagnosis. Relevant statements are:

Students should be able to integrate material from all parts of the undergraduate curriculum to demonstrate knowledge and understanding in a number of areas and topics including:

Paragraph 2.2 Integration of human body systems, normal homeostasis and mechanisms of responses to insults including trauma and disease

Paragraph 2.3 Oral biology, to include detailed knowledge of the form and function of teeth and associated structures, in health and disease

Paragraph 2.5 Human diseases and pathogenic processes, including genetic disorders, and the manifestation of those diseases which are particularly relevant to the practice of dentistry

Paragraph 2.6 Diseases and disorders of the oral cavity and associated structures, their causes and sequelae together with the principles of their prevention, diagnosis and management

Paragraph 2.7 Sources of infection and the means available for infection control

Paragraph 2.19 The broad principles of scientific research and evaluation of evidence that are necessary for an evidence-based approach to dentistry.

Further European directives govern undergraduate curriculum and competences (European Commission 1988; 1998). Dental undergraduates must participate in a course that covers the concepts of neoplasia, epidemiology, development and natural history of cancer, prevention, treatment and research, oral squamous carcinoma and premalignant lesions and conditions and other non-squamous malignancies (European Commission 1988). The related competencies are defined elsewhere and listed in detail in the chapters on oral surgery and oral medicine.

The GDC, QAA and EU learning outcomes are all minimum acceptable standards and most courses will exceed these minimum criteria and may set course-specific competencies. Many requirements in oral pathology are specified by knowledge and the limits of the expected knowledge remain undefined. Because none of the governing agencies have defined the knowledge base of the competent graduate, a national consensus minimum curriculum of oral pathology topics has been published by the British Society for Oral Pathology (Odell *et al.* 2004).

In order to meet the competencies defined by all these agencies, the student would be required to study pathological processes affecting:

♦ The jaws, teeth and periodontium

♦ Temporomandibular joint

♦ Sinuses and nasal cavity

♦ Oral, pharyngeal and lip mucosa

♦ Salivary glands

♦ Tonsils and lymph nodes of the head and neck

♦ Skin, soft tissues, nerves and vessels of the head and neck and the development of these tissues as relevant.

The list is not exhaustive and for systemic diseases, knowledge of the disease process at remote sites such as thyroid gland, kidney or heart will be essential.

Intended learning outcomes

Table 2.10.1 Intended learning outcomes and competencies for oral pathology

Be competent at	Have knowledge of	Be familiar with
Undertaking minor soft tissue surgery (including biopsy)	The role of laboratory investigations in diagnosis	The diagnosis of oral cancer and the principles of tumour management
Obtaining a detailed history of the patient's dental state (application of pathological knowledge)	The pathogenesis and classification of oral diseases	The pathogenesis of common oral medical disorders and their treatment
Obtaining a relevant medical history (application of pathological knowledge)	The aetiology and processes of oral diseases	
Using laboratory and imaging facilities appropriately and efficiently	Matters relating to infection control	
Arranging appropriate referrals (application of pathological knowledge)	The causes and effects of oral diseases needed: for their prevention, diagnosis and management	

The QAA Benchmark Statement on Dentistry also defines specific competencies. Relevant statements are:

Graduating dentists should have the ability to perform the following skills and possess the following attributes:

Paragraph 3.5: Describe and understand prevalence of oral diseases in the United Kingdom adult and child populations

Paragraph 3.6 Recognize predisposing and aetiological factors that require intervention to promote oral health

Paragraph 3.7 Apply their knowledge of the aetiology and processes of oral diseases in prevention, diagnosis and treatment

Paragraph 3.8 Obtain and record a relevant medical history which identifies as both the possible effects of oral disease on medical well-being and the medical conditions that affect oral health or dental treatment

Paragraph 3.8 Assess and appraise contemporary information on the significance and effect of drugs and other medicaments, taken by the patient, on their dental management

Paragraph 3.13 Assess patient risk for dental caries and non-bacterial tooth surface loss and be able to provide dietary counselling and nutritional education for the patient relevant to oral health and disease, based upon knowledge of disease patterns and aetiology

Paragraph 3.17 Understand the importance of and procedures for submitting specimens for laboratory diagnosis and demonstrate the ability to interpret diagnostic reports.

There is consensus in UK schools that students require the knowledge to classify diseases and lesions. They are expected know a synopsis for each disease entity or lesion that would include:

◆ Epidemiology

◆ Aetiology

◆ Genetics and molecular biology

◆ Microbiology

◆ Transmission

◆ Immunology and innate host defences

◆ Pathogenesis

◆ Structural changes at the macroscopic and microscopic levels

◆ Sequelae and complications.

The depth of knowledge required for each individual disease varies and is not defined. A greater amount and depth of knowledge is expected for diseases that are either common or carry significant health implications for patients, such as malignancy. Students should also study rarer diseases relevant to general professional training and hospital practice at SHO level because oral pathology is not formally required within vocational training or general professional training. A minimum curriculum list of diseases for the UK is published and most, if not all, schools aspire to exceed it (Odell *et al.* 2004).

The competent student would be able to use knowledge from pathology to meet the competencies of other clinical specialties. Specifically they should be able to identify the interrelationships between disease processes and use the knowledge in diagnosis, patient management and to predict prognosis. Knowledge of diseases and lesions should inform and focus history taking, examination and the process of differential diagnosis and provide an evidence base for the selection of investigations and their interpretation in all subjects. The graduate must be able to perform an oral biopsy, handle the specimen correctly, submit it for the tests required and interpret the result. They must also identify diseases and lesions for which biopsy is contraindicated and those for which biopsy in general dental practice is inappropriate.

There is inconsistency across the UK in the teaching of oral pathology with microscopes. Diagnostic histopathology is a postgraduate specialty and most teachers of oral pathology in the UK consider that detailed diagnostic histopathology is inappropriate for the undergraduate dental curriculum. However, understanding the microscopic appearances of disease is often helpful in gaining an appreciation of the relevance of the disease process to diagnosis, treatment or complications (Nash *et al.* 2001) and all UK schools and the GDC continue to require an understanding of the microscopic basis of disease, whether using microscopes, pictures or digital resources. Students need to seek local guidance on specific competences required for microscopy and these are likely to reflect those required in courses of basic sciences and general pathology. Use of a microscope should be considered a useful generic skill because microscopy is integral to several undergraduate subjects, many research areas and increasingly in clinical endodontics. Histology of oral tissues is considered core knowledge across Europe (DENTED).

Effective communication with patients, other dentists and health care workers is a key objective of the GDC. This requires competence in pathological terminology, classifications and spelling of technical terms including the names of diseases (Odell *et al.* 2004).

A series of competencies required of new graduates in the European Union (European Commission 1998) has recently been published by the EU Advisory Committee on the Training of Dental Practitioners. There is considerable variation in emphasis on pathology and clinical expectations of students from dental and stomatological schools across Europe. The following prerequisites for competences are listed:

> **Paragraph a** Having a sufficient understanding of the basic, biological, behavioural and medical sciences on which modern oral health care and maintenance of health is based.
>
> **Paragraph e** Knowledge of the aetiology, principles of the molecular biological processes, pathogenesis, demographic features, prevention and treatment of oral and dental diseases.

Specific competencies in disease recognition and diagnosis are listed in sections 1.1–1.7. The competencies are broadly based, define only a minimum standard and specifically are not intended to reflect 'the full range of competence required by a modern dentist'. The GDC and QAA requirements exceed and encompass these newer EU requirements.

Underpinning knowledge

The learning outcomes outlined in this chapter build on those of other subject areas including human disease and therapeutics (Chapter 1.8 this volume) and also some excluded from this book, notably physiology, anatomy, pharmacology and general pathology including immunology, microbiology and virology. A document listing core knowledge and understanding in these areas has been published by DENTED, the Thematic Network Project Achieving Convergence in Standards of Output of European Dental Education (DENTED), though these recommendations have no formal status.

References and further reading

Commission of the European Communities (1998) *Advisory Committee on the Training of Dental Practitioners. Report and recommendations concerning clinical competences required for the practice of dentistry in the European Union*. Document XV/E/8316/8/93. Brussels, European Commission.

Commission of the European Communities (1988) *A curriculum in oncology for dental students in Europe*. Commission of the European Communities V-241/91/9EC Report from the European Workshop on Dental Education in Oncology and Prevention of Cancer, Copenhagen, 1990 and Advisory Committee on the Training of Dental Practitioners 1988 III/D/886/3/88-EN.

DENTED document: core knowledge and understanding. Available at: http://www.dented.org/parse.php3?file=content/knowledge.html

GDC (2002) *The First Five Years. A framework for undergraduate education*, 2nd edn. London, General Dental Council. Also available at http://www.gdc-uk.org/pdfs/first_five_years_2002.pdf

Nash J. R. G., West K. P. and Foster C. S. (2001) The teaching of anatomic pathology in England and Wales: A transatlantic view. *Human Pathology* 32, 1154–6.

Odell E. W., Farthing P. M., High A., Potts J., Soames J., Thakker N., Toner M. and Williams H. K. (2004) British Society for Oral and Maxillofacial Pathology UK Minimum Curriculum in Oral Pathology. *Eur J Dent Education* 8, 177–84.

QAA (2000) *Subject overview report on dentistry*. Gloucester, Quality Assurance Agency. Also available at http://www.qaa.ac.uk/revreps/subj_level/qo6_00.pdf

QAA (2002) *Academic Standards – dentistry* Subject benchmark statements. Gloucester, Quality Assurance Agency 2002. Also available at http://www.qaa.ac.uk/crntwork/benchmark/phase2/Dentistry.pdf

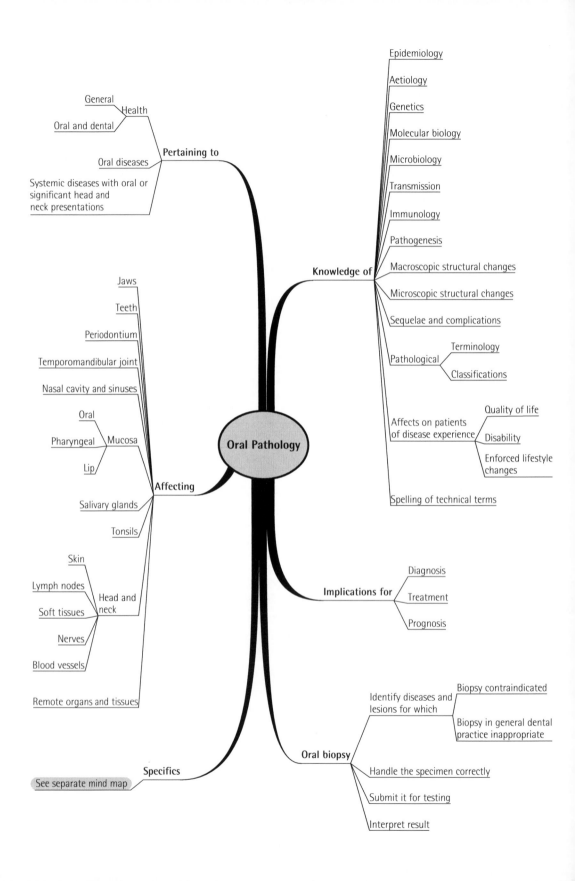

Oral Pathology

Pertaining to
- Health
  - General
  - Oral and dental
- Oral diseases
- Systemic diseases with oral or significant head and neck presentations

Knowledge of
- Epidemiology
- Aetiology
- Genetics
- Molecular biology
- Microbiology
- Transmission
- Immunology
- Pathogenesis
- Macroscopic structural changes
- Microscopic structural changes
- Sequelae and complications
- Pathological
  - Terminology
  - Classifications
- Affects on patients of disease experience
  - Quality of life
  - Disability
  - Enforced lifestyle changes
- Spelling of technical terms

Affecting
- Jaws
- Teeth
- Periodontium
- Temporomandibular joint
- Nasal cavity and sinuses
- Mucosa
  - Oral
  - Pharyngeal
  - Lip
- Salivary glands
- Tonsils
- Head and neck
  - Skin
  - Lymph nodes
  - Soft tissues
  - Nerves
  - Blood vessels
- Remote organs and tissues

Implications for
- Diagnosis
- Treatment
- Prognosis

Oral biopsy
- Identify diseases and lesions for which
  - Biopsy contraindicated
  - Biopsy in general dental practice inappropriate
- Handle the specimen correctly
- Submit it for testing
- Interpret result

Specifics
- See separate mind map

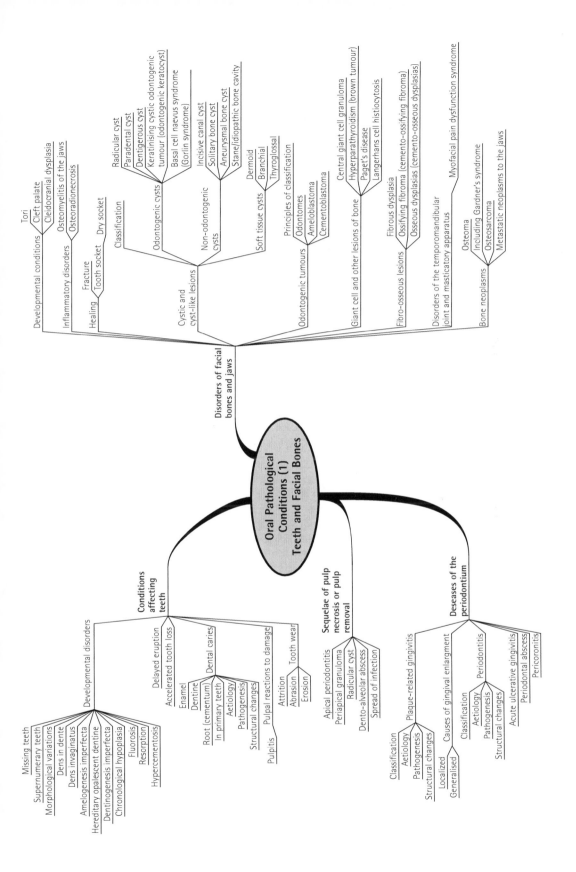

Oral Pathological Conditions (1) Teeth and Facial Bones

Conditions affecting teeth

Developmental disorders
- Missing teeth
- Supernumerary teeth
- Morphological variations
- Dens in dente
- Dens invaginatus
- Amelogenesis imperfecta
- Hereditary opalescent dentine
- Dentinogenesis imperfecta
- Chronological hypoplasia
- Fluorosis
- Resorption
- Hypercementosis

Delayed eruption
Accelerated tooth loss

Dental caries
- Enamel
- Dentine
- Root (cementum)
- In primary teeth
- Aetiology
- Pathogenesis
- Structural changes

Pulpal reactions to damage
- Pulpitis

Tooth wear
- Attrition
- Abrasion
- Erosion

Sequelae of pulp necrosis or pulp removal
- Apical periodontitis
- Periapical granuloma
- Radicular cyst
- Dento-alveolar abscess
- Spread of infection

Deseases of the periodontium

Plaque-related gingivitis
- Classification
- Aetiology
- Pathogenesis
- Structural changes

Causes of gingival enlargment
- Localized
- Generalised

Periodontitis
- Classification
- Aetiology
- Pathogenesis
- Structural changes
- Acute ulcerative gingivitis
- Periodontal abscess
- Pericoronitis

Disorders of facial bones and jaws

Developmental conditions
- Tori
- Cleft palate
- Cleidocranial dysplasia

Inflammatory disorders
- Osteomyelitis of the jaws
- Osteoradionecrosis

Healing
- Fracture
- Tooth socket
- Dry socket

Cystic and cyst-like lesions
- Classification

Odontogenic cysts
- Radicular cyst
- Paradental cyst
- Dentigerous cyst
- Keratinising cystic odontogenic tumour (odontogenic keratocyst)
- Basal cell naevus syndrome (Gorlin syndrome)

Non-odontogenic cysts
- Incisive canal cyst
- Solitary bone cyst
- Aneurysmal bone cyst
- Stane/idiopathic bone cavity

Soft tissue cysts
- Dermoid
- Branchial
- Thyroglossal

Odontogenic tumours
- Principles of classification
- Odontomes
- Ameloblastoma
- Cementoblastoma

Giant cell and other lesions of bone
- Central giant cell granuloma
- Hyperparathyroidism (brown tumour)
- Paget's disease
- Langerhans cell histiocytosis

Fibro-osseous lesions
- Fibrous dysplasia
- Ossifying fibroma (cemento-ossifying fibroma)
- Osseous dysplasias (cemento-osseous dysplasias)

Disorders of the temporomandibular joint and masticatory apparatus
- Myofacial pain dysfunction syndrome

Bone neoplasms
- Osteoma
- Including Gardner's syndrome
- Osteosarcoma
- Metastatic neoplasms to the jaws

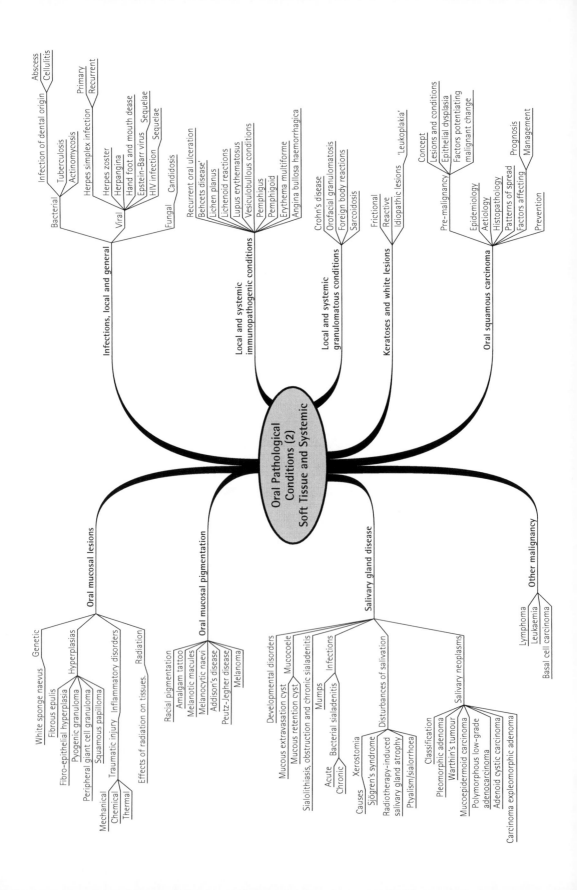

Oral Pathological Conditions (2)
Soft Tissue and Systemic

Infections, local and general

Bacterial
- Infection of dental origin — Abscess, Cellulitis
- Tuberculosis
- Actinomycosis

Viral
- Herpes simplex infection — Primary, Recurrent
- Herpes zoster
- Herpangina
- Hand foot and mouth dease
- Epstein–Barr virus — Sequelae
- HIV infection — Sequelae

Fungal — Candidosis

Local and systemic immunopathogenic conditions

- Recurrent oral ulceration
- Behcets disease'
- Lichen planus
- Lichenoid reactions
- Lupus erythematosus
- Vesiculobullous conditions
- Pemphigus
- Pemphigoid
- Erythema multiforme
- Angina bullosa haemorrhagica

Local and systemic granulomatous conditions

- Crohn's disease
- Orofacial granulomatosis
- Foreign body reactions
- Sarcoidosis

Keratoses and white lesions

- Frictional
- Reactive
- Idiopathic lesions 'Leukoplakia'
- Concept
- Lesions and conditions
- Epithelial dysplasia
- Factors potentiating malignant change

Oral squamous carcinoma

- Pre-malignancy
- Epidemiology
- Aetiology
- Histopathology
- Patterns of spread
- Factors affecting — Prognosis, Management
- Prevention

Oral mucosal lesions

- White sponge naevus — Genetic
- Fibrous epulis
- Fibro-epithelial hyperplasia
- Pyogenic granuloma
- Peripheral giant cell granuloma — Hyperplasias
- Squamous papilloma
- Traumatic injury — Inflammatory disorders
  - Mechanical
  - Chemical
  - Thermal
- Effects of radiation on tissues. — Radiation

Oral mucosal pigmentation

- Racial pigmentation
- Amalgam tattoo
- Melanotic macules
- Melanocytic naevi
- Addison's disease
- Peutz–Jeher disease
- Melanoma

Salivary gland disease

- Developmental disorders
- Mucous extravasation cyst — Mucocoele
- Mucous retention cyst
- Mumps — Infections
- Bacterial sialadenitis
- Sialolithiasis, obstruction and chronic sialadenitis
  - Acute
  - Chronic
- Xerostomia
- Sjögren's syndrome — Disturbances of salivation
- Radiotherapy-induced salivary gland atrophy
- Ptyalism/sialorrhoea
- Classification
- Pleomorphic adenoma
- Warthin's tumour
- Mucoepidermoid carcinoma — Salivary neoplasms
- Polymorphious low-grade adenocarcinoma
- Adenoid cystic carcinoma
- Carcinoma expleomorphic adenoma
- Causes

Other malignancy

- Lymphoma
- Leukaemia
- Basal cell carcinoma

3.1 Key skills in integrated dental care

Gareth Holsgrove, David Stirrups, Peter Mossey and Elizabeth Davenport

Introduction

Key skills are the skills that are commonly needed for success in a range of activities in education and training, work and life in general. They are the generic, transferable skills which all students develop during the course of their academic studies. Other skills, not covered elsewhere in this book, are also needed for successful clinical practice and will be discussed towards the end of this chapter.

Generic key skills can be contemplated under the following headings:

- Application of numbers
- Improving one's own learning and performance
- Information technology
- Problem-solving
- Communication
- Working with others.

Communication skills and team working are covered elsewhere in this book.

In the GDC's *The First Five Years* they state that undergraduate dental education should:

> **Paragraph 17** Promote acquisition of the skills and professional attitudes and behaviour that facilitate effective and appropriate interaction with patients and colleagues; foster the knowledge, skills and attitudes that will promote effective lifelong learning and support professional development.

and

> **Paragraph 19** Acquire a wide range of skills, including research, investigative, analytical, problem-solving, planning, communication, presentation and team skills; use contemporary methods of electronic communication and information management.

They suggest that the dental graduate needs the following attributes.

> **Paragraph 20** Approaches to teaching and learning that are based on curiosity and exploration of knowledge rather than its passive acquisition; a desire for intellectual rigour, ...an awareness of personal limitations, a willingness to seek help as necessary, and an ability to work effectively as a member of a team; respect for patients and colleagues that encompasses, without prejudice, diversity of background and opportunity, language and culture.

In relation to information technology they advise:

> **Paragraph 31** The university will also provide library facilities and information technology resources. These should be sufficient to enable all dental students to undertake guided self-learning. Formal instruction should be given in the use of personal learning techniques, such as computer-assisted learning, with emphasis on the developing area of health informatics.

Further advice on expectations on information technology is given in paragraph 70.

> Progress in information technology and particularly health informatics will continue to accelerate and become an important and integral part of dental practice. These technologies provide access to clinical and educational information in a wide variety of formats. Ideally students should enter the dental school equipped with sufficient skills to be able to use these from the start of the programme. During their clinical years they should develop an understanding of the advantages and limitations of electronic sources of health information, the electronic patient record, electronic decision support systems and teledentistry. They should have an opportunity to use information and communication technologies for research, healthcare provision and health promotion. They must become aware of the law as it relates to data protection and patient confidentiality.

On graduation dental students are expected to:

> Be familiar with the need for lifelong learning and professional development;
> Be competent at using information technology;
> Be familiar with the mechanisms of knowledge acquisition, scientific method and evaluation of evidence.

Team-working and communication skills are covered elsewhere in this book: the key skills covered in this chapter are:

- Application of numbers and information technology
- Improving one's own learning and performance

- Personal and professional development
- Problem-solving.

Application of numbers and information technology

Most dentists work in general dental practice: these are small businesses and basic numeracy skills are essential to running the financial aspects. More advanced numeracy is required to evaluate the scientific advances that will be made in dentistry during the practising lifetime of a dentist. The dentist is bombarded with product promotion literature and without an understanding of the simpler statistical methodologies and methods of data presentation is liable to make costly mistakes by buying misleadingly promoted, under-evaluated materials and equipment. There is a link from numeracy to IT skills in that spreadsheets are now the usual way of managing business finances, for profit and loss projections and providing information for business planning. Numeracy skills use are required to make successful spreadsheets.

During dental education, practical experimental projects provide a vehicle for enhancing numerical skills. With the use of spreadsheets and computer presentation packages IT skills can also be developed. The level of attainment in information technology that is expected of the dental graduate is that of the European Computer Driving Licence. The syllabus for that qualification covers all the aspects of information technology (IT) required of a graduating dental student. These are:

- Basic concepts of IT
- Using the computer and managing files
- Word processing
- Spreadsheets
- Database
- Presentation
- Information and communication.

Personal and professional development

Improving own learning and performance

The writing style of the following is to address directly the reader in dealing with a number of key concepts.

Finding information

- Electronic databases. You need to know how to access computer-based bibliographic databases and how to search them for references, such as by using keywords, truncation, Boolean and field searching.
- Library search skills are the steps which should be taken to ensure finding all relevant information for a project or essay. You need to be able to put together a search strategy by defining terms, identifying keywords, generating broader and narrower terms, finding synonyms and related terms.
- Survey, Question, Read, Recall, Review.

Taking and making notes

This is an important skill to develop in doing your research for essays and other assignments. Good note-taking will help you decide on appropriate information to include in your projects, as well as helping you to get the most from lectures and seminars. Good referencing is also vital.

Managing your reading

There may be extensive information available on the subject you have been asked to cover for an assignment. It will often take time to go through this information and prioritize the relevant pieces. Try to ensure that you allocate enough time to do this properly.

Deciding what to read

You can get a good overview of how useful a text might be by using some of the following tactics:

♦ Looking for abstracts and summaries in journal articles

♦ Checking the date of publication – is the information still relevant?

♦ Scanning the contents page

♦ Scanning the index pages

♦ Looking for a 'Foreword' or 'Preface' introducing the content

♦ Reading the first and last paragraphs of chapters.

It is useful to keep asking yourself what you want to find out from a source – this helps you to avoid getting lost in interesting but irrelevant information. You should already have specific questions in mind for your reading to answer.

Having chosen your sources, you can begin to read through them. You can narrow the text down to relevant sections by using differing reading strategies:

♦ Skimming – reading for the general thrust of a passage or chapter

♦ Scanning – reading quickly to find specific information

♦ Search reading – scanning with attention to the meaning of specific items

♦ Reading in depth – reading the text fully and taking appropriate notes.

Try not to start noting everything indiscriminately – pick out the relevant points for your notes. If you are going to quote from a source, make sure you have taken down the quotation accurately.

As you read and make notes, reflect on what you have read. Decide on the most appropriate information. Reflect on other information which might relate closely to what you're studying. One way of recalling, and later reviewing, what you have read is by using notes.

Referencing is nearly always required in assignments, usually, you need to know the name of the book, journal or other source you are referring to, the author(s) or editor(s), and place and date of publication. Record the reference information down before you begin to make any notes. Note down the page numbers you refer to in your notes – always do this when quoting directly from a source.

Summarizing and *paraphrasing* information are important skills which will help you in making notes from other sources. Summarizing a piece of text means cutting it to about one third of its original length, and using your own words – paraphrasing – where possible.

If you find it difficult to cut large chunks of information down to size, these suggestions might help:

+ Photocopy what you're reading and number the main points in each paragraph

+ Write down the key words from these points to build up your summary or write a short sentence to convey the meaning of each of your numbered points.

+ Remove descriptive words to reduce your points to the bare essentials

+ If the summary is for your own use only, try using bullet points or diagrams showing how the points interrelate.

Critical thinking

This involves considering issues from a range of perspectives and draw upon appropriate concepts and values in arriving at a critical assessment. It includes reasoning, problem-solving, analysis, synthesis, and evaluation. The skills or tasks involved in may include:

+ Developing a logical argument;

+ Identifying the flaws or weaknesses in an argument;

+ Making relevant connections or links across disciplines, or from theory to practice;

+ Analysing the material in a range of sources and synthesizing it;

+ Applying theory to particular cases.

Critical thinking skills help you decide what to believe about an issue, how to defend what you believe, and how to evaluate the beliefs of others. The skills used include:

+ Being as clear as possible

+ Focusing on a question or issue

+ Taking into account the whole problem

+ Considering all relevant alternatives

+ Being as precise as possible

+ Being aware of your biases and assumptions

+ Being open-minded

+ Withholding judgement until you have sufficient information

+ Reasoning logically

+ Defining clearly and reasonably

- Concise presentation
- Stating and defending assumptions
- Being well informed
- Using identified and credible sources
- Using reasonable generalizations
- Using sound hypotheses and predictions
- Examining alternative views
- Being fair and open-minded
- Being convincing.

Active learning and reflection

This is a willingness to take an active role in learning and recognizing the responsibility for life-long learning. Key skills in active learning are review and reflection.

The processes of review and reflection are important. Reflection combines ideas of reviewing, thinking, rehearsing, reworking and so on, but reflection is not an end in itself. The outcomes of structured reflection might include a new way of doing things, the development of a new skill, the resolution of a problem or the consolidation of effective learning – recognizing that you have done something really well and resolving to do it like that in the future. The reflective process consists of:

- **Thinking about what you have done:** This involves thinking back over an activity. What you did and how well you did it. It also involves looking at the outcome as critically/objectively as possible; considering any feedback that you received; recognizing your achievements and giving yourself a pat on the back when you deserve it!

- **Identifying your learning:** This involves looking beyond the concrete product of the task and thinking about the less tangible outcomes. What additional skills have you acquired? What have you learnt about yourself and what sorts of strategies worked or didn't work well for you?

- **Thinking about your next task:** Once you are aware of what you have done, how you have done it and how well you have done it, you are in a good position to adapt what you have learnt to help tackle the next task.

In other words, generalize from your learning experience by identifying the general principles and applying them to new situations. Becoming more aware of the process of learning and the skills you have used makes it more likely that you can build on your knowledge and skills in tackling different but related tasks. It builds problem-solving skills that enable development of strategies for overcoming obstacles in pursuing an objective. It enables you to evaluate your own strengths, values, weaknesses, progress and future learning objectives.

Time management and self-discipline

This involves prioritizing, as there is usually not sufficient time to achieve all your goals in a particular time frame. If this is the case, it is vital that you prioritize your goals. It is not the quantity of what you do, but the quality and value of it that is important.

Aids to achieving this can be as simple as:

◆ Planning everything out on a big piece of paper and tick off items as they are completed

◆ Prioritizing using the following system:

◆ Have three trays and a waste bin. Allocate one tray for each of 1, 2, 3 above and throw category 4 into the bin

1. Urgent and important	Do it now
2. Urgent and **not** important	Do it if you can
3. Important but not urgent	Start it before it becomes urgent
4. Not important and not urgent	Don't do it

◆ Make out a list with the most important things first

◆ Identify which are your strongest and which are your weakest subjects. Should you allocate equal time to each, or more to the weaker one? Possible dangers include avoiding giving time to topics you dislike or feel weak at, or spending so much time on them you neglect areas you are good at

◆ Is the time you are spending on something equal to its importance?

◆ Build in breaks – a coffee, a walk around the block, watching the news

◆ Reward yourself with a treat when you have achieved a target (or part of a target)

◆ Allow for unforeseen circumstances, e.g. a long queue at the library etc., and build in leeway

◆ Make quick decisions about what action to take. Repeatedly picking up the same piece of paper wastes time.

◆ Minimize timewasters. Timewasters may be self-inflicted or arise from external sources:

Examples of self-inflicted time wasters	**Example of external time wasters**
Procrastination	
Perfectionism	Intrusions (i.e. visitors, or phone calls)
Lack of self-discipline	Television
Worrying	Travelling
Personal disorganization	Waiting

Examples of self-inflicted time wasters	Example of external time wasters
Lack of priorities	Idle conversations
Over-commitment (inability to say 'No')	Crises
Indecisiveness	Not being able to contact people
Socializing	

General study skills: online resources

John Ramsay's website (University of Staffordshire)
http://www.staffs.ac.uk/schools/business/bsadmin/staff/s3/jamr.htm
Key Skills (Canterbury Christchurch University College)
http://keyskills.cant.ac.uk/
Study Skills Online (Brunel University)
http://www.brunel.ac.uk/%7Emastmmg/ssguide/sshome.htm
Study Skills Self-Help Information (Virginia Polytechnic and State University, USA)
http://www.ucc.vt.edu/stdysk/stdyhlp.html
Study Skills Tipsheets (University of Wolverhampton)
http://www.wlv.ac.uk/lib/systems/gt-tips.htm

Problem–solving

1. Identify the issues, especially time constraints.

2. Gather available information. There is rarely all the information you would like to have: decide whether any additional information is essential and whether and how it can be obtained and if it can be obtained in time.

3. Decide whether a solution is needed. Do not put off those problems which have to be addressed but also do not waste time on trying to solve those problems for which time may provide more information or alter the constraints and where the solution cannot be yet implemented.

4. Break the problem down into small components.

5. Identify the order in which they need to be solved: this may not be linear and some aspects may need to be addressed in parallel.

6. Identify the feasible options for each sub-problem.

7. Identify the effect of each option on the chain of component sub-problems to identify the best available solution. Some parts of the solution chain may be closed off or opened up by the effect of earlier actions.

8. Check this solution and identify critical aspects. Where resources are limited (time, financial, people etc.) target resources at the critical aspects.

9. Accept that partial or suboptimal solutions may need to be considered where information or resources are lacking.

10. Be prepared to revise the solution in the light of new information or unexpected events.

Other skills

Practice management

Successful clinical practice depends on managing the business of dentistry as well as the delivery of high standard clinical care. The business of dentistry is affected by the socio-economic arrangements under which it is provided. It may be state funded, part state funded, insurance based, or patient funded or a mix of those options. Within the United Kingdom these arrangements are in a state of flux with differing arrangements developing in England and Wales, Scotland and Northern Ireland. A textbook would be well out of date before it was published if it attempted, at this time of uncertainty, to define key skills in relation to practice management. Any such definitions would be so country-specific as to be valueless. All dental schools should have practice management modules that are relevant and contemporaneous for the circumstances in which their graduates will predominately practice. Information is available from the professional associations such as the British Dental Association and in the dental press. Students are advised to keep themselves informed of developments in this rapidly changing situation.

However, in any sphere of clinical practice the standards of care provided are dependent on all members of the dental team taking responsibility for ensuring this is as high as is achievable. This is delivered through the process of clinical governance.

Clinical governance

This is the term used for the concept that anyone working in a health service delivery is accountable for continuously improving the quality of their services and safeguarding high standards of care by creating an environment in which excellence in clinical care will flourish. This involves sharing ideas on good practice and practice improvement within and between health care teams. For dentistry this includes all the dental team members, and is the rationale for defining responsibilities and accountability. It is delivered through targeted staff training, development of local and other care guidelines and work protocols, monitoring their use and ensuring they are up to date, relevant and being used appropriately. Monitoring is usually achieved through reports to team meetings. The information that underpins and provides the evidence base for these reports is clinical audit.

Clinical audit

This is described as a cycle:

1. A standard is defined for an aspect of care,

2. Performance of the dental team is measured against that standard,

3. Deficiencies, or otherwise, are identified

4. A programme of changes instituted in order to raise the standard of deliver of that aspect of care

5. Performance is re-measured to check that the desired improvements were achieved.

The cycle of steps two to five is repeated, as necessary, until the desired standard is reached. At this stage the standard can be raised or a monitoring process instituted to ensure that the standard is maintained.

All dental staff are expected to be involved in clinical governance and audit and an understanding of the processes involved is essential for the new graduate. On registration with the General Dental Council, periodic information and updates will be forwarded automatically, and these will provide important information with respect to regulation, clinical governance and professional responsibilities. This information, contained in the GDC guidance document 'Standards for Dental Professionals' came into effect on 1 June 2005, and may also be obtained on the GDC website (available at http://www.gdc-uk.org/News+publications+and+events/).

Checklist 53 **For a written assignment**

Clear?	Could what is written be interpreted in more than one way?
Accurate?	Are statements factually correct?
Precise?	Is there sufficient detail to be meaningful?
Relevant?	Does all the content relate to the question being answered?
Breadth?	Have you answered the question too narrowly or have you included peripheral information with too little relevance to the topic?
Depth?	Is the writing superficially addressing the subject or is there too much minutiae?
Logical?	Does the linkage between ideas build consistently to the points you wish to make?
Ownership?	Is this your own work?

Checklist 54 **Self-management checklist**

Specify a clear cut goal you want to accomplish	Be very specific
Specify when you will do it	Today, weekly etc.
Record your hit rate	Keep a record of your successes and your failures
Make a public commitment	Tell someone what your goals and your deadline are. Ask them to monitor you
Add an explicit penalty for failure, if you need to	Keep the penalty small, otherwise you are liable to fib a bit
Think small	Don't try to make up for your past in a single day
Specify the amount of product you are going to produce	If simply specifying the amount of time you are going to log in doesn't do the trick, specify the number of pages you're going to read etc.
Get a timer that beeps every five minutes and chart whether you are on task, if you find yourself drifting off too much	This is especially good when you might have trouble measuring the amount of the product
Arrange for regular contact with your monitor, daily or weekly as needed	It helps to put your self-management project on the agenda with someone you meet with regularly
Get rid of distractions	Try to do your work when and where no one can bother you
Recycle	Self-management may not work the first time you try it and will certainly occasionally fail

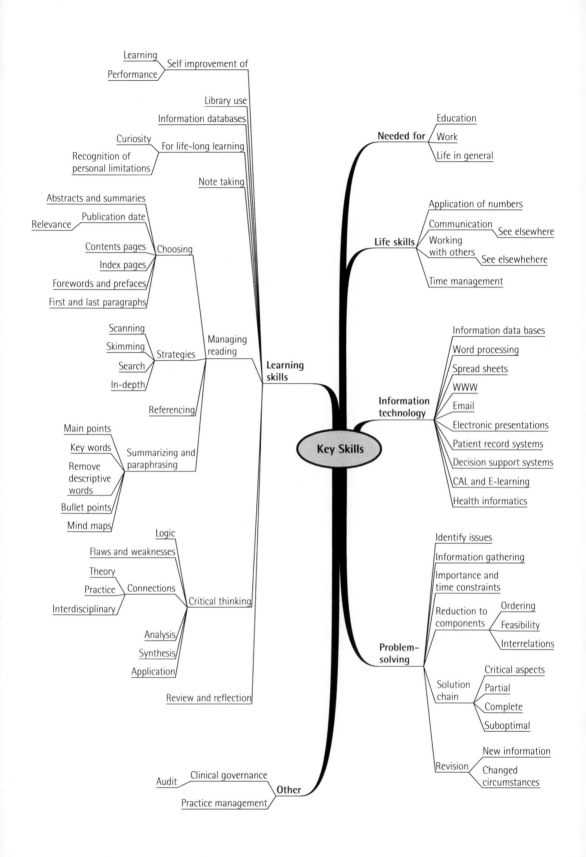

3.2 Assessment

Gareth Holsgrove, Peter Mossey, Elizabeth Davenport and David Stirrups

Key points

- In setting out the requirements of assessment, both the General Dental Council in *The First Five Years* (2002) and the Quality Assurance Agency (QAA) Benchmarking Statement for Dentistry (2002) independently produced their recommendations. Combining both sources enables consensus on the aims and objectives of assessments that should be adopted in dental schools.

- Assessment should enable students to demonstrate their understanding, level of attainment and to demonstrate a full range of clinical and other abilities.

- Methods of assessment should encourage integration of knowledge, understanding, clinical and communication skills and attitudes, and should encourage reflection and self-assessment.

- Assessment should be appropriately documented and should not only reflect student progression through the programme, but also lead to accurate, constructive feedback to students on their performance.

- Assessment should provide information for programme organizers on the quality of provision, allow the participation of external examiners, and engage in mechanisms of quality assurance.

- Ultimately assessment should reliably indicate whether a student has reached an appropriate standard.

Introduction

The first two sections of this book describe competencies that the student can be expected to achieve at graduation. This chapter on assessment describes the qualities that the assessments themselves must have and how assessment can assist with the delivery of the intended learning outcomes. Assessment is an issue that is relevant to course organizers, examiners and students, and this chapter aims to:

1. Identify the purposes of assessment;

2. Outline some basic principles of effective assessment;

3. Describe some of the more commonly used assessment methods;

4. Describe the concept of and methods of standard-setting;

5. Contribute to a quality assurance process for assessments.

Throughout this chapter, the educational principles that form the foundations of good assessment will be elaborated on with students, course organizers, and examiners in mind.

Teaching, learning and assessment

The following section reproduces the information and guidance provided by GDC's *The First Five Years* (2002) and QAA Benchmarking (2002) in the context of undergraduate dental education.

Section 4 of the QAA Benchmarking on Teaching and learning states that:

Teaching and learning in undergraduate programmes in dentistry use a variety of different approaches including:

- Lectures

- Tutorials/seminars/workshops

- Practical and laboratory classes

- Group work and problem-oriented learning

- Projects

- Directed self-study

- The use of communications and information technology

- The acquisition and development of practical clinical skills

- Observation and treatment of patients

- Reflective practice and integration of learning

The emphasis on different approaches is dependent upon the philosophy of each individual curriculum, but direct clinical treatment of patients is central to all.

Paragraph 4.1 Traditional lectures provide a means for delivering core information and an introduction to issues, themes or relevant clinical aspects of subjects to be studied. Lectures are used to develop student skills in listening, note taking, understanding and reflection. Such 'formal' presentations can be increased in value by the incorporation of varied presentation techniques, such as encouragement of student participation and planned activity within lectures. *Mindmaps may be seen by students as a useful learning tool and a method of organising material logically to assist learning and recall.*

Paragraph 4.2 Tutorials, seminars and workshops are often related to clinical issues or problems and are designed to provide an interactive focus for learning. They are concerned with the development of skills such as communication, teamwork, reasoning and critical appraisal.

Paragraph 4.3 Practical and laboratory classes are an important means of reinforcing deeper understanding of topics as well as developing skills in scientific methodology and in methods of observation relevant to diagnosis and treatment.

Paragraph 4.4 Student engagement in group work or specific educational approaches such as problem-based learning (PBL) fosters skills such as the location, sifting and organisation of information, time management, task allocation, team working and preparation of reports. *PBL can be used effectively to explore disease states which have clinical relevance to the practice of dentistry that both engages and stimulates students.*

. Section 4.10 of the QAA Benchmarking on Assessment states that:

Assessment is recognized as an important factor in the way in which students learn and manage their time. There should be both formative and summative assessments. Summative assessments can be used formatively. The process of assessment should be transparent: explicit criteria facilitate effective learning and allow for the provision of effective and meaningful feedback. In the development of knowledge, skills and attitudes appropriate to the clinical practice of dentistry, the importance of student progression during the programme must be acknowledged. Whilst, in a global sense, competence is seen to be achieved at the threshold level of graduation, students and teachers must see the value of 'staging posts' along the way.

The attainment of learning outcomes should be demonstrated by clear links with methods of both teaching and learning, with methods of assessment, and with the specific tasks of assessment.

Methods of assessment adopted in dental schools should:

- ◆ Be relevant to the purposes of undergraduate dental education
- ◆ Reflect student progression through the programme
- ◆ Encourage integration of knowledge, understanding, skills and attitudes
- ◆ Enable students to demonstrate their understanding, level of attainment and to demonstrate a full range of clinical and other abilities
- ◆ Provide accurate, constructive feedback to students on their performance
- ◆ Indicate whether a student has reached an appropriate standard

- Examine student's communication skills
- Allow records of student academic and clinical performance to be collated
- Allow the participation of external examiners
- Engage in mechanisms of quality assurance
- Provide information for course and programme organizers on the quality of provision
- Reflect the intended learning outcomes of a course.

In setting out the requirements of assessment, *The First Five Years* and the QAA Benchmarking booklets are very similar in content, but the GDC also comments on in-course assessment and examinations in paragraphs 123 to 125 as follows:

IN-COURSE ASSESSMENT

Paragraph 123 Schools should make regular formative assessments of their students, feeding back the results and discussing them with each student. In-course assessment systems may be used to establish the progress of students toward achievement of attitudinal objectives as well as testing knowledge and skills objectives.

Paragraph 124 Schools are required to have effective systems of progressive monitoring of student progress in all clinical disciplines so that students have been adequately assessed with regard to their clinical skills and acumen before proceeding to the final examination. In addition students should take practical examinations in the course of those assessments and external examiners should be given an opportunity to attend and participate. The assessment of students in this part of the course should include an evaluation of awareness of limitations, of situations in which to refer patients and the importance of clinical governance, including peer review and audit.

EXAMINATIONS

Paragraph 125 Candidates' knowledge and understanding of the subjects studied must be effectively tested. It is not necessary that there should be a separate paper or other examination in each subject. It is preferable that subjects should be appropriately grouped and that the examination in each group should take place soon after the completion of the relevant courses. At least two examiners should participate in the adjudication of all parts of the examinations when possible and appropriate. In assessing a candidate's performance both external and internal examiners should be empowered to take into account the records of the work done by the candidate throughout the course of study in the subject of the examination.

The six key questions about assessment

The intended learning outcomes listed above are not discrete entities but have varying degrees of overlap. This means that they can probably best be covered in an integrated way by considering six basic questions about assessment:

1. What?

2. Why?

3. Who for?

4. When?

5. How?

6. To what standards?

What is assessment?

Assessment throughout the UK education system has traditionally been biased towards knowledge. Knowledge can be fairly easy to assess, but the information derived is of comparatively limited use. It is usually more efficient to assess the application of knowledge, on the grounds that if someone can apply knowledge then they must possess it. Moreover, application is a higher level of functioning than simply knowing something. Performance is at a higher level still, so if assessments can focus on what a student can do (or even better, what they actually do in their daily work), then the information yielded is likely to be even more useful.

> As a general rule, the higher the level of performance that can be assessed the more valid and useful the assessment will be.

Levels of performance have been described in a number of ways. Bloom (1956) described a taxonomy of six levels of cognitive performance. Knowledge was the most basic, the next was comprehension, then application, analysis, synthesis, and finally evaluation.

> Dental assessments should aim to allow students to demonstrate their highest levels of performance in knowledge-based and skills-based competencies, as well as in their personal qualities.

Why is assessment necessary?

A major purpose of assessment is to ensure that a required standard has been achieved. This might be before progressing to the next part of the course, or to graduate at the end of it. Assessment of this kind is called *summative assessment*. This is a measure of attainment that might carry major implications for the students concerned and for their future patients, too. In the USA these are referred to as 'high-stakes' assessments. Summative assessments still tend to be quite formal, often taking the form of traditional exams. However, they need not all be formal and imaginative informal methods of summative assessment are coming into use in dental education. In view of their importance, summative assessments, whether formal or informal, must have robust and demonstrable qualities in respect of the things that are assessed, the ways in which they are assessed, and the reliability of decisions made on the evidence the assessment provides.

> Summative assessments provide the evidence on which important decisions are made. They can be formal or informal, but must be reliable, valid, feasible and fair.

In contrast to the strict requirements for summative assessment, *formative assessments* do not need to have a high degree of reliability, and can be planned or opportunistic, but are characteristically informal and often short. The most effective formative assessments tend to focus on personal attributes and competencies such as procedural skills, rather than knowledge in isolation. Their purpose is to provide feedback to individual students and their teachers about progress. Formative assessment helps fulfil the GDC and QAA requirements that assessment must be appropriate to the relevant learning outcomes, reflect student progression through the programme, provide accurate, constructive feedback to students on their performance, provide information for course and programme organizers on the quality of provision, and encourage reflection and self-assessment.

> Formative assessments provide information on progress, which is fed back to the student and their teachers. It is usually very informal, often opportunistic, and focuses on skills and attributes.

Somewhere between summative and formative assessment comes *diagnostic assessment*, which aims to identify specific weaknesses. It is particularly useful in highly complex situations such as dentistry, because a student who is identified either in summative or formative assessment to be weak in a particular area can be encouraged, through a diagnostic assessment, to identify exactly what the problem is and then be given specific help to overcome it.

> Diagnostic assessments help a student and their teachers to identify specific learning problems and agree a strategy to overcome them.

Who is assessment for?

As the preceding section shows, *formative* and *diagnostic* assessments are principally to help and guide individual students, while *summative* assessments are to provide evidence on which decisions are made by others concerning the student's progress. Decisions made on the evidence of summative assessment usually carry the potential for major consequences. For example, a student judged to be not ready to progress to the next stage of the course will be held back for the sake of their own learning, and for patient care. Therefore, these decisions should be made collectively by an Examination Board, which includes external representation in the form of external examiners.

> Formative and diagnostic assessments are carried out for the benefit of the students. Summative assessments safeguard a student's progress through the course and ensure that institutional and national standards are met in order to protect the profession and the public.

When should assessment be carried out?

Although the traditional pattern of summative assessment has been to have a final examination at the end of each year, or each phase of the course, dental schools are increasingly taking advantage of in-course assessment. In-course summative and formative assessment can be continuous or at predetermined points throughout the course.

Incorporation of *in-course assessment* is compatible with the GDC and other 'quality' requirements, in a way that relying exclusively on annual examinations is not. This system makes it easier to reflect student progression through the programme; encourage integration of knowledge, understanding, skills and attitudes; enable students to demonstrate their understanding, level of attainment; and to demonstrate a full range of clinical and other abilities. Formative assessments can usefully be undertaken fairly frequently during the course. They might be timetabled, impromptu, or ideally both. It is important that they are kept quite short and essential that they are highly relevant to what the student is doing. It is also essential that they result in feedback to the student.

In-course assessment allows continuous monitoring of student academic and clinical performance and indicates whether a student has reached an appropriate standard in clinical and communication skills. It may also be used to encourage reflection and self-assessment. Other advantages are that the information it provides is useful to course and programme organizers, and contributes to quality assurance. As in summative examinations, participation of external examiners is possible.

Diagnostic assessments are undertaken as and when they can contribute usefully to an individual student's progress.

> In-course summative assessment is an effective alternative, or at least supplement, to major annual examinations. Formative and diagnostic examinations should always be in-course.

How is assessment carried out?

There are many assessment methods applicable to the undergraduate dental curriculum. New ones are being added to the list from time to time and most are described well in the literature: *The Good Assessment Guide* (Jolly and Grant 1997) and *Assessing in Competence* (Mossey *et al.* 1999) are particularly recommended for those who wish to look at methods in more detail.

The essential principles in assessment are to identify what needs to be assessed and then to select appropriate methods; and to use a variety of methods, because no single method is capable of assessing all the key aspects of dental practise. It is also necessary to bear in mind that summative assessment must be able to withstand public scrutiny and, if necessary, legal challenge. This means that it must be provably reliable, valid, feasible and fair.

The following is a selection of methods of assessing (a) knowledge, (b) application and (c) performance of clinical skills:

Assessment of knowledge and understanding

+ Essays and modified essays
+ Multiple-choice questions
+ Short answer questions
+ Extended matching questions
+ Structured *viva voce*.

Assessment of application

+ Review of case notes and other records
+ Standardized patient management problems
+ Objective Structured Clinical Examination (OSCE)
+ Communication skills assessment
+ Review of significant incidents such as medical emergencies/CPR.

Assessment of clinical performance

+ Validated self-assessment
+ Clinical supervision

- Direct observation
- Peer review
- Clinical logbook
- Case presentations
- Objective Structured Clinical Examination (OSCE)
- Structured Clinical Operative Test (SCOT).

Assessment of knowledge and understanding

Essays and modified essays

Essays are no longer a universal assessment instrument, and for good reason. They do provide an opportunity to assess the ability to synthesize information from a variety of sources, to construct and justify a logical case, and to organize and present written material in an interesting and accessible way. However, they are time-consuming to write and to mark, are vulnerable to plagiarism, are not particularly valid and are often unreliable.

Modified essays are designed to test understanding as opposed to 'knowledge'.

Short answer questions

Short answer questions are frequently used to assess breadth of knowledge either in conjunction with essays or as a replacement for them. They tend to be used to test factual knowledge but if carefully worded they can be used to assess understanding.

They lend themselves to objective marking schemes since the topics are usually limited in breadth, and the use of such marking schemes maximizes inter and intra examiner reproducibility. Differential weighting can then be applied to create a marking scheme. In some places erroneous or inappropriate content can be penalized by negative marks but this is not recommended by professional test developers for a number of good reasons.

A typical short answer examination consists of a limited choice from a number of questions, such as 5 from 7. This creates the problem that some questions will inevitably be easier than others. An element of fairness is then lost and this can be overcome by removing choice so that all questions have to be answered.

Multiple choice questions

These exist in a variety of formats, and the best type (and probably the only type worth using) is the single best answer type, in which a question stem is followed by a set of five options, of which one is a much better answer than the other four. Candidates have to identify the best answer. Useful rules are:

- Whenever possible, the question stem should be a clinical vignette.
- Do not waste time testing simple factual recall.
- Options should be short (e.g. just one or two words) and homologous (e.g. all antibiotics).

◆ Options must be arranged in a logical order (e.g. alphabetic, ascending numeric).

◆ The 'correct' answer must be clearly better than any of the others, although these can be partially correct – they do not have to be 'false'.

◆ It is best to avoid deducting marks for incorrect answers (negative marking, or penalty scoring) as this introduces an uncontrollable variable – each candidate's attitude towards giving an answer when they are less than 100 per cent sure.

To achieve good reliability, a testing time of about two and a half hours is required. Good MCQs are extremely reliable and reasonably valid. Poorly written ones are neither valid nor reliable.

Extended matching questions

Extended matching questions (EMQs) are a development of MCQs that could go on to replace them completely in some exams. Typically, the question stem is more detailed than in an MCQ and is usually in the form of a clinical scenario. The stem is followed by a list of options (more than 5, usually 10 to 20, but might be more). Candidates select a specified number (which can be more than one) of responses from the option list. These tend to be more valid than MCQs, can be very reliable, and it is possible to assess processes of clinical reasoning using EMQs (Beullens *et al.* 2005).

Structured viva voce

The '*viva*' remains part of the summative examination at the end of each year in some UK Dental schools, and on occasion these are even employed in the assessment of borderline 'pass/fail' situations. It is something of an irony that having used a range of educational tools, presumably selected for their reliability, validity and fairness to assess a candidate's performance, the bluntest tool is then used to assist with the final decision.

It is no longer acceptable to conduct unstructured *viva voce* examinations because of their subjectivity, poor reliability and potential for bias. It is recommended that structured *viva voce* examinations should be reserved only for circumstances whereby the objective is to differentiate grades of academic performance, and not to determine sufficiency in terms of competence.

Assessment of application

Objective Structured Clinical Examination (OSCE)

OSCEs have been developed as a method of summatively assessing a range of defined clinical skills in medicine and dentistry. An OSCE consists of a number of stations through which the candidates rotate. Each presents a different task for the candidates and they have a set time at each. Stations can use real or simulated patients, referral letters, lab reports, radiographs etc to pose a clinical challenge, or might feature a piece of specialist equipment (e.g. an articulator) which the candidates demonstrate how to use correctly. The Dental OSCE can either be designed (a) to minimize the burden on supervision, and typically few stations will have an examiner present, or (b) create high fidelity clinical simulations with manned stations (Mossey *et al.* 2001). The marking is according to predetermined criteria/answers.

While the stations are set by examiners in different specialties, they can be multidisciplinary and of between 5 and 10 minutes duration. It is important with OSCEs not to waste valuable testing time on trivia or things that can be tested better in other types of examination. Well designed OSCEs are reliable, have high validity, and are seen to be fair because of their objectivity.

Communication skills testing

Systems for testing communication skills continue to evolve through study and discussion, and various methods, both formative and summative have been devised. Like other clinical skills, both formative and summative assessment is important, and direct observation of communication skills based on a set clinical scenario is the preferred model. To ensure reliability, it is regarded as appropriate to include two assessors using an agreed checklist and making independently, with appropriate aspects assessed by the patient or simulated patient. Communication skills can also be assessed in authentic clinical chairside scenarios (see SCOTs below).

Medical emergency/CPR Skills

It would not be possible or appropriate to carry out assessments on real emergency scenarios or cardiopulmonary resuscitation (CPR). Nevertheless these life support skills are essential skills and the accepted method of examination of student competence in these situations is to use mannequins or simulated patients (trained actors). Difficulties remain with the standard setting and marking of such scenarios, though there are well-developed scenarios and marking schedules for CPR (e.g. by the Resuscitation Council UK).

Assessment of clinical performance

Validated self-assessment

Self-assessment is a valuable component in learning because it requires a person to accurately assess both the quality of their performance and also their own strengths and weaknesses. It is not self-marking (or guessing at the mark that their supervisor might assign) but making judgements about whether performance of a task or its component parts was of a satisfactory standard. These judgements and reflections can be recorded in a logbook. The self-assessment can be validated through feedback at the end of the procedure or session with the supervising member of staff.

Clinical supervision

This is clearly an important component of in-course assessment – one which focuses on day to day clinical work. This method is used in 'continuous assessment' for assessing technical, procedural and other demonstrable skills. It is not generally suitable for assessing reasoning skills since this would interrupt the clinical process. In assessments made through clinical supervision, evidence may be obtained by direct observation by the educational supervisor, or through peer review.

Clinical logbook

The clinical logbook contains specific details of clinical work undertaken. This will include information on cases managed and procedures carried out. It will also record the degree of involvement and responsibility – for example, it will record whether the student simply observed an activity, assisted in a minor way, assisted to a substantial degree, or undertook the task themselves under supervision. The logbook also provides the means to reflect on treatment provided, success, satisfaction etc.

Case presentations

Case presentations enable students to consolidate their own learning. They offer opportunities to assess some skills that might be difficult to assess by other methods, such as presentation skills, the ability to synthesize various aspects of a case and present it in a logical, coherent way. Summaries and feedback from assessments of case presentations can be incorporated in the clinical logbook.

Patient management problems

This method assesses clinical problem-solving using a patient-based scenario which the student has to work through, answering specific questions at each stage. Patient management problems (PMPs) are most usually computerized or answered on paper. Typically, the scenario might start with comparatively little information, followed by an instruction such as 'identify the most appropriate course of action to take at this stage'. The answer might be written in or selected from a list of options. Having provided an answer (or declined to answer) the student is given a further piece of information followed by another question.

Structured Clinical Operative Test

As with the OSCE, the Structured Clinical Operative Test (SCOT) utilizes a checklist for the assessor to employ while observing the student completing an authentic clinical procedure in the clinical setting (Mossey and Newton 2001). The SCOT is a form of practise-based assessment that has high validity but involves procedures on different patients and therefore is not entirely objective. It is particularly suitable for invasive procedures such as administration of local anaesthesia, extraction of or restoration of teeth, or taking an impression. Performance in the SCOT can be assessed at any time suitable to the student and assessor. Procedures suitable for SCOTs must be completed in a short space of time to ensure that it is feasible in a clinical setting. Longer tasks may be broken down into component parts. The checklist should be clear and unambiguous to the student and assessor. Each checkpoint should be short and concise for ease of use. Between 10–20 checkpoints are advisable. It is crucial that the checklist represents agreed best clinical practice.

Checklists are a flexible tool that can facilitate assessment of competencies in either a formative or summative manner. They may be used freely as formative (or diagnostic) assessments, but for summative assessment they must be validated for inter-examiner reliability.

To what standard?

Section 5 of the QAA Benchmarking Statement on Standards states that:

> Upon successful completion of the undergraduate programme of study, graduating dentists are eligible to apply for registration with the General Dental Council and then to practise without supervision. Graduating dentists, therefore, will have the professional qualities, attitudes and attributes necessary for this role. As a minimum they will have demonstrated a systematic understanding of the knowledge outlined in the previous parts of this statement. They will be able to apply the key and professional skills gained during the undergraduate programme, being aware of their limited experience and able to develop new skills to a high level.

Standard-setting generally refers to establishing the pass mark for an examination. The issue of standard-setting is important, particularly in summative assessment, and is particularly sensitive in considering quality of care and maintaining standards. The aim in summative examinations for dentistry is that all who have reached the required standard should pass. This requires what is known as an absolute standard to be set. Accepted standard setting methods in this context are the Angoff (1971), Ebel (1972) and borderline (Wilkinson *et al.*. 2001; Kramer *et al.*. 2003) methods.

Summary

The essential principles in assessment are to identify what needs to be assessed and then to select appropriate methods: and then to use a variety of methods, because no single method is capable of assessing all the key aspects of dental practise. Also summative assessment must be able to withstand public scrutiny and, if necessary, legal challenge. This means that it must be provably reliable, valid, feasible and fair.

References and further reading

Angoff, W. H. (1971) Scales, norms and equivalent scores. In R. L. Throndike (ed.) *Educational Measurement*, pp. 508–600. Washington, DC, American Council on Education.

Beullens J., Struyf E. and Van Damme B. (2005) Do extended matching multiple-choice questions measure clinical reasoning? *Medical Education* **39**(4), 410–17.

Bloom, B. S. (1956) *Taxonomy of Educational Objectives. Handbook 1: Cognitive Domain*. New York, Longman, Green and Co.

Davenport E. S, Davis J. E. C., Cushing A. M., and Holsgrove G. (1998) An innovation in the assessment of future dentists. *Br Dent J* 184, 192–5.

Davenport E. S, Fry H., Pee B., and Woodman T. (2003) Learning throughout life: Can a progress file help? *Br Dent J* 196, 101–10.

Ebel, R. L. (1972) *Essentials of Educational Measurement*. Englewood Cliffs, NJ: Prentice-Hall.

Holsgrove G. (1997) 'Principles of assessment' in P. Campion *et al* (ed) *Teaching Medicine in The Community*, 183–5. Oxford, Oxford University Press.

Holsgrove G. (1997) 'Assessing knowledge' in P. Campion *et al* (ed) *Teaching Medicine in The Community*, 186–94. Oxford, Oxford University Press.

Holsgrove G. (1997) 'Assessing clinical skills' in P. Campion *et al* (ed) *Teaching Medicine in The Community*, 195–7. Oxford, Oxford University Press.

Holgrove G., Bowler, G. and Elzubeir M. (1997) 'Developing written assessments for use in Advanced Life Support couses' in A. Scherpbier *et al* (eds) *Advances in Medical Education*, 363–5.

Holgrove G. and Elzubeir M. (1998) Imprecise Terms in UK Medical Multiple-Choice Questions: what examiners think they mean. *Medical Education*, 32(4), 343–50.

Holgrove G. and Kauser Ali S. (2004) Quality assurance, standard-setting and item banking in professional examinations. *Journal of the College of Physicians and Surgeons Pakistan*.

Jolly, B. and Grant J. (eds) (1997) *The Good Assessment Guide*. London, Joint Centre for Education in Medicine.

Kramer A., Muijtjens A., Jansen K., Dusman H., Tan L. and van der Vleuten C. (2003) Comparison of a rational and an empirical standard setting procedure for an OSCE. *Medical Education* 37, 132–9.

Morris, Z. S., Bullock, A. D., Belfield, C. R., Butterfield, S. and Frame, J. W. (2001) Assessment in postgraduate Dental Education: an evaluation of strengths and weaknesses. *Medical Education* 35, 537–43.

Mossey P. A., Newton J. P. and Stirrups D. R. (1997) Defining, conferring and assessing the skills of the dentist. *British Dental Journal* 182(4), 123–5.

Mossey P. A., Newton J. P., Mason A. and Stirrups D. R. (eds) (1999) *Clinical competencies in Dentistry: Assessing in competence*. Publication produced by Queen Mary and Westfield College (September 1999).

Mossey P. A. and Newton J. P. (2001) The Structured Clinical Operative Test (SCOT) in dental competency assessment. *British Dental Journal* 190(7), 387–90.

Mossey P. A., Newton J. P. and Stirrups D. R. (2001) Scope of the OSCE in the assessment of clinical skills in dentistry. *British Dental Journal* 190(6), 323–6.

Nunally J. C. Jr (1978) *Psychometric Theory*, 2nd edn. New York, McGraw Hill (cited in Streiner and Norman, 1995).

Scott B. J. J., Evans D. J. P., Drummond J. R., Mossey P. A. and Stirrups D. R. S. (2001) An investigation into the use of a structured clinical operative test for the assessment of a clinical skill. *European Journal of Dental Education* 5, 31–7.

Streiner D. L. and Norman G. R. (1995) *Health Measurement Scales: a practical guide to their development and use*, 2nd edn. Oxford, Oxford University Press.

Wilkinson T. F., Newble D. I. and Frampton C. M. (2001) Standard setting in an objective structured clinical examination: use of global ratings of borderline performance to determine the passing score. *Medical Education* 35, 1043–9.

Woods R. (1991) *Assessment and Testing: a survey of research*. Cambridge, University of Cambridge Local Examination Syndicate.

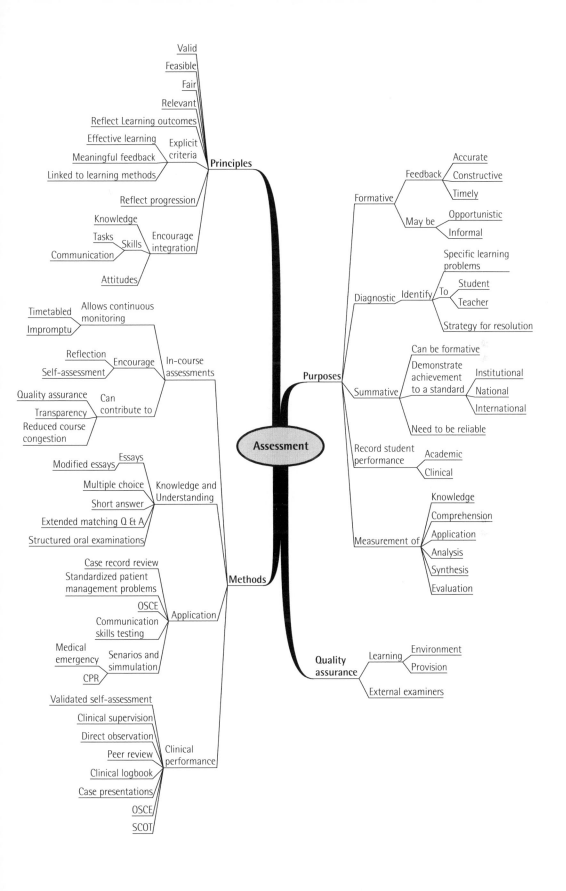

Assessment

Principles
- Valid
- Feasible
- Fair
- Relevant
- Reflect Learning outcomes
- Explicit criteria
  - Effective learning
  - Meaningful feedback
  - Linked to learning methods
- Reflect progression
- Encourage integration
  - Knowledge
  - Skills
    - Tasks
    - Communication
  - Attitudes

Purposes
- Formative
  - Feedback
    - Accurate
    - Constructive
    - Timely
  - May be
    - Opportunistic
    - Informal
- Diagnostic — Identify
  - Specific learning problems
  - To
    - Student
    - Teacher
  - Strategy for resolution
- Summative
  - Can be formative
  - Demonstrate achievement to a standard
    - Institutional
    - National
    - International
  - Need to be reliable
- Record student performance
  - Academic
  - Clinical
- Measurement of
  - Knowledge
  - Comprehension
  - Application
  - Analysis
  - Synthesis
  - Evaluation

Quality assurance
- Learning
  - Environment
  - Provision
- External examiners

Methods
- In-course assessments
  - Allows continuous monitoring
    - Timetabled
    - Impromptu
  - Encourage
    - Reflection
    - Self-assessment
  - Can contribute to
    - Quality assurance
    - Transparency
    - Reduced course congestion
- Knowledge and Understanding
  - Essays
  - Modified essays
  - Multiple choice
  - Short answer
  - Extended matching Q & A
  - Structured oral examinations
- Application
  - Case record review
  - Standardized patient management problems
  - OSCE
  - Communication skills testing
  - Senarios and simmulation
    - Medical emergency
    - CPR
- Clinical performance
  - Validated self-assessment
  - Clinical supervision
  - Direct observation
  - Peer review
  - Clinical logbook
  - Case presentations
  - OSCE
  - SCOT

3.3 Teamwork

Elizabeth Davenport, Gareth Holsgrove,
Peter Mossey and David Stirrups

Key points

- Describe what is meant by a team.
- Identify four characteristics of teams in general dental practice.
- Highlight the key policy, operational and strategic issues in managing integrated dental care.
- Differentiate between leadership and management, and outline the dentist's role in each.
- Summarize the roles of clinical and management teams.
- Teamwork will help you to progress towards achieving professional competence in leading and working within multi-skilled teams, as set out in GDC and QAA documents.

Introduction

The dental team has evolved over many years, in response to many influences such as the growing complexity in terms of techniques and technical aids and public demand. Legislation, four-handed dentistry, infection control, clinical governance, management of practices, and professionals complementary to dentistry have also influenced the demand and need for an effective and efficient dental team working together. Hence the need for undergraduate students to be fully conversant with the demands of leadership and team work.

The General Dental Council has outlined its expectations (GDC 2002, paragraph 14). These are that 'the dentist has a role as a team leader and is responsible for diagnosis, treatment planning and the quality control of the treatment provided', and that 'dental students and professionals complementary to dentistry should have the opportunity to learn and work together'. An important first step in understanding the weight the GDC gives to inter professional education in dentistry.

The First Five Years document (GDC 2002) supports the requirement that:

Paragraph 36 The dental student on graduation should understand the techniques and principles which enable the dentist to act as the leader of the dental team consisting of PCDs (dental hygienists, dental nurses, dental technicians, dental therapists, and any other groups which are created in the future). That will involve task analysis, scheduling, delegation, authorisation and monitoring of results. The collaboration of the dental student and DCPs must be a feature of the dental curriculum. The dental student should be made aware that being a leader if a dental team carries onerous responsibilities in terms of professional conduct. With increasing emphasis being placed on DCPs, there is a need for the undergraduate to have experience of working as an integral part of the greater dental team. All members of the team benefit by becoming aware early on of the contribution each can make in the provision of oral healthcare. This also assists in the development of a team approach. Other elements for inclusion include managing a team, leadership, motivating others and delegation.

In addition, 'dental students must learn the principles and practice of assisted operating dentistry, which is the normal method used in clinical practice to ensure safety and provision of high-quality care for patients...' (paragraph 37). Dental students should also be aware of their professional and legal responsibilities to all staff (paragraph 38).

Whilst considering dental domains, specific mentions of management and teamwork are listed in six different learning outcomes, such as those associated with professional and personal development, appropriate attitudes, ethical understanding and legal responsibilities, and communication. It is clear that teamwork is as an important aspect of modern dentistry and that on graduation dentists are expected to be both knowledgeable and competent in working within dental teams. Specific dental domains extend the requirement beyond understanding the principles to being able to competently and effectively apply in practice four different domains: communication; appropriate attitudes, ethical understanding and legal responsibilities; professional development; and personal development.

To achieve the required level of knowledge and competence when working with dental teams, it is important to have some insight into teams, leadership and management. While the skills of teamwork are largely developed, as so many are in dentistry, through observation, modelling and practice, this chapter aims to provide information that will contribute to developing an understanding upon which these skills can be based. An appropriate starting point would be to consider what we mean by a team, to look at the roles and composition of dental teams and outline how they have developed over recent years, and to consider what makes a successful team and how to recruit team members.

Benchmark

In addition to the GDC guidelines, the QAA Subject Benchmark for Dentistry suggests that the undergraduate programme should encompass the development of key skills, which underpin life-long learning. That is to communicate effectively at all levels in

Table 3.3.1 Intended learning outcomes for teamwork

Be competent at	Have knowledge of	Be familiar with
Communication with patients, other members of the dental team and other health professionals	The permitted duties of DCPs	The work of health care workers
Working with other members of the dental team	Working as part of the dental team	The place of dentistry in the provision of health care
Communicating effectively with patients, their families and associates, and with other health professionals involved in their care	Providing a comprehensive approach to oral care	The responsibility and demonstrate the ability to share information and professional knowledge verbally and in writing
An awareness of personal limitations, a willingness to seek help as necessary, and an ability to work effectively as a member of a team	How to prescribe effectively (verbally and in writing) to the dental therapist, dental hygienist and laboratory technician	Management of circumstances where the patient's wishes are considered by the dental team not to be in his or her best interests
Communicating, debating, interacting with clinical tutors and peers in a professional manner, both verbally and in writing	How to communicate with all members of the dental team in an appropriate manner which inspires confidence, motivation and teamwork	
	How to communicate with future fellow professionals verbally and in writing, in a manner that is effective and inspires confidence and respect	
	How to communicate effectively (verbally and in writing) with referral bodies, and a willingness to seek advice where necessary	

Table 3.3.1 Intended learning outcomes for teamwork *– continued*

Be competent at	Have knowledge of	Be familiar with
How to arrange and use the working practice environment in the most safe and efficient manner for all staff and patients	The broader issues of dental practice, including ethics, medico-legal considerations, and the maintenance of a safe working environment	
	The need to interact with the dental team and peers without discrimination	

both the scientific and professional contexts using verbal, non-verbal and written means, analyse and resolve problems, work effectively as member of the team, display appropriate behaviour towards all members of the dental team, recognize the responsibility, and demonstrate the ability to share information and professional knowledge verbally and in writing and looking out for health and safety and each other.

Teams and teamwork

A defining characteristic of a team is that members voluntarily coordinate their work in order to achieve group objectives (Bennett 1997, p. 168). It is perhaps easiest to recognize this in relation to a sports team, but in fact there are very few human activities that do not involve some kind of teamwork, either directly or indirectly. Human society is, after all, collective and often co-operative, both of which are important team characteristics. These qualities can also be identified in national, local, and family life, business, and public services. So we are all members of teams, sometimes very briefly, others more or less permanently. It is clear that the roles we play may vary considerably from team to team, and the purpose and organization of the teams themselves are likely to cover a very wide range, too.

The modern approach to assembling and leading teams, and the management role within organizations, has significant implications for the delivery of integrated dental care, especially for the dentist, or senior dentist in a partnership, who might traditionally have been the 'boss'.

A factor that stimulated an interest in teamwork was the fundamental research into the nature, structure and behaviour of teams and provides insight into issues such as designing teams, optimal team size, leadership, and dealing with dysfunctional teams (Belbin 1981).

Dental teams

In a general dental practice, there are usually two different types of teams working simultaneously. Furthermore, they are often composed of almost the same people. One is the service-delivery team, the other the management team. Both are technically known as process teams, which consist of individuals convened to provide a service. The focus for undergraduate dental education (GDC 2002) is clearly the service delivery.

In most dental practices the dentist is likely to be the leader of both the clinical and management teams, although a practice manager might be appointed to take charge of the management team – a concept which is common in general medical practice and is becoming increasingly so in dental practice.

As dentistry has developed, chair-side assistants (dental nurses) have become important team members in helping to ensure safe and effective delivery of oral health care. The support that the dentist requires also extends to include booking appointments and managing paperwork, and this role has become the receptionist's domain. Practice managers and other qualified and highly skilled personnel are also found in dental practice teams, that might consist of many or all of the following: principal dentist, associate dentist(s) dental hygienist, dental therapist, practice manager, dental nurse(s) and receptionist (Bridges 2002).

It is important to the efficient management of the practice that team members are skilled and committed to the success of the practice. This should mean that they have a considerable amount to contribute to its management and development. An important aspect of leadership is to ensure that this happens. It must be recognized, though, that the involvement of members of staff, let alone the delegation of management functions to them, can be a challenge for many dentists. This is partly because of the long and strong tradition of having only dentists in the top positions – they deliver the service and run the operation. However, such are the advantages of management teams, rather than management by a boss, that it is a tradition well worth moving away from. It means that there is a broader input into discussion, decision-making, learning, and planning within the organization. It enables all team members to become actively involved, rather than simply be passive recipients of instructions. In a professional environment this is an important factor. However, a team still needs a leader for their vision, provision of direction, and motivation skills.

Leadership and management

A dental practice should have strong clinical and management teams. There should be good leadership and management. Since these two terms, leadership and management, are often confused, it is worth clarifying what we mean by them.

It is important to designate roles and authority appropriately; this is where the distinction between manager and leader is important because both are likely to have different contributions to make to the team. A manager makes plans and works out detail, sets up and monitors structures to produce results, whereas leaders have vision, provide direction and inspire and motivate team members and produce change (Kotter 2001). These distinct but complementary roles are sometimes summarized by saying that the manager does the right things, whereas the leader does things right. Therefore, we can see that the vision for an organization is usually provided by the leader, who will also be responsible for creating the right connections, motivation etc. Implementation and the day-to-day functioning of the organization is the job of the managers. Because of this distinction between roles, in most organizations the management function would not usually be undertaken by the leader.

It is clear to see that, in the present climate particularly, effective leadership might result in quite dramatic changes which benefit the team.

The manager's task (doing things right) is to implement the leader's vision and strategy and deal with day-to-day issues. They will also be in close contact with the major stakeholders (in our case the patients, health authority, equipment suppliers, and so on) and will co-ordinate the logistics and delivery of the service, or the particular aspect of the service for which they are responsible.

Leadership and management in dental teams

We have described two quite different types of teams in a dental practice – the team that delivers the service and the one that has a management function. There are practical and clinical reasons why dentists should play a prominent role in both teams, particularly since 'the dentist has the role of team leader and is responsible for diagnosis, treatment planning and the quality control of the treatment provided' (GDC 2002, paragraph 14).

Leadership involves analysis, scheduling, delegation, authorization and monitoring of results. This, in its turn, requires a detailed knowledge of the role of each member of the team and the ability to plan an efficient, integrated service. In developing appropriate skills and insights for this to be achieved, the GDC requires that 'the collaboration of the dental student with DCPs must be a feature of the dental curriculum' (GDC 2002, paragraph 36).

Managing integrated dental care

The management of a service providing integrated dental care needs to consider management issues, such as the headings of policy, operations, and strategy.

Policy issues

In the National Health Service, many policy issues are strongly influenced by legislation, regulations and guidelines. However, management, whether by a team or an individual, must ensure that policies are adhered to and that audit trails and clinical governance are in place to ensure the best possible care for the patient. Policy documents and guidelines set out the legal and ethical requirements, employment law and issues of health and safety at work to take into account by and for the dental team.

Operational aspects

The operational areas in a dental service are complicated and often interdependent. They include the following five areas:

1. **Composition of the practice teams:** This will involve the mix of skills and expertise within the team, identifying any specific requirements, and deciding on how to address them – for example, by recruiting, training or obtaining them from external sources.

2. **Workload:** This is concerned with working patterns, balancing those of full and part-time employees, covering for leave etc. It will also drive the range of services that the practice offers, the number of patients it can support and other work-related issues.

3. **Practice administration:** This is a topic of growing importance, covering routine and special administration issues, procedures and efficiency. There is a powerful interrelationship between administrative matters and clinical service, and this is one of the reasons why it is advantageous to have certain people in the practice involved with both the clinical and management teams.

4. **Finance:** Clearly, the practice will not survive long as a business unless it has properly managed financial and cash-flow arrangements. In this aspect of management, the practice is very likely to benefit from external support and advice from the accountant, bank manager etc.

5. **Premises and equipment:** The premises represent a costly but essential component of the practice. Dental equipment and materials are expensive, in terms of usage, maintenance and replacement. Both the clinical and management teams are involved in planning and managing premises, equipment and consumables.

Practical implications

In this chapter we have suggested that there is almost certainly more room for manoeuvre in an integrated dental service than has traditionally been the case. We can review aspects of team dynamics and consider some characteristics that are associated with successful, effective teamwork.

Leadership

Time and again we have seen and heard evidence, or perhaps even had personal experience, that the quickest and most successful way to improve a failing organization is to replace the person at the top. An important practical implication for a general dental practice is that the person at the top may be difficult or impossible to replace. It is, therefore, particularly important that in this situation the person at the top has, or develops, good leadership qualities. In many respects these qualities are fairly obvious, though some are more subtle. It requires someone with good vision and organizing ability, who is approachable, experienced, calm under pressure, has excellent interpersonal skills etc. Perhaps even more important than these, though, is someone who has a leadership style that suits their personality, because leadership is not about role-play. The qualities of a leader, both obvious and subtle, and styles of leadership are well described in the quality business literature and will not be reiterated at length here.

Successful teams

In addition to having a good leader, which is an essential prerequisite, there are other characteristics associated with successful teams.

Characteristics can be seen as a combination of personal attributes, which in our context will include specific clinical skills, and the corporate attitude and disposition of the team. Leaving aside specific clinical skills and competencies, which are dealt with in the rest of this book and elsewhere, there are various personal attributes that should be represented in dental teams. It is always an advantage to any team to have at least one member who is particularly clever and creative – Belbin (1981) calls this type of team worker a 'plant'. Indeed, apart from the leader, this might be the most important person to have in the team. However, it is not practical to have too many people with similar attributes in a team – Belbin also found in his teamwork research that successful teams also often had a spread of personal attributes which gave wide coverage across the eight types of team roles he identified. These include positive features such as enthusiasm, a capacity to follow things through to a conclusion, and a capacity for communicating well with people.

Two important aspects of the disposition of the team as a whole are motivation and trust. An important factor in fostering these is for every team member to have a good knowledge of what everyone else in the team does and what everyone's role in the team is. Educational and training standards for DCPs are well established, and an integrated approach ensures that people are much more aware of each other's roles. Each person's team role should be identified and known, and for a team to work effectively everyone must feel that they have a positive part to play and that they should also respect the contribution of others. Excessive overlap of roles, a feeling of not really being part of the team, that one is not expected to become actively involved in the team's business, or that contributions from certain individuals are not appreciated are all signs of dysfunctional teamwork.

Recruitment

The principal aim of a good dental practice must be the delivery of a high-quality clinical service, which has taken priority in both recruitment and practice management. The practice leader must ensure that a proper balance is achieved between clinical and management issues, particularly since several members of the practice will be involved in both.

Practice management

A management team can be more effective than an individual manager. For example, a team can bring a range of ideas and experience that probably would not be possessed by an individual. Learning can be disseminated in a team, and can then be used constructively in planning and policy decisions. Teams can also be very effective in the management of change – a topical issue throughout both business and health care.

There are important roles for teams within a dental practice, extending far beyond their traditional functions. Careful selection, leadership and management are important if either the clinical or management teams are to be successful, but the effort expended in making sure that the practice does the right things, and that things are done right, is sure to pay dividends in today's challenging, highly professional and fast-changing environment.

Dental care professionals

Dental care professionals (DCPs) are people in the dental team who are not dentists. DCPs include dental hygienists, dental therapists, dental nurses, dental technicians, clinical dental technicians and orthodontic therapists. All DCPs will be required to be registered with the GDC in the near future. Each DCP is governed by their remit, out-lined in 'Developing a dental team'.

The dental student on graduation should understand the techniques and principles which enable the dentist to act as the leader of a dental team consisting of DCPs (dental hygienists, dental nurses, dental technicians, dental therapists and any other group which are created in the future). This will involve task analysis, scheduling, delegation, authorization, and monitoring results. The collaboration of the dental student with DCPs must be a feature of the dental curriculum. The dental students should be made aware that being a leader of the dental team carries onerous responsibilities in terms of professional conduct. With increasing emphasis being placed on DCPs, there is the need for undergraduate to have experience of working together as an integral part of the greater dental team. All members of the team benefit by becoming aware early on of the contribution each can make in the provision of oral health care. This also assists in the development of a team approach. Other elements for inclusion include managing a team, leadership, motivating others and delegation (GDC 2002, paragraph 36).

In addition the undergraduate should be familiar with the need to communicate effectively with a dental technician, so that indirect restorations and fixed and removable prosthesis can be constructed (paragraph 76).

Four-handed dentistry

For a clinician and dental nurse work effectively together and achieve the highest standard of patient care, they should work together as a team which will bring benefits to both the patient and operator, such as increasing patient comfort and reducing the stress and strain on the clinician.

The dental nurse and clinician should be seated properly, with good posture and in comfort. The dental nurse should be seated in a stable position with feet on the chair platform and 10 cm above the clinician to ensure good vision. It is also important that the dental nurse can reach and transfer instruments, materials, and suction equipment safely. The clock concept enables four-handed dentistry to be practiced in reasonable comfort. This uses four zones: a static zone located behind the patient; the dental nurse zone; the transfer zone where dental instruments and materials are passed over the patient's chest (care must be taken not to transfer over the patient's face as this can be dangerous); and the operator zone where the clinician works.

It is important that dental students come to appreciate the different roles within the dental team, take on the most appropriate role themselves, are able to identify the principles of patient care, and become familiar with areas of responsibility within the team. When the roles and responsibilities are clearly defined in a well led and properly managed dental team, it will result in increased patient comfort, reduced treatment time, and a decrease in stress and fatigue for the clinician (Paul 1991).

References and further reading

Belbin R. M. (1981) *Management Teams.* Oxford, Butterworth-Heinmann.

Bennett R. (1997) *Organisational Behaviour,* 3rd edn. Harlow, UK, Pearson Education.

Bennis W. (1989) *On Becoming a Leader.* Menlo Park, CA, Addison-Wesley.

Bridges G. (2002) An update on interaction between dental team members. *Teamwork: changing roles in the dental team.* London, Faculty of General Dental Practitioners (UK), Royal College of Surgeons of England.

GDC (2002) *The First Five Years: a framework for undergraduate dental education,* 2nd edn. London, The General Dental Council.

GDC (2004) *Developing the Dental Team. Curricula frameworks for registrable qualifications for professionals complementary to dentistry.* London, The General Dental Council.

Kotter J. P. (2001) What leaders really do. *Harvard Business Review.* Best of HBR. Reprint R0111F.

Paul E. (1991) *Chairside Procedures and Management.* London, Martin Dunitz Ltd.

QAA (2002) *Dentistry: academic standards.* Subject benchmark statements. Gloucester, Quality Assurance Agency for Higher Education.

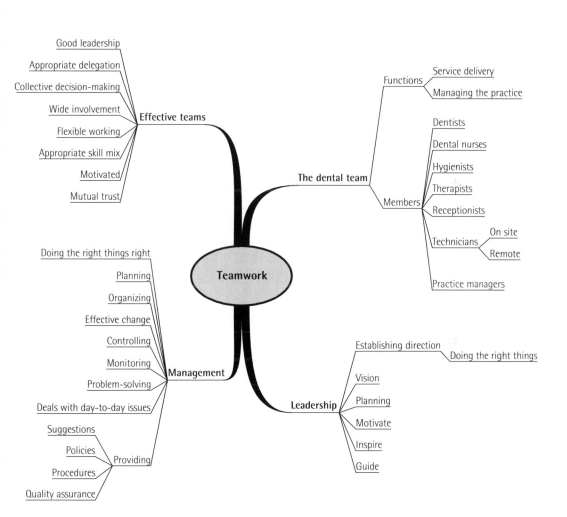

Effective teams
- Good leadership
- Appropriate delegation
- Collective decision-making
- Wide involvement
- Flexible working
- Appropriate skill mix
- Motivated
- Mutual trust

Management
- Doing the right things right
- Planning
- Organizing
- Effective change
- Controlling
- Monitoring
- Problem-solving
- Deals with day-to-day issues
- Providing
  - Suggestions
  - Policies
  - Procedures
  - Quality assurance

Teamwork

The dental team
- Functions
  - Service delivery
  - Managing the practice
- Members
  - Dentists
  - Dental nurses
  - Hygienists
  - Therapists
  - Receptionists
  - Technicians
    - On site
    - Remote
  - Practice managers

Leadership
- Establishing direction
  - Doing the right things
- Vision
- Planning
- Motivate
- Inspire
- Guide

Index

abfraction 343
abrasion 343
abscesses 377, 424, 425
abuse 2, 90
  substance 2, 90, 443, 451
access to oral health care 82
accidents and RIDDOR 51
acrylic 211
acrylic splint therapy 449
action potential, ionic basis 113
acute infection 424
Addisonian collapse 87
adhesive restorations 195
  isolation and moisture control 197–8
advanced sedation techniques 119
advertising 80
Advisory Committee on the Training of Dental
  Practitioners (ACTDP) 441, 464
aerosol and splatter 64
aesthetic restorative dentistry 224–5
agar 210
AHA Evidence Evaluation Conference 89
airway, protection 24, 86
Akinosi–Vazirani technique 116
alcohol intake 30, 103
alginate 210, 211, 404
allergies 6, 103, 448
  to latex 199, 200, 201
  to local anaesthetics 117
alveolar bone
  level 156
  support 156
  surgery to 423, 426
Alvesalo, H. *et al.* 138
amalgam 221–2, 239
  safety 221, 222, 237
amalgam tattoo 445
ambivalence and resistance 141
*American Dental Education Association
  Competencies for the New Dentist* 335
American Society of Anesthesiologists (ASA),
  Physical Status Classification 87–8, 88, 119,
  122

amnesia 119
amphotericin 446
anaesthetic techniques 114–17
  injection techniques 114–16
  topical/surface anaesthesia 114
analgesics 427
anaphylactic reaction 86
angina bullosa haemorrhagica 448
Angoff, W.H. 493
angular cheilitis 446, 448
antecubital fossa 119
antibiotics 319, 425, 427
antibody titres 445, 450
antimicrobials 446
antipsychotic agents 451
anxiety *see* dental anxiety
anxiolysis 119
apexification (root-end closure) 380
apexogenesis (root development) 380
appearance of patient 2
approach to practice 179
area-specific curettes 321
arthrocentesis 431
arthroscopy 431
aseptic storage 65
Aspergillus spp. 62
aspiration 114, 115, 116
assault 23
assertive behaviour 42
assessment of students 481–95
  assessment of
    application 488, 490–1
    clinical performance 488–9, 491–2
    knowledge and understanding 488, 489–90
  case presentations 489, 492
  clinical logbook 489, 492
  clinical supervision 488, 491
  communication skills testing 488, 491
  direct observation 489
  essays and modified essays 488, 489
  examinations 484
  extended matching questions (EMQs) 488, 490
  The First Five Years on 482–3

assessment of students *continued*
  in-course assessment 484, 487, 488
  medical emergency/CPR skills 491
  methods 489–93
  mind map 495
  multiple choice questions 488, 489–90
  Objective Structured Clinical Examination
    (OSCE) 488, 489, 490–1
  patient management problems 492
  peer review 489
  reasons for 485–6
  review of case notes and other records 488
  self-validated self-assessment 488, 491
  short answer questions 488, 489
  standardized patient management problems
    488
  standards 493
  Structured Clinical Operative Test (SCOT) 489,
    492
  structured *viva voce* 488, 490
atraumatic restorative treatment (ART) 341,
  342
attitudes 100
attrition 343
atypical facial pain 448, 449
autoclaves and pressure vessels 65
  health and safety 52–3
autonomy of the patient 24–5, 144
AVPU (Alert, Verbal response, Pain response, or
  Unresponsive) 89
avulsion 276
Ayliffe, G.A. *et al.* 64

bacteraemia 254
bacteria 62
bacterial sialadenitis 448
basic periodontal examination (BPE) 338
Batt bur 265
beam-aim devices 153, 157
behaviour modification 42
  model of behaviour change 42
behavioural management of dental anxiety
  132–4, 148–9
  alternative methods 146
  biofeedback 146
  and conscious sedation 120
  desensitizing hierarchy 145
  hypnosis 146
  iatrosedation 144
  mind map 148, 148–9
  psychological issues 136–8
  relaxation 146
  tell-show-do 144
behavioural sciences 100
Belbin, R.M. 504

Bennett, R. 500
benzoates (E210–E219) 450
Beullens, A. *et al.* 490
bimanual palpation 9
bimaxillary surgery 430
biofeedback 146
biomaterial safety 182
biopsy 423, 426, 430
  incisional and exisional 444, 449
  of mucosal lesions 445
bitewing 153, 156
  indications for 156
Blinkhorn, A.S. 235
blood count 445
blood glucose 442
blood pressure 104, 120
  taking 88
blood-borne viruses 61–2
Bolam Test 23
bone augmentation 431
Bradnock, G. and Morris, J. 72
bridges, 501
bridgework 333, 352
British Association for the Study of Community
  Dentistry (BASCD) 79
British Dental Association (BDA), infection
  control booklet 62
British National Formulary 93, 318, 451
British Orthodontic Society 155
British Society for Oral Pathology 461
British Society of Paediatric Dentistry 233, 253
British Society of Periodontology 322, 326
British Society for Restorative Dentistry 211,
  335
Brocklebank, L.M. 155, 157, 162, 163
buccal/lingual expansion 156
Buckley's Formocresol 251, 252, 253
bupivacaine 113
Burke, F.J.T. and Freeman, R. 136
burning mouth syndrome 448, 449

CAD CAM 215, 227
calcium hydroxide 226, 261, 263, 266
Calgary–Cambridge Guide, on interview skills
  101–3
cancer *see* oral cancer
Candida spp. 62
candidosis 62, 446, 448, 451
carbamazepine 451
cardiac arrest 86, 89
cardiopulmonary resuscitation (CPR) 85,
  89–90, 491
  sequence for an adult 92–3
cardiovascular physiology 119
care, primary, secondary and tertiary 82

caries 178, 180, 182
  assessment of operative management 356–7
  detecting dyes 341
  management 340, 341
  in primary dentition 233–4
  in primary molars 252
Carson, P. and Freeman, R. 144
case notes 1, 3
case study, human science and ethics 30–2
cavity bases 226–7
cavity linings 226
CCD (charge-coupled device) 154
cellulose pads 202
central giant cell granuloma 318
cerebral trauma 274
cerebrovascular accident 87
cervical nodes 104
Chambers, D.W. xii
chemomechanical caries removal 341
chemosensory disorders 443, 450–1
chest problems 6
Child Fear Survey Schedule 138, 142
child patient see paediatric dentistry
Children Act 23
chlorhexidine 318, 321
chlorhexidine solution 265
cicatrial pemphigoid 319
cinnamon 450
cleft palate 157
  surgery 431
clefting 421
clinical attachments 100
clinical audit 477–8
clinical diary 99
clinical empathy 5
clinical evaluation 163
clinical examination, restorative dentistry 338
clinical governance 477
clinical logbook 489
clinical materials, and the postal system 65, 67
clinical photography 443, 450
clinical records see record keeping
clinical supervision 488
clinical trials 91
clinical waste, disposal of 65
CMOS (complementary metal-oxide semiconductor) 154
co-operation and behaviour management, in special needs dentistry 292
collapse
  causes of 86–7
  management of the collapsed patient 91
communication 469
  and teamwork 499

communication skills 20, 21, 37–47, 95, 101, 179
  assertive behaviour 42
  case study 32
  case used in OSCE assessment 44–5
  checking understanding 41
  and children 135–6
  and dental anxiety 133, 134–6, 141
  educational guidelines 38–9
  elderly patients 350
  empathy 5, 12, 32, 40
  factors impeding communication 40
  giving information 41
  learning outcomes 39
  listening skills 41, 134–5
  mind map 47
  non-verbal communication 40, 134
  patient-centred communication 39
  questions 41
  testing 488
  therapeutic relationship 43–4
  verbal communication 134
  and vulnerable patients 100
community dentistry see dental public health
community oral health see dental public health
community-based outreach programmes 75–6
community-based preventive measures 81
competence ix–x
Competencies Required for the Practice of Dentistry in the European Union 460
complaints 29, 30, 43
complete dentures
  master impressions 394
  preliminary impressions 393–4
compomer 227, 239
composite 239
concussion 276
condyle 431
confidentiality 22, 25, 30
connective tissue disease 448
conscious sedation 111, 117–21
  airway management 120
  and behaviour management 120
  consent 120
  GDC definition 117
  instructions for patient at end of appointment 120
  monitoring 120
  potential drug interaction 119
consciousness, assessing level 89
consent 19, 23, 25, 26–9
  and children 26–7, 29
  conscious sedation 120
  and general anaesthesia 122
  practical and ethical considerations 21

consent *continued*
and professionalism 19–35
and restorative dentistry 340
and sedation 120
stages in process of obtaining, checklist
27
and surgical procedures 426
UK Department of Health guidance 26
value of informed consent 28
written 26, 28
consultation, shape of 40–1
contact sports 174
continued professional education 327, 329,
470
continuing medical education (CME) 313
contracting for dental services 82
Control of Substances Hazardous to Health
Regulations (1988) 51
copper 222
copy dentures 215, 397–8
Corah, N.L. 138
Coriat, I.H. 136
COSHH assessments of substances 53
cotton wool 202, 262, 263
Cow–Gates technique 116
coxsackie group viruses 451
cracked teeth 377
cranial nerves 443, 444
criminal charges 23
critical appraisal framework 76–7
critical thinking 473–4
Crohn's disease 319
cross-cultural communication 28, 43
cross-infection control 24
and medical emergencies 90
radiography 158, 160–1
crowding/rotated teeth 322
crowns 333, 352
preparation of tooth 353
cryotherapy 442, 452
cultural competence 43
cultural groups 79
cystic lesions 156
cysts 423, 427

data, evaluation 76–7
Data Protection Act 23, 29, 32
Dearing Report x
deciduous teeth, extraction 251
deficient restoration margins 322
demastication 343
dental anxiety
ambivalence and resistance 141
assessing anxiety using psychological
inventories 137–8

Child Fear Survey Schedule 138, 142
and communication 134–6
definition of 136
Dental Anxiety Scale (DAS) 138, 139
diagnosis 137
difficulties in clinical management 143–4
HAD scale 450
learning outcomes 131–2, 133
management 118
with behavioural techniques 141–3
and surgical procedures 426–7
Modified Dental Anxiety Scale (MDAS) 138,
140–1
pharmacological management 111–29
presenting symptomatology 136
and psychological issues 136–7
readiness to change 142–3
referrals based on assessment 138, 141
scope and precipitating factors 119
Dental Anxiety Scale (DAS) 138, 139
dental audit 20
dental care professionals (DCPs) 20, 29, 75,
179, 181, 313, 499, 505
dental conditions, in the UK 77–9
dental defence organizations 20
Dental Directives document 441
Dental Guidance Notes 167
dental health education 180
dental health surveys 77
dental implants 340, 356
dental materials science 219–31, 342
cavity bases 226–7
cavity linings 226
dental amalgam 221–2
dental porcelains and aesthetic restorative
dentistry 224–5
extra coronal restorations 221, 223–4
glass-ionomer cement and its derivatives
223
ideal posterior filling material 221
impression materials 221, 225
luting cements 227–8
luting and lining cements 221
mind map 230–1
plastic restorations 221
resin-based composites 222
Dental National Formulary (DNF) 91
dental nurse 505–6
dental pain 424
dental panoramic radiography (DPR) 157
dental phobia 136–7, 138
diagnosis 137
and patients with learning difficulties 137
dental porcelains and aesthetic restorative
dentistry 224–5

Dental Practice Board for England and Wales 195, 207, 235
dental public health 71–84, 174
  assessment methods 77
  The First Five Years on 72–3
  learning outcomes for 73–4
  mind map 84
  patient's response to dental care 73
  role of dentist 73
  social and economic trends 73
dental radiology and imaging 151–71
  assessment of students 157–63
  cross-infection control 158, 160–1
  diagnosis 152
  direct digital radiographic procedures 154
  dose reduction 167
  The First Five years on 151–2
  guidelines 155–6
  hazards and regulations 152, 167
  image receptors 153–4
  indications and contraindications 155–7
  indirect digital systems 155
  intra-oral film 153, 161–2
  intra-oral radiographic examination 158–9
  learning outcomes 152–7
  legal responsibilities 167
  mind map 170–1
  orthodontics 300
  panoramic radiographic examination 159–61
  and pregnancy 155–6
  processing 154–5, 161–3
  radiographic examination in oral medicine 450
  radiographic interpretation 163–5
    assessment of students 165–7
  radiographic reports 152, 163–5
  radiographic views
    extra-oral 153
    intra-oral 153
  radiographs
    checklist and order for examination 164–5
    periodontology 322
    prosthodontics 391–2
  radiography, and pulp therapy in the primary dentition 257
  restorative dentistry 338–9
  safelight testing 155, 162–3
  test film 162
dental teams 501
  leadership and management 502
dental trauma 340, 345–7
  diagnosis 345–6
  maintenance 347
  treatment planning and strategies 346
dental trauma in children *see under* paediatric dentistry

'DentEd' xii 464
dentigerous cyst 167
dentin 226
Dentists Act 22, 23
dento-alveolar injuries 276
dento-facial deformities 421
dentopantogram 300
denture insertion 396–7
  checklist 409
denture rebase 215
denture reline 215
denture-induced stomatitis 389
dentures 388
  complete dentures 392–7
Department of Health directives 23
desensitizing hierarchy 145
developing teeth 156
devitalization 380
diabetes 6, 103, 448
diabetic collapse 86
diagnostic assessment 486
diagnostic histopathology 463–4
diazepam 119
dietary control 173, 178, 180–1, 182, 342
  checklist for diet history and advice 184
  periodontology 323
digit sucking habit 303, 305
digital imaging techniques 152
diphtheria 63
direct digital radiographic procedures 154
direct observation 489
direct pulp capping, checklist 383
disability awareness 285, 286–8
  checklist 287–8
  definition of disability 283
Disability Discrimination Act 20, 285
disclosing tablets 323
disease, standardizing measurement 75
disease prevention 80–1, 178
disinfection 65
dislocation 431
displacement (luxation) 276
disposal of clinical waste 65
distraction osteogenesis 430
Djemal, S. 193
DMFT (Decayed, Missing, Filled Teeth) index 76
Down's syndrome 290
drug and alcohol use, by dentists 29, 30
drug information courses 93
drugs 90–1, 97
  cultural use 103
  effects of 2
  evaluation of new drugs 113
  in oral medicine 443, 451

duties of care 24, 59
dysplastic lesions 451

Ebel, R.L. 493
edentulousness 31, 386–7
elderly patients 2, 30–2, 333, 334, 335
  communication with 350
  epidemiology of oral health 347
  maintenance 351
  mind map 366–7
  oral effects of aging 348–9
  oral health 348
  restorative care 347
  systemic aging 348
  treatment 350–1
  treatment goals and planning 349–50
electric pulp test 276
electric pulp testers 322
Electricity at Work Regulations (1988) 51
electronic databases 471
Eley, B.M. 237
emergency treatment 28
empathy 5, 21, 32, 40
employment law 21
Endo-Z bur 265
endocarditis 103
endodontic emergencies 380
endodontic treatment 156, 195
endodontic views 153
endodontics 371–84
  checklist for skills 373
  clinical examination 375–6
  definition 371
  diagnostic statement 376
  direct pulp capping, checklist 383
  history taking 373–5
    standards 373–4
  indirect pulp capping/stepwise excavation,
    checklist 382
  isolation and moisture control 198
  learning outcomes 372
  mind map 384
  root canal obturation, checklist 381–2
  root canal preparation, checklist 380–1
  rubber dam in 378
  treatment 378–83
  treatment plan 377–8
epidemiology 71–84, 319
  oral health in elderly patients 347
epilepsy/epileptic fit 87
Epstein–Barr virus 451
erosion 343
erupted teeth, extraction 425
erythroplakia 447
ethics and law 19–35, 100

applying dental ethics to a case 30–2
case study 31–2
ethical principles 24–5
The First Five Years on 20–2
health and safety obligations 50–3
law applied to dentistry 22–4
learning outcomes 22
mind map 14–15
orthodontics 306
special care dentistry 285
ethyl chloride 276, 322
European Academy of Paediatric Dentistry 176,
  235
European Commission 155, 461
European Commission Advisory Committee on
  the Training of Dental Practitioners 2, 3
European Computer Driving Licence 471
European Federation of Periodontology 315,
  326
*European Guidelines on Radiation Protection in
  Dental Radiography* 155
European Society of Endodontology 196, 198,
  199, 371, 372
evaluating data, standards 76–7
evidence-based approach 72, 182
examination 8–11, 104
  blood pressure 104
  checklist for competence 13
  examination of hands 104
  format of 1, 10–11
  general examination 104
  lymph nodes 104
  periodontology 321–2
  pulse 104
  temperature 104
exodontia (uncomplicated), checklist 432
exostosis 445
exposed furcations 322
extended matching questions (EMQs) 488,
  490
extra-coronal restorations 221, 223–4
extra-oral examination 10
extra-oral implants 431
extra-oral radiographic views 153
extraction
  erupted teeth 425
  roots 426
  unerupted teeth 426
eye protection 64

facial deformity 423, 427, 428
  surgery 421, 430
facial pain 443
  of dental and non-dental origin 448
facial skeleton 444

Faculty of General Dental Practitioners 155, 157
fainting, on receiving local anaesthetic 117
Falster, C.A. *et al.* 259
family history 7–8, 103
  in letter of referral 191–2
Family Law Reform Act 23
Farooq, N.S. *et al.* 259
Fayle, S.A. *et al.* 233
ferric sulphate 262
fibre-optic transillumination (FOTI) 341
fibro-epithelial polyp 445
film holders 153, 157
The First Five Years on
  assessment 482–3
  communication skills 38
  control of anxiety and pain 111–12
  dental anxiety 131–2
  dental materials 219–20
  dental public health 72–3
  dental radiology 151–2
  dental trauma 273–4
  history taking 2
  impression making 207–8
  infection control 59–60
  key skills 469–70
  law, ethics and professionalism 20–2
  medical emergencies 85–6
  oral medicine 441–2
  oral pathology 459
  oral surgery 422
  orthodontics 297–8
  paediatric dentistry 234, 252
  patient referral 189
  periodontology 314
  preventive dentistry 174–5
  prosthodontics 386–7
  restorative dentistry 334–5
  teamwork 195–6, 497–8
The First Five Years x 2, 38
fissure sealing 173, 178, 180, 236, 241, 244
fissured tongue 445
fixed prostheses 353–4
flabby ridge 215
fluconazole 446
flumazenil 119
fluoride 73, 81, 173, 178, 181, 182–3, 184
  checklist for assessment of need and provision
    of therapy 185
folic acid 445
foreign objects 156
formaldehyde 251, 252
formalin-fixed paraffin-processed material 449
formative assessments 486
four-handed dentistry 505–6

fractures
  facial bones 274
  roots 377
Frankfort plane 302
free end saddle 215
fucidic acid 446
functional appliance occlusal record 310
fungal infection 445
fungi 62
furcation lesions 322

gag reflex 201
gauze 202
general anaesthesia 29, 121–3
  GDC on 121
  learning outcomes 121
  management of patients under 122
  patients at risk 427
  problems with 6
General Dental Council 19, 23, 29, 100, 101, 251
General Dental Council Requirements 23
General Professional Training (GPT) xi
general study skills, online resources 476
geographic tongue 445
Gillick *v* West Norfolk and Wisbech HA (1985) 27
gingivae 10
gingival blood supply, and crevicular fluid (GCF) 318
gingival inflammation 314, 322
gingival recession 322, 348
gingival retraction 212
glass-ionomer cement and its derivatives 223, 226, 227, 239, 260
gold alloy 223, 224
'Golden Standard' for European Undergraduate teaching 176
Gordon, P.H. 235
government initiatives 80
graduated pocket measuring probe 320
The Guidance Notes for Dental Practitioners on the Safe Use of X-ray Equipment 153
Guidance on Professional and Personal Conduct 60
Guidelines for Crown and Bridge 335
gutta percha 211

HAD scale of anxiety and depression 450
haemangioma 445
haematinic deficiency 448
haematological investigations, venepuncture 444, 445
haematology 450
haemorrhage 87
hairy leukoplakia 448

hand, venepuncture site 119
hand protection 63–4
hands, examination of 104
Harris, R.V. *et al.* 76
health 79
health authorities, commissioning and
  performance monitoring of dental services 82
health care, in the community and in hospital
  81–2
health economics 72
health promotion 72, 73, 75, 80–1, 100, 178
Health Protection Agency 153, 167
health and safety 29, 30, 49–57
  checklist 53
  ethical and legal obligations 50–3
  General Dental Council guidance 49–50
  learning outcomes 50
  mind map 56–7
  people 51–2
  premises 52–3
  substances 53
  in the workplace 49–50
Health and Safety at Work Act (1974) 50
Health and Safety (Display Screen Equipment)
  Regulations 51
Health and Safety (First Aid) Regulations
  (1981) 51
Health and Safety Regulations 23
health service organization 72
heart problems 6
Helsinki Declaration 27, 29
hepatitis B, vaccination 52, 63
hepatitis B, C, G and TTV 61, 62
herpes simplex 62, 446–7, 451
Hibiscrub 66
histopathology 449
history taking 1–14, 96, 100, 101
  checklist 103, 106
  checklist for competence 11
  endodontics 373–5
  family history 7–8, 103
  The First Five Years on 2
  history of presenting complaint 6, 106
  learning outcomes 2
  medical history 6
  mind map 16–17
  oral medicine 444
  oral pathology 462
  in orthodontics 299
  in paediatric dentistry 236, 238–9
  past dental history 7
  periodontology 321
  prosthodontics 391
  pulp therapy in the primary dentition 255–6
  restorative dentistry 337–8

social history 7, 103–4
  taking the history 4–8
  see also medical history
HIV/AIDS 62, 64, 448
hoes 321
host-modulating drugs 318
human disease, mind map 109
human disease and therapeutics 95–109
  attitudes 100
  The First Five Years on 96–7
  history taking 101
  knowledge and understanding 99–100
  learning outcomes 98–101
  skills 100–1
human herpes virus 8 451
human papilloma virus 451
Human Rights Act 20, 23, 285
human science, applying to a case 30–2
Humphris, G.M. 138
hyperalgaesic pulp 259, 263–4
hypersensitivity 448
  reactions 86
  testing 443, 450
hypertension 103
hypnosis 146
hypodontia 305, 307
hypoglycaemia 86

iatrosedation 144
Ibricevic, H. and Al-Jame, Q. 259
image receptors 153–4
immature permanent molar in mixed dentition
  241–3
immediate dentures 403–5
  impressions 404
  instructions to patient 405
  recording the occlusion 404
  review 405
immunization 63
immunofluorescence 450
immunology 318
impairment
  definition 283
  understanding of 290–2
implants 406
impression compound 210, 211
impression materials 221, 225, 340
impression trays 211
impression making 207–17
  disinfection 214
  evaluation of impressions 213
  impression techniques 212
  learning outcomes 208
  mind map 216–17
  occlusal registration 213

prescription writing 214–15
properties of impression materials 210
reasons to make impressions 209
shade selection 213–14
soft tissue management and moisture control 212
special impression techniques 215
incisive nerve 115
index of orthodontic treatment need (IOTN) 299, 300, 306–7
indices 74
  to measure disease 76
indirect fixed restorations, mind map 360
indirect pulp capping/stepwise excavation, checklist 382
indirect pulp therapy 259–61
indirect restorations 340, 352–4
indirect technique, inferior alveolar nerve block 116
infection
  diagnosis and treatment 424–5
  distinguished from neoplastic disease 424
infection control 59–70
  The First Five Years on 59–60
  learning outcomes 61
  and medical history 62–3
  microorganisms 61–2
  mind map 68–70
  and surgery design 65
  and surgical procedures 427
  training in 65
  universal precautions 63–7
inferior alveolar nerve block 115
  Akinosi–Vazirani technique 116
  Cow–Gates technique 116
  indirect technique 116
infiltration 115
inflammatory bowel disease 448
information sources 471
information technology 469, 470, 471
inhalational sedation 119, 121
inherited disease 7–8
injection techniques
  general considerations 114–15
  infiltration 115
  regional anaesthesia 115–16
innoculation injuries 63, 64
inpatient ward and operating theatre practices 431
instrumentation, periodontology 319–21
integrated dental care
  composition of practice teams 503
  finance 503
  key skills 469–80
  managing 502–3

practice administration 503
premises and equipment 503
workload 503
interceptive orthodontics 305–6
International Agency for Research on Cancer (IARC) 252
International Endodontic Journal 371
interproximal cleaning 323
intra-bony pathological conditions 427, 429
intra-oral examination 9
intra-oral film, processing 161–2
intra-oral radiographic examination, checklist 158–60
intra-oral radiographic views 153
  bitewings 153
  occlusals 163
  periapicals including endodontic views 153
intra-osseous anaesthesia
  via the direct approach 117
  via the periodontal approach 117
intramuscular injection 90
intrapapillary anaesthesia 117
intrapulpal anaesthesia 117
intravascular injection, minimizing risk 114
intravenous sedation 119, 120–1
  monitoring 120
  reversal agents 119, 120
  titration of sedative agent 120
intravenous techniques 90
ionizing radiation 151
  hazards and regulations 167
Ionizing Radiation (Medical Exposure) Regulations (2000) 51, 151
isolation and moisture control 195–205
  and adhesive restorations 197–8
  consequences of inadequate 198
  endodontics 198
  learning outcomes 196, 197
  mind map 204–5
  reasons to undertake 196–7
isolation techniques 199–202
  cellulose pads 202
  cotton wool 202
  gauze 202
  rubber dam 199–201
  suction 202

jaundice 6, 62, 103
jaw movements 10, 13
jaw relationships
  recording 400–1
  checklist 407–8
jaws 421
  lateral oblique views 153
Journal of Prosthetic Dentistry 207

Kakehashi, S. *et al.* 371
Kaposi's sarcoma 448
Kennedy classification 399
key skills
  The First Five Years on 469–70
  integrated dental care 469–80
  mind map 480
Kilpatrick, N. 235
Kilpatrick, N.M. *et al.* 237
Kotter, J.P. 502
Kramer, A. *et al.* 493

labial gland biopsy 442, 450
laboratory work 355–6
laser and photodynamic therapy 452
lateral cephalogram 304
lateral cephalometric radiography 153,
  157
  indications for 157
lateral oblique views of jaws 153
latex allergy 199, 200, 201
law *see* ethics and law
leadership 503–4
leadership and management 501–2
  in dental teams 502
*Learning Outcomes for Undergraduate Training in
  Paediatric Dentistry* 255
learning and performance improvement 469,
  471–4
  checklist for a written assignment 478
  critical thinking 473–4
  note taking 472
  reading 472–3
Ledermix ™ 263, 264
legislation 23
  special care dentistry 285, 288, 289
lesions 8
letter of referral 290
  mind map 194
  orthodontics 306
leukaemia 448
leukoplakia 447
library search skills 471
lichen planus 447
  steroid therapy 451
lidocaine 113
life support 86, 90
life-long education 29, 98, 470
lingual nerve 115
lips 10, 13
  and oral mucous membranes 444
listening skills 41, 134–5
liver enzyme levels 445, 451
Llewelyn, D.R. 252
local anaesthesia 111, 112–17

administration of a local anaesthetic injection,
  checklist 123
anaesthetic techniques 114–17
anatomy and physiology 113
effects of drugs 113
foundation knowledge and understanding 113
mind map 128–9
pharmacology 113
physicochemical properties of LA drugs 113
psychological support 114
supplemental anaesthetic techniques 116–17
vasoconstrictors 113
local anaesthetic problems 117
  allergy 117
  failure to achieve local anaesthesia 117
  local post-anaesthetic problems 117
  systemic problems 117
local antimicrobial delivery systems 325
Loh, A. *et al.* 262
long buccal nerve 115
loosening (subluxation) 276
luting cements 227–8
luxation injuries 380
lymph node and thyroid examination, checklist
  107
lymph nodes 104, 256, 317, 321, 429, 443,
  444

McGoldrick, P.M. and Pine, C.M. 146
Maguire, A. 234, 253, 255
Maintaining Standards 20, 60, 112, 121
malocclusion, evaluation 299–300
Management of Health and Safety at Work
  Regulations (Framework Regulations) 51
mandibular fractures 431
mandibular osteotomy techniques 430
Manual Handling Operations Regulations 51
masks 64
masticatory muscles 429
maxillary antrum 428–9
maxillary labial fraenectomy 426
maxillary osteotomy techniques 430
maxillofacial implants 431
maxillofacial trauma 421, 423, 427, 428, 431
Maximum Exposure Limits (MELS) 53
medical emergencies 59, 85–94
  cardiopulmonary resuscitation 89–90, 92–3
  and cross-infection 90
  emergency drugs 88
  initial assessment 89
  learning outcomes 87
  management 90
  management of the collapsed dental patient 91
  mind map 94
  skills 87–8, 491

medical history 6, 97, 101–4
  allergies 103
  and anaesthetic techniques 114
  Calgary–Cambridge Guide: A Guide to the Medical Interview 101–3
  and general anaesthesia 122
  gynaecological and obstetric history 103
  and infection control 62–3
  interview structure 101
  in letter of referral 190–1
  medication 103
  in orthodontics 301
  past medical history 103
  patient-centred interview 101, 102
medical sciences 100
medication 107
membrane pemphgoid 448
mental and emotional state of patient 5
Mental Health Act 23
mental nerve 115
mepivacaine 113
mercury 53, 221
methicillin resistant *Staphylococcus aureus* (MRSA) 62
miconazole 446
microbial flora 64
microbiological investigations, mucosal disease 443, 445
microbiological sampling techniques 376
microorganisms, and infection control 61–2
microscopy 463–4
midazolam 119
Milburn, A. 96
mind maps
  assessment of students 495
  behavioural management of dental anxiety 148–9
  communication skills 47
  dental materials science 230–1
  dental public health 84
  dental radiology and imaging 170–1
  elderly patients 366–7
  endodontics 384
  ethics and law 34–5
  human disease 109
  indirect fixed restorations 360
  isolation and moisture control 204–5
  key skills 480
  letter of referral 194
  local anaesthesia 128–9
  mucosal disease 456–7
  oral medicine, skills 458
  oral pathology 466
    conditions
      soft tissue and systemic 468
      teeth and facial bones 467
  oral surgery
    skills 438–9
    underpinning knowledge 436–7
  orthodontics 311
  paediatric dentistry 247–9
  periodontology 331
  pharmacological management of pain and anxiety 126–9
  prosthodontics
    clinical and technical procedures 411
    complete dentures 412–13
      copy technique 414
    immediate complete dentures 415
    overview 410
    partial dentures
      clinical tasks 418–19
      design 416
  pulp therapy in the primary dentition 270–1
  restorative dentistry
    general skills 363–5
    topics 365, 368–9
  special care dentistry 296
Mitchell and Mitchell 157
mixed dentition 234
mobile teeth 322
MOCDO system 307
modified Bass technique 323
Modified Dental Anxiety Scale (MDAS) 138, 140–1
Mofidi, M. *et al.* 100
moisture contamination 195
Morris, A.J. *et al.* 314
Mortazavi, M. and Mesbahi, M. 259
Mossey, P.A. *et al.* 491
motivational interviewing 141
motor nerve paralysis 116
mouth mirrors 9
mouthrinse/toothpastes 321
mucocele 448
mucoperiosteal flap 423, 426
mucosa hyperplasia 448
mucosal disease 443, 444
  angular cheilitis 446
  candidosis 446
  herpes simplex 446–7
  lichen planus 447
  localized lesions 445
  microbiological investigations 443, 445
  mind map 456–7
  recurrent aphthous stomatitis (recurrent oral ulceration) 446
  traumatic ulceration 445
  vesiculo-bullous disorders 448
  see also oral cancer

mucous membrane pemphigoid 448
mumps 448
mylohyoid nerve block 116
myocardial infarction 86

Nadin, G. *et al.* 262
nasal fractures 431
Nash, J.R.G. *et al.* 464
nasopalatine nerve block 116
necrosis 376
necrotizing periodontitis 448
necrotizing ulcerative gingivitis (NUG) 318
necrotizing ulcerative periodontitis (NUP) 318
needlestick injuries 64, 114
negligence 23, 25
neonatal teeth 305
neoplastic disease, distinguished from infection 424
nerve blocks 115–16
neutral zone impressions 396
neutral zone technique 392, 395
nitrous oxide 119
nitrous oxide/oxygen inhalational sedation 121
nociception 113
non-accidental injury 274
non-dental medication 90–1
non-surgical root canal treatment 379
non-surgical root surface debridement 324–5
non-verbal communication 40, 134
non-vital pulp therapy 259, 264–6
numbers, application of 469, 471
Nuttall, N. *et al.* 333
nystatin 446

Objective Structured Clinical Examination (OSCE) 488
  assessment of communication skills 44–5
oblique lateral (lateral oblique) 157
O'Brien, M. 233, 251
obturators 215
occlusal
  oblique 156
    indications for 156
  true or cross-sectional, mandible only 156
occlusal faults 397
occlusal registration 213
occlusals 153
occlusion, assessment of 322
Occupational Exposure Standards (OES) 53
Odell, E.W. *et al.* 463, 464
Okamoto, Y. and Horibe, T. 221
open root surface debridement (surgery) 325–6
oral cancer 176, 193, 348, 423, 444, 447
  diagnosis 425
  management 451

potentially malignant lesions 447
  treatment planning and outcomes 429–30
oral conditions, recording 76
oral and dental disease, special needs dentistry 292
oral disease, in the UK 73
oral health
  elderly patients 348
  impact of poor oral health 75
oral health care, access to 82
oral health promotion 175
oral health-related behaviours 79
oral hygiene 173, 178, 180, 321
  checklist for instruction to patients 183
  failure to maintain 325–6
  instruction in periodontology 323
  periodontology 326–7
oral malodour disorders 443, 450–1
oral medicine 441–58
  aetiology and management of orofacial disease 451
  clinical examination 444
  The First Five Years on 441–2
  histopathology 449
  history taking 444
  learning outcomes 442–4
  mind map 454–5
  radiographic examination 450
  referral 452
  skills, mind map 458
oral microbiology 175
oral pathology 175, 459–68
  conditions
    soft tissue and systemic, mind map 468
    teeth and facial bones, mind map 467
  diseases covered 463
  The First Five Years on 459
  history taking 462
  learning outcomes 462
  mind map 466
  referrals 462
  Subject Benchmark Statements for Dentistry (QAA) on 460–1, 462–3
oral soft tissue, surgery to 423, 426
oral surgery 421
  skills, mind map 438–9
  underpinning knowledge, mind map 436–7
oral ulceration 448
oral/dental conditions seen with impairments 292–5
orbital fractures 431
organ transplantation 327
orofacial tissues, innervation 113
orthodontic emergencies 308
Orthodontic Radiographs Guidelines 155

orthodontic wire 274
orthodontics 175, 297–311
  clinical examination 299–200, 302–3, 308–9
  diagnostic statement 304–5
  ethical/legal implications 306
  evaluation of malocclusion 299–300
  history taking 299, 300–2
  index of orthodontic treatment need (IOTN)
    299, 300, 306–7
  interceptive orthodontics 305–6
  learning outcomes 298–9
  making referrals 306
  medical history in 301
  mind map 311
  radiography in 300
  special investigations 300, 303–4
orthognathic surgery 157
orthopantomogram 322
osseo-integrated implants 389
Ottawa Charter (WHO) 80
overdentures 406
Oxford Handbook of Clinical Dentistry 157
oxygen 90, 121

paediatric dentistry 24, 174, 233–49, 251–72
  child dental health 232
  clinical examination 236, 238–9, 243
  communicating with children 135–6
  consent 26–7, 29
  dental trauma 272–81
    acid-etched retained composite tip on an
      interior tooth 279
    learning outcomes 274–8
    mind map 281
    radiography 278
    splinting of anterior teeth 274, 276, 277
    vitality assessment of anterior teeth 275–6,
      277–8
  The First Five Years on 234, 252
  history taking 236, 238–9, 243
  immature permanent molar in mixed dentition
    241–3
  learning outcomes 234–5
  mind maps 247–9
  non-surgical endontics for deciduous and
    immature teeth 380
  preventive dentistry 176
  primary teeth with symptoms of toothache or
    abscess 240–1
  restoration of deciduous dentition 236–7,
    239–41
  restoration of immature permanent dentition
    237
  restorative competency test 245
  tell-show-do 144

treatment plans 236
  see also pulp therapy in primary dentition
Page, J. 235
pain 424
  management of 95
  pharmacological management 111–29
pain history, checklist for competence 12
Panoramic or Dental Panoramic Radiograph
  (DPR) 153
  indications for 157
panoramic radiographic examination 159–61
Papillon-Lefevre syndrome 319
parafunctional activity 322
pathological lesions 156
patient care, and surgical procedures 423,
  426–7
patient examination *see* examination
patient investigations 105
patient management 105
  psychological intervention 444
patient management problems 492
patient referral *see* referral
patient-centred communication 39, 182
patients
  with complex medical conditions 327
  with learning difficulties 137
Paul 506
peer review 489
pemphigus 448
percussing teeth 9
periapical lesions 156
periapical periodontitis 254
periapicals 153, 156
  including endodontic views 153
  indications for 156
periodontal disease 178, 180
periodontal tissues 10
periodontal unit clinical competency assessment
  328
periodontal–endodontic lesions 318, 322, 327
periodontitis 314
periodontology 313–31
  anatomy 317–18
  competency tests 329
  continued professional education 327, 329
  curriculum guidelines 317–28
  dental hygienist 326
  diagnosis 323
  dietary analysis and advice 323–4
  epidemiology 319
  examination 321–2
  The First Five Years on 314
  history taking 321
  immunology 318
  instrumentation 319–21

periodontology *continued*
  learning outcomes 315–16, 320
  local antimicrobial delivery systems 325
  microbiology 318
  mind map 331
  monitoring treatment outcome 325
  mouthrinse/toothpastes 321
  natural history of disease 318–19
  non-surgical root surface debridement 324–5
  open root surface debridement (surgery)
    325–6
  oral hygiene, failure to maintain 326–7
  oral hygiene instruction 323
  pathology 318
  patients with complex medical conditions 327
  periodontal unit clinical competency
    assessment 328
  pharmacology and therapeutics 319–23
  physiology 318
  radiographs 322
  referral 326
  sites requiring further treatment 324
  smoking cessation advice 324
  study models 322
  supportive care programme 326
  systemic antimicrobial therapy 325
  systemic diseases 319
  treatment planning 323
  vitality testing 322
periradicular tissues 377
personal protection 63–4
  training in 63
Personal Protective Equipment at Work
  Regulations 51
pertussis 63
pharmacological management of pain and
  anxiety 111–29
  The First Five Years on 111–12
  learning outcomes 112–13
  mind map 126–9
pharmacology and therapeutics 90–1
photodynamic therapy 442
physicochemical properties of LA drugs 113
pigmentary changes 448
Pine, C.M. and Harris, R.V. 71
plaque control 180
plaster of Paris 211
plastic restorations 221
pocket chart 322, 324, 325
pocket depth 318
Poison and Drug Information Units 93
poliomyelitis 63
polycarboxylate 227
polyether 211
polymerization 222

polysilicone, condensation and addition 211
polysulphide 210, 211, 225
population health science 72
portable suction apparatus 86
post-trauma 156
poverty 79
practice management 477, 504–5
  ethical and legal issues 21
pre-extraction evaluation 156
pregnancy 448
  and dental radiology and imaging 155–6
pregnancy epulis 445
prescriptions, writing 91, 93
Pressure Systems and Transportable Gas
  Containers Regulations (1989) 51
prevention and interception 173–87
  clinical skills 178
  The First Five Years on 174–5
  learning outcomes 176–83
  mind map 187
primary dentition
  dental caries in 233–4
  pulp therapy in 251–72
primary medical care team 82
primary molars, dental caries 252
principles of parallax 166
priolocaine 113
prions 59, 62
prioritizing 475
problem-solving 469, 476–7
Prochaska, J. and DiClemente, C.C. 42
professional attitude xii–xiii
professional duties of care 24, 25
professional indemnity 29
professional misconduct 23
professional relationships 20, 37, 45
professionalism 29–30, 179–83
Propofol 119
prosthetic appliances 348
prosthodontics 385–419
  advice to patient 397
  anatomy 389
  clinical and technical procedures, mind map
    411
  complete dentures 392–7
    copy technique, mind map 414
    key skills 393
    mind map 412–13
  copy dentures 397–8
  denture insertion 396–7
  dentures 388
  diagnosis 392
  examination 391
  The First Five Years on 386–7
  gerontology 390

history taking 391
immediate complete dentures, mind map 415
immediate dentures 403–5
implants 406
instrumentation 390
learning outcomes 387–9
materials 390
microbiology 389
overdentures 406
overview, mind map 410
partial dentures, design, mind map 416
radiographs 391–2
recording jaw relations, checklist 407–8
relines and rebases 405–7
removable partial dentures 398–403
removable prosthodontics, learning outcomes 389
and systemic disease 390
treatment planning 392
trial dentures 396
vitality testing 392
protection of life and health 24
protective clothing 51–2
Provision and Use of Work Equipment Regulations 51
proximal carious lesions 156
pseudomembraneous candidosis 448
PSP (photo stimulable phosphor or SPP storage phosphor plates) 154
psychological disease, systemic drug therapy in 451
psychological intervention, in patient management 444, 451
psychological inventories, to assess dental anxiety 137–8
psychological investigations 450
psychological issues, in behavioural management of dental anxiety 136–8
psychology 38
 case study 31
pulp capping 379, 380
pulp therapy in the primary dentition 251–72
 carious exposure in an uncooperative child 263–4
 clinical examination 256–7
 clinical and radiographic signs 254
 criteria for success 255–67
 diagnosis of pulp status 258
 history taking 255–6
 indications and contraindications 253–4
 learning outcomes 253
 mind map 270–1
 monitoring 267
 and radiography 257
 special investigations 257–8

 symptoms 254
 treatment planning 259
 vital pulp therapy 259–64
pulpal disorders 156
pulpal status 240, 256
 diagnosis 258
pulpectomy 264–6
 one visit pulpectomy (irreversible inflammation) 265–6
 problems 264–5
 two visit pulpectomy (necrotic pulps or without peri-radicular infection) 266
pulpitis 241, 376
pulpotomy 379
pulse 104, 120
pulse oximeter 120
pulse rate 88
pupil size 88
pus 424
Putman, S. and Lipkin, M. 39
pyogenic granuloma 445

Quality Assurance Agency (QAA 2002) 2
questions, asking and inviting 41

Raadal, M. *et al.* 235
radicular cyst 166
radiography *see* dental radiology
radiopaque calculi 156
RAST (antibody test) 450
re-certification xi 29
recession 318
record keeping 3, 21, 22, 29
recording oral conditions, standards 76
rectangular collimation 153, 157
recurrent aphthous stomatitis (recurrent oral ulceration) 446
referral 108, 120, 122, 189–94
 and dental anxiety 138, 141
 learning outcomes 190, 191
 letter of referral 190–3
 mind map 194
 oral medicine 452
 oral pathology 462
 orthodontics 306
 and periodontal problems 314
 periodontology 326
 tooth wear 345
referral of pain 8
reflective approach 29, 30
reflective listening 134–5
regional anaesthesia 115–16
regional lymph nodes 9, 10
relaxation 146
relines and rebases 405–7

removable appliances 308, 309
removable partial dentures 398–403
  design 399–400
removable prosthodontics, learning outcomes
  389
resin composite 227
resin-based composites 222
respect 37
respiratory arrest 87
respiratory obstruction 87
respiratory physiology 118
respiratory rate 88
respiratory viruses 62
restorative dentistry 175, 193, 314–15, 333–69
  clinical examination 338
  communication of maintenance protocol 340
  consent 340
  dental implants 356
  dental materials 344
  dental trauma 345–7
  diagnosis 339, 341
  The First Five Years on 334–5
  fixed prostheses 353–4
  general skills, mind map 363–5
  histopathology 341–2
  history taking 337–8
  indirect fixed restorations, mind map 360
  laboratory work 355
    assessment 358
  learning outcomes 220, 335–7
  radiographs 338–9
  restoration evaluation 357
  study casts 339
  temporary restorations 354–5
  tooth preparation for crowns, assessment
    357–8
  tooth preparation for indirect restorations
    352–4
  tooth wear 342–5
  topics, mind map 365, 368–9
  treatment 341–2
  treatment plan 339–40
  veneers 353
  vitality tests 339
restorative excesses and defects 156
review 173
rheumatic fever 103
Roberts, J.F. and Sheriff, M. 237
Rogers, C. 43
Rollnick, S. 141
root canal obturation, checklist 381–2
root canal preparation, checklist 380–1
root grooves 322
root resorption 377
root surface explorers 321

roots
  extraction 426
  removal of retained roots, checklist 433
Rosenstiel, S.F. *et al.* 224, 227
rubber dam 198, 199–201
  checklist for placement 202
  disadvantages 199–200
  in endodontics 378
  modification 200–1
  in paediatric dentistry 237
rubella 63

safe dental practice 49
safelight testing 155, 162–3
safety issues 22
saliva 390
saliva substitutes 342
salivary flow rate 442, 450
salivary gland diseases 448
salivary glands 10, 424, 428, 444
salivary neoplasia 448
salivary scintiscanning 450
salivary stone 448
sarcoidosis 319
scaling and prophylaxis 324
scavenging 119
Schirmer tests 442, 450
Scotland, incapacity law 26, 29
screening programmes 76
secondary caries 156
segmental techniques 430
Selection Criteria in Dental Radiography 155
self-management checklist 470
self-validated self-assessment 491
Seow, W.K. and Thong, Y.H. 264
serum ferritin 445
service delivery 501
sharps injuries 64
Shillingburg, H.T. *et al.* 224
sialography 450
sialosis 448
single visit ferric sulphate pulpotomy 259,
  261–2
sinus lift procedures 431
Sjögren's syndrome 448, 451
Smith, D.C. and Ruse, N.D. 227
smoking 103, 318, 321
smoking cessation 80
smoking cessation advice, periodontology 324
social history 7, 103–4
  in letter of referral 191
sociology 38
  case study 31
sodium hydrochlorite solution 265
soft tissue inclusions 274

soft tissue injuries 431
soft tissue surgery 462
soft tissues 10
space maintainers 308
special care dentistry 283–96
 co-operation and behaviour management 292
 disability awareness 285, 286–8
 and ethics 285
 legislation 285, 288, 289
 management of oral/dental conditions seen
  with impairments 292–5
 mind map 296
 preventive dental care 292
 public health aspects 285
 safe handling and moving 288, 289–90
 understanding of impairments 290–2
special tests 11
specialization xii
Specialist Training Advisory Committee (STAC)
 xii
splinting of anterior teeth 274, 276, 277
split case mounting technique 395
squamous cell papilloma 445
SSRI 451
stainless steel crowns 237, 239, 240, 252
standards
 assessment of students 493
 evaluating data 76–7
 professional conduct 30
 for recording oral conditions 76
Standards for Dental Professionals 20
Standing Dental Advisory Committee (SDAC) xi
stereotyping 79
sterilization 65
steroid therapy, lichen planus 451
Stewardson, D.A. and McHugh, E.S. 198
stress 30
Structured Clinical Operative Test (SCOT) 489
study casts, restorative dentistry 339
study models, periodontology 322
Subject Benchmark Statements for Dentistry
 (QAA) 50, 60, 73, 86, 97–8
 assessment 483–4
 dental anxiety 132–3
 dental public health 73
 dental radiology and imaging 151–2
 endodontics 371
 human disease and therapeutics 97–8
 infection control 60
 isolation and moisture control 196
 medical emergencies 86
 oral pathology 460–1, 462–3
 paediatric dentistry 234, 252
 prevention and interception 175–6
 prosthodontics 387

restorative dentistry for the elderly 335
 surgical dentistry 422
 teamwork 498, 500
submucous fibrosis 425, 447
suction 202
suction apparatus 86
summative assessments 486
Summitt, J.B. 195, 198
superior alveolar nerves 116
supernumerary or supplemental teeth 156, 305
support classification 399
supra and subgingival deposits 313
surgery clothing 64
surgery design, and infection control 65
surgical dentistry 421–39
 competence at graduation 424–7
 diagnosis and treatment planning 424–5, 427–9
 inpatient ward and operating theatre practices
  431
 knowledge at graduation 427–30
 learning outcomes 422–3
surgical procedures
 and consent 426
 control of pain and anxiety 426–7
 and infection control 427
 and patient care 423
surveys of dental health, checklists 77, 78
swelling 9, 10
syringes 114
systematic hand wash technique 64
systemic antimicrobial therapy 325
systemic diseases 101, 319
 oral manifestations 448
systemic drug therapy, in psychological disease
 451
systemic lupus erythematosis 319

team-based approach 99, 179, 181, 313
teamwork 497–507
 communication 44
 defining characteristics of teams 500
 dental teams 501
 The First Five Years on 195–6, 497–8
 integrated dental care, managing 502–3
 leadership 503–4
 leadership and management 501–2
 learning outcomes 499–500
 mind map 507
 practice management 504–5
 recruitment 504
 successful teams 504
tell-show-do 144
temperature 104
 taking 88
temporary restorations 354–5

temporomandibular disorders, construction of appliances for 432
temporomandibular joint dysfunction syndrome 448
temporomandibular joint (TMJ) 13, 302, 423, 429, 443, 444
  pain 449
  problems 421, 427
  surgery 431
tetanus 63
therapeutic agents 91
therapeutic relationship 43–4
Thompson, S. *et al.* 285
time management and self-discipline 475–6
tooth loss 390
tooth wear 178, 180, 340, 342–5, 348
  diagnosis 343–4
  maintenance 344–5
  referral 345, 347
  treatment planning 344
  topical/surface anaesthesia 114
training
  in infection control 65
  in personal protection 63
transillumination 275
transmissible diseases 59, 60
transmissible spongiform encephalopathies (vCJD) 62
trauma 117
traumatic ulceration 445
treatment planning, periodontology 323
trial dentures 396
  checklist 408
tricyclics 451
trigeminal nerve 113
trigeminal neuralgia 448–9
trismus 117
trust 20, 44, 45
tuberculosis 62, 63, 64, 103, 319
two dots technique 395

UK
  dental conditions in 77–9
  oral disease in 73
UK Adult Dental Health Survey 314, 333
UK Child Dental Health Survey 251
ulcerative gingivitis 448
ulcers 9, 10
ultrasonic/or sonic scaler 320
unconsciousness 90
undergraduate dental training x–xi
  Europe and USA xii
unerupted teeth 156
  extraction 426
universal curettes 321

universal precautions
  checklist 66–7
  concept 59, 61, 63–5
urinalysis 442, 450

vaccination, hepatitis B 52
varicella zoster virus 451
vascular epulis 318
vasoconstrictors 113
vasovagal attack 87
veneers 353
venepuncture 120, 443
  for haematological investigations 444, 445
venepuncture sites 119
venous cannula 90
venous plasma glucose 445
vertex occlusal view 156
vesicullo-bullous disease 451
vital pulp therapy 259–64
vital signs 88, 90
  monitoring 119
vitality testing 9
  periodontology 322
  prosthodontics 392
vitality tests, restorative dentistry 339
vitamin B12 445
Vitapex 266
vocational training (VT) xi
vulnerable patients 25, 43
  and communication skills 100

Warfarin 327
Wassel, R.W. *et al.* 213
Waterhouse, P.J. *et al.* 252
Watson, N. 283
wax 211
Weinstein, M. *et al.* 223, 224
Welbury, R.R. 237, 274
West, R. *et al.* 80
White, D.A. 193
WHO probe 320
Wilkinson, T.F. 493
Willis gauge 395
working with others 469
Workplace (Health Safety and Welfare) Regulations 51

xerostomia 318, 334, 336, 341, 342, 448
  in the elderly 348

yeasts 451

zinc oxide and eugenol 210, 211, 226, 262, 266
zinc phosphate 226, 227
zygomaticus implants 431